THE
HUMAN
BRAIN
BOOK

THE HUMAN BRAIN BOOK

RITA CARTER

SUSAN ALDRIDGE

MARTYN PAGE

STEVE PARKER

CONSULTANTS Professor Chris Frith, Professor Uta Frith, and Dr. Melanie Shulman

CONTENTS

NO ORDINARY ORGAN 6

INVESTIGATING THE BRAIN 8
LANDMARKS IN NEUROSCIENCE 10
SCANNING THE BRAIN 12
A JOURNEY THROUGH THE BRAIN 14

THE BRAIN AND THE BODY 36
BRAIN FUNCTIONS 38
THE NERVOUS SYSTEM 40
THE BRAIN AND THE NERVOUS
SYSTEM 42
BRAIN SIZE, ENERGY USE, AND
PROTECTION 44
EVOLUTION 48

BRAIN ANATOMY 50
BRAIN STRUCTURES 52
BRAIN ZONES AND PARTITIONS 56
THE NUCLEI OF THE BRAIN 58
THE THALAMUS, HYPOTHALAMUS,
AND PITUITARY GLAND 60
THE BRAINSTEM AND CEREBELLUM 62
THE LIMBIC SYSTEM 64

THE CEREBRAL CORTEX 66
BRAIN CELLS 68
NERVE IMPULSES 72
BRAIN MAPPING AND
SIMULATION 74

THE SENSES 76
HOW WE SENSE THE WORLD 78
THE EYE 80
THE VISUAL CORTEX 82
VISUAL PATHWAYS 84
VISUAL PERCEPTION 86
SEEING 88
THE EAR 90
MAKING SENSE OF SOUND 92
HEARING 94
SMELL 96
PERCEIVING SMELL 98
TASTE 100
TOUCH 102
THE SIXTH SENSE 104
PAIN SIGNALS 106
EXPERIENCING PAIN 108

LONDON, NEW YORK, MELBOURNE,
MUNICH, AND DEHLI

SENIOR EDITOR Peter Frances
SENIOR ART EDITOR Maxine Lea
PROJECT EDITORS Nathan Joyce,
Ruth O'Rourke, Miezan van Zyl
EDITORS Salima Hirani, Katie John,
Rebecca Warren
US EDITOR Jill Hamilton
PROJECT ART EDITORS Alison Gardner,
Siân Thomas, Francis Wong
DESIGNER Riccie Janus
EDITORIAL ASSISTANT Elizabeth Munsey
INDEXER Hilary Bird
PROOFREADER Polly Boyd

PICTURE RESEARCHER Liz Moore
JACKET DESIGNER Duncan Turner

SENIOR PRODUCTION CONTROLLER
Inderjit Bhullar
PRODUCTION EDITOR Tony Phipps
CREATIVE TECHNICAL SUPPORT
Adam Brackenbury, John Goldsmid

MANAGING EDITOR Sarah Larter
SENIOR MANAGING ART EDITOR
Phil Ormerod
PUBLISHING MANAGER Liz Wheeler
REFERENCE PUBLISHER Jonathan Metcalf
ART DIRECTOR Bryn Walls

ILLUSTRATORS
Medi-Mation, Peter Bull Art Studio

MOVEMENT AND CONTROL 110
REGULATION 112
THE NEUROENDOCRINE SYSTEM 114
PLANNING A MOVEMENT 116
EXECUTING A MOVEMENT 118
UNCONSCIOUS ACTION 120
MIRROR NEURONS 122

EMOTIONS AND FEELINGS 124
THE EMOTIONAL BRAIN 126
CONSCIOUS EMOTION 128
DESIRE AND REWARD 130

THE SOCIAL BRAIN 132
SEX, LOVE, AND SURVIVAL 134
EXPRESSION 136
THE SELF AND OTHERS 138
THE MORAL BRAIN 140

LANGUAGE AND COMMUNICATION 142
GESTURES AND BODY LANGUAGE 144
THE ORIGINS OF LANGUAGE 146
THE LANGUAGE AREAS 148
A CONVERSATION 150
READING AND WRITING 152

MEMORY 154
THE PRINCIPLES OF MEMORY 156
THE MEMORY WEB 158
LAYING DOWN A MEMORY 160
RECALL AND RECOGNITION 162
UNUSUAL MEMORY 164

THINKING 166
INTELLIGENCE 168
CREATIVITY AND HUMOR 170
BELIEF AND SUPERSTITION 172
COGNITIVE ILLUSIONS 174

CONSCIOUSNESS 176
WHAT IS CONSCIOUSNESS? 178
LOCATING CONSCIOUSNESS 180
ATTENTION AND CONSCIOUSNESS 182
THE IDLING BRAIN 184
ALTERING CONSCIOUSNESS 186
SLEEP AND DREAMS 188
TIME 190
THE SELF AND CONSCIOUSNESS 192

THE INDIVIDUAL BRAIN 194
NATURE AND NURTURE 196
INFLUENCING THE BRAIN 198
PERSONALITY 200
BRAIN MONITORING AND STIMULATION 202
STRANGE BRAINS 204

DEVELOPMENT AND AGING 206
THE INFANT BRAIN 208
THE ADULT BRAIN 212
THE AGING BRAIN 214
THE BRAIN OF THE FUTURE 216

DISEASES AND DISORDERS 220
THE DISORDERED BRAIN 222
DIRECTORY OF DISORDERS 224–49

GLOSSARY 250
INDEX 256
ACKNOWLEDGMENTS 264

REVISED EDITION

SENIOR EDITOR Peter Frances
SENIOR ART EDITOR Anna Hall
PROJECT EDITOR Ruth O'Rourke-Jones
US ASSOCIATE MANAGING EDITOR Allison Singer
US EDITOR Jill Hamilton

PICTURE RESEARCHER Liz Moore
PRE-PRODUCTION PRODUCER Francesca Wardell
SENIOR PRODUCER Alice Sykes

MANAGING EDITOR Angeles Gavira Guerrero
MANAGING ART EDITOR Michelle Baxter
PUBLISHER Sarah Larter
ART DIRECTOR Phil Ormerod
ASSOCIATE PUBLISHING DIRECTOR Liz Wheeler
PUBLISHING DIRECTOR Jonathan Metcalf

DVD-ROM minimum system requirements

PC Windows XP or later; sound card; 24-bit color display; screen resolution 1,366 x 768

Macintosh OS 10.6.8 or later; sound card; 24-bit color display; screen resolution 1,344 x 768

The publisher cannot take responsibility for the performance of this DVD-ROM on operating systems released after the time of going to print.

First American edition, 2009
This revised edition published in 2014

Published by DK Publishing, 4th floor, 345 Hudson Street, New York, New York, 10014

14 15 16 17 18 10 9 8 7 6 5 4 3 2 1

001–192892–Mar/2014

Copyright © 2009 and 2014
Dorling Kindersley Limited

Published in Great Britain by Dorling Kindersley Ltd.

The Human Brain Book provides information on a wide range of medical topics, and every effort has been made to ensure that the information in this book is accurate. The book is not a substitute for medical advice, however, and you are advised always to consult a doctor or other health professional on personal health matters.

A catalog record for this book is available from the Library of Congress.

ISBN 978-1-4654-1602-5

DK books are available at special discounts when purchased in bulk for sales promotions, premiums, fund-raising, or educational use. For details, contact: DK Publishing Special Markets, 345 Hudson Street, New York, New York 10014 or SpecialSales@dk.com.

Printed and bound in China by South China Printing Co. Ltd.

Discover more at www.dk.com

NO ORDINARY ORGAN

The human brain is like nothing else. As organs go, it is not especially prepossessing–3lb (1.4kg) or so of rounded, corrugated flesh with a consistency somewhere between jelly and cold butter. It doesn't expand and shrink like the lungs, pump like the heart, or secrete visible material like the bladder. If you sliced off the top of someone's head and peered inside, you wouldn't see much happening at all.

SEAT OF CONSCIOUSNESS

Given this, it is perhaps not surprising that for centuries the contents of our skulls were regarded as relatively unimportant. When they mummified their dead, the ancient Egyptians scooped out the brains and threw them away, yet carefully preserved the heart. The Ancient Greek philospher, Aristotle, thought the brain was a radiator for cooling the blood. René Descartes, the French scientist, gave it a little more respect, concluding that it was a sort of antenna by which the spirit might commune with the body. It is only now that the full wonder of the brain is being realized.

The most basic function of the brain is to keep the rest of the body alive. Among your brain's 100 billion neurons, some regulate your breathing, heartbeat, and blood pressure and others control hunger, thirst, sex drive, and sleep cycle. In addition to this, the brain generates the emotions, perceptions, and thoughts that guide your behavior. Then it directs and executes your actions. Finally, it is responsible for the conscious awareness of the mind itself.

THE DYNAMIC BRAIN

Until about 100 years ago, the only evidence that brain and mind were connected was obtained from "natural experiments"–accidents in which head injuries created aberrations in their victims' behavior. Dedicated physicians mapped out areas of the cerebral landscape by observing the subjects of such experiments while they were alive–then matching their deficits to the damaged areas of their brains. It was slow work because the scientists had to wait for their subjects to die before they could look at the physiological evidence. As a result, until the early 20th century, all that was known about the physical basis of the mind could have been contained in a single volume.

Since then, scientific and technological advances have fueled a neuroscientific revolution. Powerful microscopes made it possible to look in detail at the brain's intricate anatomy. A growing understanding of electricity allowed the dynamics of the brain to be recognized and then, with the advent of electroencephalography (EEG), to be observed and measured. Finally, the arrival of functional brain imaging machines allowed scientists to look inside the living brain and see its mechanisms at work. In the last 20 years, positron emission tomography (PET), functional magnetic resonance imaging (fMRI), and, most recently, magnetic encephalography (MEG) have among them produced an ever more detailed map of the brain's functions.

LIMITLESS LANDSCAPE

Today we can point to the circuitry that keeps our vital processes going, the cells that produce our neurotransmitters, the synapses where signals leap from cell to cell, and the nerve fibers that convey pain or move our limbs. We know how our sense organs turn light rays and sounds waves into electrical signals, and we can trace the routes they follow to the specialized areas of cortex that respond to them. We know that such stimuli are weighed, valued, and turned into emotions by the amygdala–a tiny nugget of tissue that punches well above its weight. We can see the hippocampus retrieve a memory, or watch the prefrontal cortex make a moral judgment. We can recognize the nerve patterns associated with amusement, empathy– even the thrill of *schadenfreude* at the sight of an adversary suffering defeat. More than just a map, the picture emerging from imaging studies reveals the brain to be an astonishingly complex, sensitive system in which each part affects almost every other. "High level" cognition performed by the frontal lobes, for instance, feeds back to affect sensory experience–so what we see when we look at an object is shaped by expectation as well as by the effect of light hitting the retina. Conversely, the brain's most sophisticated products can depend on its lowliest mechanisms. Intellectual judgments, for example, are driven by the body reactions that we feel as emotions, and consciousness can be snuffed out by damage to the humble brainstem. To confuse things further, the system doesn't stop at the neck but extends to the tips of your toes. Some would argue it even goes beyond–to encompass other minds with which it interacts.

Neuroscientific investigation of the brain is very much a work in progress and no one knows what the finished picture will look like. It may be that the brain is so complicated that it can never understand itself entirely. So this book cannot be taken as a full description of the brain. It is a single view, from bottom to top, of the human brain as we know it today–in all its beauty and complexity. Be amazed.

Rita Carter

INVESTIGATING THE BRAIN

THE BRAIN IS THE LAST OF THE HUMAN ORGANS TO GIVE UP ITS SECRETS. FOR A LONG TIME, PEOPLE WERE NOT EVEN ABLE TO UNDERSTAND WHAT THE BRAIN IS FOR. THE DISCOVERY OF ITS ANATOMY, FUNCTIONS, AND PROCESSES HAS BEEN A LONG AND SLOW JOURNEY ACROSS THE MILLENNIA, AS HUMAN KNOWLEDGE ABOUT THIS MYSTERIOUS ORGAN HAS DEVELOPED AND ACCUMULATED.

EXPLORING THE BRAIN

The brain is particularly difficult to investigate because its structures are minute and its processes cannot be seen with the naked eye. The problem is compounded by the fact that its most interesting product, consciousness, does not feel like a physical process, so there was no obvious reason for our distant ancestors to associate it with the brain. Nevertheless, over the centuries, philosophers and physicians built up an understanding of the brain and, in the last 25 years with the advent of brain-imaging techniques, neuroscientists have created a detailed map of what was once an entirely mysterious territory.

USING RATS
The brains of rats are very similar to human brains. Until imaging techniques were developed, the only way scientists were able to look directly at brain tissue was by using the brains of rats and other non-human animals.

PAPYRUS

387 BCE
The Greek philosopher Plato teaches at Athens; he believes the brain is the seat of mental processes.

PLATO

DRAWING THE BRAIN

1664
Oxford physiologist Thomas Willis publishes the first brain atlas, locating various functions in separate brain "modules."

BRAIN ATLAS

1700 BCE
Egyptian papyrus gives a careful description of the brain, but Egyptians do not rate this organ highly; unlike other organs, it is removed and discarded before mummification, suggesting that it was not considered to be of any use in future incarnations.

4000 BCE
Early Sumerian writing notes the euphoric effect of poppy seeds.

450 BCE
Early Greeks begin to recognize the brain as the seat of human sensation.

1543
Andreas Vesalius, a European physician, publishes the first "modern" anatomy, with detailed drawings of the human brain.

1774
German physician Franz Anton Mesmer introduces "animal magnetism," later called hypnosis.

1848
Phineas Gage has his brain pierced by an iron rod (see p.141).

| 4000 BCE | 3000 BCE | 2000 BCE | 1000 BCE | | 1500 | 1600 | 1700 | 1800 |

2500 BCE
Trepanation (boring holes into the skull) is a common surgical procedure across many cultures, possibly used for relieving brain disorders such as epilepsy, or for ritual or spiritual reasons.

335 BCE
Greek philosopher Aristotle restates the ancient belief that the heart is the superior organ; the brain, a radiator to stop the body from overheating.

RENÉ DESCARTES

1649
French philosopher René Descartes describes the brain as a hydraulic system that controls behavior. "Higher" mental functions are generated by a spiritual entity, however, which interacts with the body via the pineal gland.

1791
Luigi Galvani, an Italian physicist, discovers the electrical basis of nervous activity by making frogs' legs twitch.

LUIGI GALVANI

TREPANNING

170 BCE
Roman physician Galen theorizes that human moods and dispositions are due to the four "humors" (liquids that are held in the brain's ventricles). The idea persists for more than 1,000 years. Galen's anatomical descriptions, used by generations of physicians, were based mainly on work on monkeys and pigs.

ARISTOTLE

GALEN AT WORK

1849
German physicist Hermann von Helmholtz measures the speed of nerve conduction and subsequently develops the idea that perception depends upon "unconscious inferences."

THE ADVENT OF IMAGING TECHNIQUES

Scientists were unable to find out much about the workings of the brain until relatively recently. The only way they were able to match functions such as sight, emotion, or speech to the locations in the brain in which they are controlled was to find a person in whom a faculty was disturbed due to injury, and then wait until they were dead in order to look at the location and extent of the brain damage. Otherwise, scientists could only guess at what was happening to the brain by observing people's behavior. Today, modern imaging techniques such as functional MRI and EEG (see p.12) allow neuroscientists to see the electrical activity in the brain as a person carries out various tasks or thought processes. This allows them to link types of actions, emotions, and so on, to specific types of activity in the brain. The freedom to observe the brain that imaging techniques have afforded has allowed for an explosion of knowledge within neuroscience, and has deepened our understanding of the brain and how it works.

MAGNETIC RESONANCE IMAGING
Brain scans can reveal damaged tissue — the red area in the MRI scan above indicates damage caused by a stroke.

Electrode "cap"

ELECTRODES
Neural activity can be measured by attaching electrodes to the scalp. These pick up electrical activity in the brain and transform it into a digital record.

1889
Santiago Ramón y Cajal proposes that nerve cells are independent elements and the basic units of the brain in *The Neuron Doctrine*. He wins the Nobel Prize in 1906.

Circa 1900
Sigmund Freud abandons an early career in neurology to study psychodynamics. The success of Freudian psychoanalysis eclipsed physiological psychiatry for half a century.

SIGMUND FREUD

1934
Portuguese neurologist Egas Moniz carries out the first leucotomy operations (later known as lobotomies, see p.11). He also invented angiography, one of the first techniques that allowed scientists to make images of the brain.

1981
Roger Wolcott Sperry is awarded the Nobel Prize for his work on the different functions of the two brain hemispheres (see pp.11 and 205).

1862–74
Broca and Wernicke (see p.10) discover the two main language areas of the brain.

1906
Santiago Ramón y Cajal describes how nerve cells communicate.

NERVE CELLS IN RODENT HIPPOCAMPUS

1919
Irish neurologist Gordon Morgan Holmes localizes vision to the striate cortex (the primary visual cortex).

2013
The United States and European Union start human brain simulation projects. The Connectome, a global cooperative endeavor, delivers its first charts of the connections between neurons.

1859
Charles Darwin publishes *On the Origin of Species*.

1874
Carl Wernicke publishes on aphasia (language disorders after brain damage).

1953
Brenda Milner describes patient HM (see p.157), who suffers memory loss after hippocampal surgery.

EGAS MONIZ

1983
Benjamin Libet writes on the timing of conscious volition (see p.11).

1900

2000

1850
Franz Joseph Gall founds phrenology (see p.10), which attributes different personality traits to specific areas of the head.

1906
Alois Alzheimer describes presenile degeneration (see p.231).

1914
British physiologist Henry Hallett Dale isolates acetylcholine, the first of the neuro-transmitters (see p.73) to be discovered. He wins the Nobel Prize in 1936.

1924
The first electroencephalograms are produced by Hans Berger.

ELECTROENCEPHALOGRAPHY

1970–80
Brain scanning is developed: PET, SPECT, MRI, and MEG all emerge during this decade.

1973
Timothy Bliss and Terje Lomo describe long-term potentiation (see p.158).

1991
Mirror neurons are discovered by Giacomo Rizzolatti in Parma (see pp.11 and 122–23).

1873
Italian scientist Camillo Golgi publishes the silver nitrate method, making it possible to see nerves in their entirety. He wins the Nobel Prize in 1906.

NERVE CELLS

1909
Korbinian Brodmann describes 52 discrete cortical areas based on neural structure. These areas are still used today (see p.67).

CORTICAL MAP

1957
W. Penfield and T. Rasmussen devise a motor and sensory homunculus (see pp.10 and 103).

EARLY MAGNETIC IMAGING

LANDMARKS IN NEUROSCIENCE

MOST OF THE KNOWLEDGE WE HAVE ABOUT THE BRAIN HAS BEEN GATHERED BY SLOW, PAINSTAKING RESEARCH INVOLVING LARGE TEAMS OF PEOPLE. HOWEVER, OCCASIONALLY THE HISTORY OF NEUROSCIENCE HAS BEEN PUNCTUATED BY DRAMATIC DISCOVERIES OR IDEAS, OFTEN ARISING FROM THE WORK OF A SINGLE SCIENTIST. SOME OF THESE SUBSEQUENTLY PROVED TO BE VALUABLE BREAKTHROUGHS WHILE OTHERS, ALTHOUGH INFLUENTIAL, PROVED TO BE DEAD ENDS.

PHRENOLOGY
Franz Joseph Gall

Gall thought that personality could be read by feeling the contours of the skull. He theorized that various faculties were localized in the brain and that the strongest were correspondingly large, making the skull bulge measurably. It was hugely popular in nineteenth-century America and Europe–nearly every town had a phrenology institute. Although nonsense, Gall's idea that brain functions are localized has turned out to be largely true. Imaging research aimed at locating brain functions is often called "modern phrenology."

PHRENOLOGY HEAD
Models such as this claimed to show the bulges on the skull that revealed a person's character. Categories included "blandness" or "benevolence."

THE MAN WHO LOST HIMSELF
Phineas Gage

This polite, well-liked American railroad foreman changed dramatically, becoming "grossly profane," after an accident destroyed part of his brain (see p.141). His case was the first to show that faculties such as social and moral judgment can be localized to the frontal lobes.

FATEFUL INJURY
This reconstruction of Phineas Gage's skull shows how an iron rod damaged the frontal lobes of his brain.

LANGUAGE AREAS
Broca and Wernicke

PAUL BROCA   **CARL WERNICKE**

In 1861, French physician Paul Broca described a patient who he named "Tan," as it was the only word "Tan" could say. When Tan died, Broca examined his brain and found damage to part of the left frontal cortex. This part of the brain became "Broca's Area" (see p.148). In 1876, German neurologist Carl Wernicke found that damage to a different part of the brain (which became known as "Wernicke's Area") also caused language problems. These two scientists were the first to clearly define functional areas of the brain.

EARLY BRAIN IMPLANT
José Delgado

Spanish neurologist Dr. José Delgado invented a brain implant that could be remotely controlled by radio waves. He found that animal and human behavior could be controlled by pressing a button. In a famous experiment, conducted in 1964, Delgado faced a charging bull, bringing it to a halt at his feet by activating the implant in its brain. In another, he put a device in the brain of a chimp that was bullying its mate. He put the control in the cage where the victim chimp used it to "turn off" the bully's bad behavior.

DELGADO AND THE BULL

MAPPING THE BRAIN
Wilder Penfield

The first detailed maps of human brain function were made by Canadian brain surgeon Wilder Penfield. He worked with patients undergoing surgery to control epilepsy. While the brain was exposed, and the patient conscious, Penfield probed the cortex with an electrode and noted the responses of the patient as he touched each part. Penfield's work was the first to reveal the role of the temporal lobe in recall and map the areas of the cortex that control movement and provide bodily sensations.

CANADIAN STAMP

MODERN MAPPING
Today advanced imaging (see above) allows neural activity to be matched to mental tasks. However, much of the basic map was established by Penfield half a century earlier.

LOBOTOMY

The first lobotomies were performed in the 1890s, but they only took off in the 1930s when the Portuguese neurosurgeon Egas Moniz found that cutting the nerves from the frontal cortex to the thalamus relieved psychotic symptoms in some patients. Moniz's work was picked up by US surgeon Walter Freeman, who invented the "ice pick lobotomy." From 1936 until the 1950s, he advocated lobotomy to cure for a range of problems, and 40,000 to 50,000 patients were lobotomized. The operation was overused and is now thought abhorrent. However, in many cases it eased suffering: a follow-up of patients in the UK found 41 percent were "recovered" or "greatly improved," 28 percent "minimally improved," 25 percent had "no change," 4 percent had died, and 2 percent were worse off.

"ICE PICK" LOBOTOMY
Walter Freeman, above, found he could perform a lobotomy under local anesthetic by hammering an ice pick above each eye of a patient and swishing the device back and forth like a windshield wiper.

ICE PICK

TREPANATION
The practice of drilling holes in the head has been used since prehistoric times as a treatment for a vast array of illnesses. The modern equivalent, craniotomy, is carried out to relieve pressure within the skull.

MAKING MEMORIES
Henry G. Molaison

In 1953, aged 27, "HM" underwent an operation in the US, to stem severe epilepsy. The surgeons, then unaware of the functions of the hippocampus, took out a large area of that part of his brain (see p.159). When he came round, he was unable to lay down new memories and remained so for the rest of his life. The tragic accident demonstrated the crucial role of the hippocampus in recall.

FROZEN IN TIME
Henry G. Molaison—generally known only as "HM"—was one of the most studied patients in the history of modern medicine.

CONSCIOUS DECISIONS
Benjamin Libet

A series of ingenious experiments by US neuroscientist Benjamin Libet (see p.191) in the early 1980s demonstrated that what we think are conscious "decisions" to act are actually just recognition of what the unconscious brain is already doing. Libet's experiments have profound philosophical implications because, on the face of it, the results suggest that we do not have a conscious choice about what we do, and therefore cannot consider ourselves to have free will.

The Volitional Brain

Towards a neuroscience of free will

Edited by:
Benjamin Libet
Anthony Freeman &
Keith Sutherland

INVESTIGATING FREE WILL

SPLIT-BRAIN EXPERIMENTS
Roger Sperry

Neurobiologist Roger Sperry conducted the split-brain experiments (see p.204) on people whose brain hemispheres were surgically separated in the course of treatment for epilepsy. They showed that, under certain conditions, each hemisphere could hold different thoughts and intentions. This raised the profound question of whether a person has a single "self."

ROGER SPERRY RECEIVES THE NOBEL PRIZE IN 1981

MIRROR NEURONS

Mirror neurons (see pp.122–23) were discovered in 1991–by accident. A group of researchers in Italy, led by Giacomo Rizzolatti, were monitoring neural activity in the brains of monkeys as they made reaching movements. One day a researcher inadvertently mimicked the monkey's movement while it was watching, and found that the neural activity in the monkey's brain that sparked up in response to the sight was identical to the activity that occurred when the monkey made the action itself. Mirror neurons are thought by some to be the basis of theory of mind, mimicry, and empathy.

MIMICKING MACAQUE
Mirror neurons produce automatic mimicry by producing a similar state in an observer's brain to the state of the person they are watching.

SCANNING THE BRAIN

BRAIN IMAGING TECHNIQUES CAN BE DIVIDED INTO TWO DIFFERENT TYPES: ANATOMICAL IMAGING, WHICH GIVES INFORMATION ABOUT THE STRUCTURE OF THE BRAIN, AND FUNCTIONAL SCANNING, WHICH ALLOWS RESEARCHERS TO SEE HOW THE BRAIN WORKS. USED TOGETHER, THESE TECHNIQUES HAVE REVOLUTIONIZED NEUROSCIENCE.

PET SCANS
These scans involve injecting a volunteer with a radioactive marker that attaches to glucose in the brain. Areas of high activity (red) attract glucose for fuel. The marker dye shows which parts of the brain are firing.

A WINDOW ON THE BRAIN

The structure of the brain is well known, but until recently the way it created thoughts, emotions, and perceptions could only be guessed at. Imaging technology has now made it possible to look inside a living brain and see it at work. The brain works by generating tiny electrical charges. Functional imaging reveals which areas are most active. This may be done by measuring electrical activity directly (EEG), picking up magnetic fields created by electrical activity (MEG), or measuring metabolic side effects such as alterations in glucose absorption (PET) and blood flow (fMRI).

PET SCANNER
Positron emission tomography (PET) scanners detect signals from radioactive markers in tissues to show activity in the brain.

FUNCTION

The brain is composed of modules that are specialized to do specific things. Functional brain imaging is largely about identifying which ones are most concerned with doing what. This has allowed neuroscientists to build a detailed map of brain functions. We now know where perceptions, language, memory, emotion, and movement occur. By showing how various functions work together, imaging also gives us a glimpse into some of the most sophisticated aspects of human psychology. For example, observing a person's brain making a decision, we see that apparently rational decisions are driven by the emotional brain. Imaging the brains of master chess players shows why expertise depends on practice. Watching the brain of a person seeing a frightened face shows that emotion is contagious.

BRAIN WAVES
Electroencephalographs (EEGs) show electrical activity caused by nerve cells firing. They record distinct "brain waves," which reflect the speed of firing in different states of mind.

Motor area

BEFORE MOVEMENT

Sensory area

MOVEMENT

REAL-TIME ACTIVITY
Magnetoencephalography (MEG) picks up magnetic traces of brain activity. It is poor at showing where activity occurs, but good at pinpointing timing. Here, a brain plans a finger movement, then 40 milliseconds later its activity shifts as the movement is made.

ANATOMY

The brain looks very different according to how it is viewed. Computed tomography (CT) imaging combines the use of a computer and fine X-rays to produce multiple "slices" of the body. It allows you to see normally obscured body tissues, such as the inside of the brain, from any angle or level, with the delicate inner structures thrown into clear relief. Artificial coloring of the areas further distinguishes one part from another. CT scans are purely structural: they show the form of the organ but not how it works. They are very good at showing contrast between soft tissues and bone, and are therefore useful in diagnosing tumors and blood clots.

STRUCTURAL DETAILS
These CT images show different tissues in detail. The image on the left shows the cerebellum and eyeballs in red, the bones in blue and green, and the sinuses and ear cavities in bright yellow. The image on the right shows a healthy brain (front at bottom). The black areas are the fluid-filled ventricles.

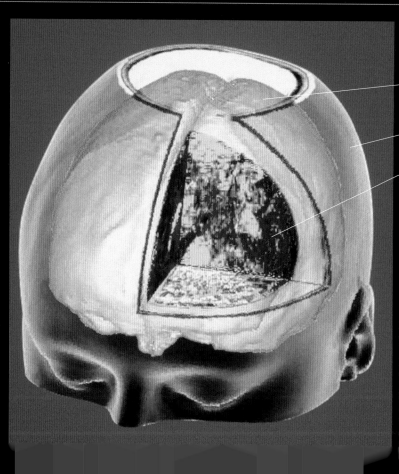

Three-dimensional brain

Computer-generated head

Inner tissue

3-D BRAIN
CT allows pictures of brains to be displayed in three dimensions, and "sliced" to reveal the inner workings. Here, the front right quarter of the brain's coverings and surface are cut away to reveal the tissues beneath.

MAGNETIC RESONANCE IMAGING

Magnetic resonance imaging (MRI) provides a better contrast between tissue types than CT. Instead of using X-rays, it uses a powerful magnetic field, which causes hydrogen atoms in the body to realign. The nuclei of the atoms produce a magnetic field that is "read" by the scanner and turned into a three-dimensional computerized image. The brain is scanned at a rapid rate (typically once every 2–3 seconds) to produce "slices" similar to those in CT scans. Increases in neural activity cause changes in the blood flow, which alter the amount of oxygen in the area, producing a change in the magnetic signal. Functional MRI (fMRI) involves showing differing levels of electrical activity in the brain, overlaid on the anatomical details.

NERVE PATHWAYS IN THE BRAIN
A refinement of MRI called diffusion tensor imaging picks up the passage of water along nerve fibers. Here, the blue fibers run from top to bottom, the green from front to back, and the red between the two hemispheres.

MOVEMENT
FMRI is very good at localizing brain activity. In this image (bottom of brain at top), the red area shows activity in the part responsible for moving the right hand. Each side of the body is controlled by the opposite hemisphere of the brain.

FIBER DETAIL
This diffusion tensor image shows another view of the nerve fibers. The green fibers link the various parts of the limbic system. The blue fibers run from the cerebellum, which joins onto the spine. The red fibers connect the two hemispheres.

INNER STRUCTURES
This MRI scan is set within an X-ray of the neck and skull. The MRI reveals the intricate folds of the brain tissue.

COMBINED IMAGING

Each type of imaging has its advantages. MRI is good on detail, for example, but is too slow to chart fast-moving events. EEG and MEG are fast but are not as good at pinpointing location. To get scans that show both fast processes *and* location, researchers use two or more methods to produce a combined image. Here (right), for example, high-resolution MRI, taking about 15 minutes to acquire, is combined with a low-resolution fMRI, which takes seconds to produce and shows the location of activity in the brain areas used in hearing language. The areas shift during a task like this that involves many aspects, and they have to work fast and in concert. The areas used in a task vary from person to person, so studies often combine data from volunteers to give an average.

STUDYING LANGUAGE
In most people, the main language areas of the brain are located in the left hemisphere, so this area shows greater activity when a person listens to spoken words. The right hemisphere is also required for complete hearing, and for distinguishing tone and rhythm.

SLICED TOGETHER
Here, a combined CT and MRI scan shows the surface folds of the brain. It also reveals the skull bones and the top vertebrae.

A JOURNEY THROUGH THE BRAIN

THE BRAIN IS THE MOST COMPLEX ORGAN IN THE BODY AND IS PROBABLY THE MOST COMPLEX SYSTEM
KNOWN TO HUMANKIND. OUR BRAIN CONTAINS BILLIONS OF NEURONS THAT ARE CONSTANTLY SENDING
SIGNALS TO EACH OTHER, AND IT IS THIS SIGNALING THAT CREATES OUR MINDS. WITH THE HELP OF
MODERN SCANNING TECHNOLOGY, WE NOW KNOW ABOUT BRAIN STRUCTURE IN GREAT DETAIL.

In the nineteenth century, much was learned about the structure of the brain by removing it from the body after death. Knowledge of the workings of the living human brain could only be gained by studying people with damaged brains, for example Phineas Gage (see p.141), but the precise location of this damage could not be known while the patient was still alive. Everything changed with the invention of brain scanners at the end of the twentieth century. In the following pages, we shall undertake a journey through the brain of a healthy, 55-year-old man revealed by magnetic resonance imaging (MRI). In these images, we can see the many components of the brain. We are starting to understand the function of some of these, but we are only at the very beginning of this journey of understanding.

The captions that accompany the scans indicate the most likely function of various brain regions. But these regions often have many functions, and these functions depend upon interactions with other brain regions. Most structures in the brain are paired, with identical counterparts in the left and right hemispheres, so structures identified in one hemisphere are mirrored in the opposite one. The scans themselves have been colored, so that the cerebrum appears in red, the cerebellum in light blue, and the brainstem in green.

Frontal lobe

Frontal-polar cortex

Orbitofrontal gyrus

Eye

Nasal cavity

Maxillary sinus

1 THE FRONTAL-POLAR CORTEX

The frontal-polar cortex is the most recently evolved part of the prefrontal cortex in the frontal lobe and is concerned with forward planning and the control of other brain regions. This slice, right at the front of the brain, also reveals other features of the skull, including the eyes, nasal cavity, maxillary sinus, and tongue.

Frontal-polar cortex

Orbitofrontal gyrus

Olfactory bulb

Optic nerve

Nasal septum

Tongue

2 THE FRONTAL LOBE

The frontal lobe, of which the prefrontal cortex is the front part, is the largest of the brain's lobes and the latest to evolve. The frontal lobe is devoted to the control of action—precise control of muscles at the back, high-level planning at the front. In this slice, the optic nerve can also be seen carrying visual information from the eye to the brain.

Superior frontal gyrus

Middle frontal gyrus

Inferior frontal gyrus

Orbitofrontal gyrus

Optic nerve

Nasal septum

Temporalis muscle

Tongue

Masseter muscle

3 THE CORTEX

The cortex, which appears on these scans as yellow lines, is heavily folded, creating a large surface area. The major ingoing folds (sulci, singular sulcus) are used as landmarks to define brain regions. The bulges between the ingoing folds are known as gyri (singular, gyrus). The major components of the frontal lobe are the superior, middle, and inferior frontal gyri.

Superior
frontal gyrus

Middle frontal
gyrus

Inferior frontal
gyrus

Orbitofrontal
gyrus

Temporalis
muscle

Nasal septum

Tongue

Masseter muscle

4 THE ORBITOFRONTAL GYRI
The orbitofrontal gyri, located at the bottom of the
brain, receive signals about smell and taste. Like the rest
of the prefrontal cortex, this area is concerned with
predicting the future, but specializes in predictions about
rewards and punishments and therefore emotions. This
area is connected with the amygdala (see slice 9, p.24).

Superior frontal gyrus

Anterior cingulate cortex

Middle frontal gyrus

Inferior frontal gyrus

Orbitofrontal gyrus

5 THE ANTERIOR CINGULATE CORTEX

Here we see the beginning of the anterior cingulate cortex, which lies between the two hemispheres. This sits alongside the limbic system. It is involved in linking emotions to actions and predicting the consequences of actions. The back part of the anterior cingulate cortex has direct connections with the motor system.

Superior frontal gyrus

Anterior cingulate cortex

Middle frontal gyrus

Lateral ventrical

Inferior frontal gyrus

Temporal lobe

Orbitofrontal gyrus

Middle temporal gyrus

Fusiform gyrus

6 THE TEMPORAL LOBES

In this slice, the temporal lobes come into view for the first time. At the very front of the temporal lobes (the temporal poles), knowledge acquired from all the senses is combined, along with emotional tone. We can also see the lateral ventricles in the middle of the slice. These are parts of a system of fluid-filled spaces in the middle of the brain.

Superior frontal gyrus

Middle frontal gyrus

Anterior cingulate cortex

Corpus callosum

Inferior frontal gyrus

Head of caudate

Lateral ventrical

Insula

Superior temporal gyrus

Optic chiasm

Putamen

Middle temporal gyrus

Nucleus accumbens

Inferior temporal gyrus

Fusiform gyrus

7 THE INSULA
The insula is a fold of cortex hidden deep in the brain between the frontal and temporal lobes. Signals about the internal state of the body—such as heart rate, temperature, and pain—are received here. Also visible in this slice is the corpus callosum, the band of nerve fibers that joins the brain's left and right hemispheres.

Superior frontal gyrus

Middle frontal gyrus

Anterior cingulate cortex

Corpus callosum

Inferior frontal gyrus

Head of caudate

Lateral ventrical

Internal capsule

Third ventrical

Insula

Superior temporal gyrus

Putamen

External globus pallidus

Middle temporal gyrus

Amygdala

Internal globus pallidus

Hippocampus

Inferior temporal gyrus

Fusiform gyrus

8 THE BASAL GANGLIA

Located in the middle of the brain, the basal ganglia include the caudate, putamen, and globus pallidus. Also known as nuclei, ganglia are clumps of gray matter (or nerve-cell bodies) surrounded by white matter. The basal ganglia are linked to the cortex, the thalamus, and the brainstem and are concerned with motor control and decision making.

Superior frontal gyrus

Middle frontal gyrus

Anterior cingulate cortex

Corpus callosum

Inferior frontal gyrus

Head of caudate

Internal capsule

Lateral ventrical

Third ventrical

Insula

Putamen

Superior temporal gyrus

External globus pallidus

Middle temporal gyrus

Amygdala

Hippocampus

Internal globus pallidus

Inferior temporal gyrus

Fusiform gyrus

9 THE AMYGDALA AND HIPPOCAMPUS
This slice includes the amygdala and the front part of the hippocampus. Both structures lie in the inner part of the temporal lobe. The amygdala is involved in learning to approach or avoid things and hence with emotion. The hippocampus has a critical role in spatial navigation and memory of past experiences, including routes between places.

Superior frontal gyrus

Middle frontal gyrus

Corpus callosum

Inferior frontal gyrus

Lateral ventrical

Third ventrical

Insula

Superior temporal gyrus

Middle temporal gyrus

Inferior temporal gyrus

Amygdala

Hippocampus

Fusiform gyrus

Ear

Spine

Anterior cingulate cortex

Head of caudate

Internal capsule

Putamen

External globus pallidus

Internal globus pallidus

Temporal horn of lateral ventrical

Pons

10 BROCA'S AREA
Here we approach the back of the frontal lobe. The bottom of the inferior frontal gyrus in the left hemisphere, just above the insula, contains Broca's area, which has a critical role in speech and language. At the bottom of the slice, we see the front of the brainstem, the pons, which joins the brain to the spinal cord.

Superior frontal gyrus

Middle frontal gyrus

Anterior cingulate cortex

Corpus callosum

Inferior frontal gyrus

Precentral gyrus

Lateral ventrical

Thalamus

Third ventrical

Insula

Putamen

Superior temporal gyrus

Middle temporal gyrus

Body of fornix

Inferior temporal gyrus

Hippocampus

Pons

Fusiform gyrus

Ear

Pyramidal tract

11 THE THALAMUS

This slice includes the thalamus, which lies between the cerebrum and the brainstem. A complex structure, the thalamus is made up of more than 20 nuclei (see p.60). The thalamus acts as a relay station, taking in information from all of the senses (except smell) and sending them on to different parts of the cerebral cortex.

Superior frontal gyrus

Middle frontal gyrus

Anterior cingulate cortex

Corpus callosum

Precentral gyrus

Lateral ventrical

Thalamus

Third ventrical

Insula

Putamen

Superior temporal gyrus

Middle temporal gyrus

Body of fornix

Temporal horn of lateral ventrical

Inferior temporal gyrus

Hippocampus

Pons

Fusiform gyrus

Cerebellum

Ear

Pyramidal tract

12 THE BRAINSTEM

The brainstem (in green) joins the brain to the spinal cord and contains a number of structures such as the pons. The brainstem has a special role in the control of basic body functions, including the control of heart rate and breathing. It also relays signals from the brain to the muscles and from senses in all parts of the body to the brain.

Posterior cingulate cortex

Precentral gyrus

Postcentral gyrus

Parietal lobe

Pulvinar of the thalamus

Cerebellum

Superior frontal gyrus

Middle frontal gyrus

Corpus callosum

Lateral ventrical

Insula

Superior temporal gyrus

Middle temporal gyrus

Temporal horn of lateral ventrical

Inferior temporal gyrus

Entorhinal cortex

Fusiform gyrus

Ear

13 THE PARIETAL LOBE

The parietal lobe includes the supramarginal gyrus and the angular gyrus (see slices 14–20, pp.29–35). The parietal lobe integrates signals from many of the senses (including visual information that arrives via the dorsal route, see pp.84–85) to estimate the position of the body and the limbs in space. This information is critical when we reach for and grasp objects.

Posterior cingulate cortex

Precentral gyrus

Postcentral gyrus

Superior frontal gyrus

Middle frontal gyrus

Corpus callosum

Supramarginal gyrus

Lateral ventrical

Superior temporal gyrus

Middle temporal gyrus

Inferior temporal gyrus

Cerebellum

Vermis

14 THE PRECENTRAL AND POSTCENTRAL GYRUS
The last part of the frontal cortex is the precentral gyrus. This contains the motor strip, where different regions send signals to control different parts of the body. The immediately adjacent part of the parietal cortex (the postcentral gyrus) has a corresponding sensory strip, where sensory signals are received from different parts of the body.

Posterior cingulate cortex

Precentral gyrus

Postcentral gyrus

Supramarginal gyrus

Lateral ventrical

Superior temporal gyrus

Middle temporal gyrus

Inferior temporal gyrus

Fusiform gyrus

Vermis

Cerebellum

15 **THE PRIMARY AUDITORY CORTEX**
The primary auditory cortex, where signals from the ears reach the cortex via the thalamus, lies along the very top of the superior temporal gyrus, in the fissure between the temporal lobe and the parietal lobe. Adjacent to the primary auditory cortex is Wernicke's area, where incoming sounds are turned into words.

Precentral
gyrus

Postcentral
gyrus

Posterior cingulate
cortex

Supramarginal
gyrus

Occipital gyrus

Vermis

Cerebellum

Lateral
ventrical

Middle temporal
gyrus

Inferior temporal
gyrus

Fusiform gyrus

16 THE FUSIFORM GYRUS
The inferior temporal gyrus and the fusiform gyrus at
the bottom of the temporal lobe are two areas concerned
with recognition of objects. Part of the fusiform gyrus, known
as the face-recognition area, is specialized for recognizing faces.
It not only identifies facial features but also scrutinizes them
for meaning, so it plays an important part in social interaction.

Postcentral gyrus

Posterior cingulate cortex

Supramarginal gyrus

Occipital gyrus

Cerebellum

Lateral ventrical

Middle temporal gyrus

Inferior temporal gyrus

17 THE CEREBELLUM
The cerebellum (colored light blue) is the highly convoluted "little brain" that sits at the back and below the main brain (also known as the cerebrum). The cerebellum is concerned with fine motor control and the timing of movements. There are many connections between the cerebellum and the motor cortex.

Postcentral gyrus

Supramarginal gyrus

Occipital lobe

Occipital gyrus

Cerebellum

Precuneus

Lateral ventrical

Angular gyrus

Inferior temporal gyrus

18 THE OCCIPITAL LOBE

The occipital lobe is concerned with vision. In the forward-most areas, signals from the primary visual cortex (see slice 20, p.35) are analyzed in terms of features such as shape and color. This information is then sent forward to the inferior temporal cortex (see slice 16, p.31), along a pathway called the ventral route, and used for object recognition.

Postcentral
gyrus

Superior parietal
lobule

Precuneus

Angular gyrus

Lateral ventrical

Occipital gyrus

Cerebellum

19 THE PRECUNEUS AND THE POSTERIOR CINGULATE CORTEX

The precuneus in the back part of the parietal lobe and posterior cingulate cortex (see slice 17, p.32) lie between the two hemispheres. These remain some of the more mysterious regions of the brain. They probably have a role in memory, especially memories about the self.

Precuneus

Superior parietal
lobule

Cuneus

Angular gyrus

Occipital gyrus

Cerebellum

Primary visual cortex

20 THE PRIMARY VISUAL CORTEX

The primary visual cortex is right at the back of the brain and lies mostly on the inside of the two hemispheres. This is the first point in the cortex where signals arrive from the eyes via the thalamus. These signals are retinotopically mapped—that is, a signal from a particular point on the retina is sent to a corresponding point on the primary visual cortex.

THE HUMAN BRAIN KEEPS US PRIMED TO RESPOND TO THE
WORLD AROUND US. IT IS AT THE HUB OF A VAST AND
COMPLEX COMMUNICATIONS NETWORK THAT CONSTANTLY
SEEKS AND COLLECTS INFORMATION FROM THE REST OF THE
BODY AND THE OUTSIDE WORLD. AS THE BRAIN INTERPRETS
THIS INFORMATION, IT GENERATES EXPERIENCES—SIGHTS
AND SOUNDS, EMOTIONS AND THOUGHTS. BUT ITS
PRIMARY FUNCTION IS TO PRODUCE CHANGES IN THE
BODY. THESE INCLUDE LIFE-SUSTAINING BASICS SUCH AS
THE REGULAR CONTRACTIONS OF THE HEART THROUGH

THE BRAIN AND THE BODY

BRAIN FUNCTIONS

THE PRIMARY TASK OF THE BRAIN IS TO HELP MAINTAIN THE WHOLE BODY IN AN OPTIMAL STATE RELATIVE TO THE ENVIRONMENT, IN ORDER TO MAXIMIZE THE CHANCES OF SURVIVAL. THE BRAIN DOES THIS BY REGISTERING STIMULI AND THEN RESPONDING BY GENERATING ACTIONS. IN THE PROCESS, IT ALSO GENERATES SUBJECTIVE EXPERIENCE.

WHAT THE BRAIN DOES

The brain receives a constant stream of information as electrical impulses from neurons in the sense organs. The first thing it does is determine whether the information warrants attention. If it is irrelevant or just confirmation that everything is staying the same, it is allowed to fade away and we are not conscious of it. But if it is novel or important, the brain amplifies the signals, causing them to be represented in various regions. If this activity is sustained for long enough, it will result in a conscious experience. In some cases, thoughts are taken one step further, and the brain instructs the body to act on them, by sending signals to the muscles to make them contract.

THE BRAIN AND BODY
The brain and spinal cord constitute the central nervous system, which is the body's main control center, responsible for coordinating all of the processes and movement in the body.

KEY FEATURES OF THE BRAIN

FEATURE	DESCRIPTION
Processing information	The brain registers a vast amount of information. However, only a very small amount of this is actually selected for processing to the point at which it enters our consciousness and can be reported. Experience that cannot be reported is not conscious. Unconscious brain processing nevertheless guides and sometimes initiates actions (see p.116 and p.191).
Sending signals	The brain consists of about 1000 billon cells. Roughly 10 percent are specialized electrical cells called neurons, which send signals to one another; this signal transmission makes brain function different from any other bodily process. Although the signals are electrical, the mode of transmission between cells is chemical—the signals are passed on by substances called neurotransmitters.
Modules and connections	The brain is modular—different parts do different things. The modules are densely interconnected, however, and none works without the support of many others (and the rest of the body). Generally, lower-level functions, such as registering sensations, are strongly localized, but higher-level functions, such as memory and language, result from interconnections between brain areas.
Individuality	The basic "blueprint" of the brain is dictated by our genes. As with any other body feature, brains share a basic anatomy, but each one is also unique. Even identical twins have visibly different brains, right from the time they are born, because the brain is exquisitely sensitive to its environment. The differences between individual brains result in each person having a unique personality.
Plasticity	Brain tissue can be "strengthened" and built up like a muscle, according to how much it is exercised. So, if a person learns and practices a skill, such as playing a musical instrument or doing mathematics, the part of the brain concerned with that task will grow physically bigger. It also becomes more efficient and enables the person to perform the task more skillfully.

HOW THE BRAIN DOES IT

No one knows exactly how electrical activity turns into experience. That remains a famously hard problem, which has yet to be cracked (see p.179). However, much is now known about the brain processes that turn incoming information into the various components of subjective experience, such as thoughts or emotions. Much depends on where the information comes from. Each sense organ is specialized to deal with a different type of stimulus–the eyes are sensitive to light, the ears to sound waves, and so on. The sense organs respond to these stimuli in much the same way–they generate electrical signals, which are sent on for further processing. But the information from each organ is sent to a different part of the brain, and then processed along a different neural pathway. Where information is processed therefore determines what sort of experience it will generate.

ACTIONS
Certain brain areas are specialized to produce body movement. Brainstem modules control automatic internal actions, such as the lung and chest movements needed for breathing, the beating of the heart, and the constriction or dilation of blood vessels to control blood pressure. In conscious activities, the primary motor cortex sends messages (via the cerebellum and basal ganglia) to the muscles of the limbs, trunk, and head to create gross movements.

MEMORIES
Some of the experiences we have change brain cells in such a way that the pattern of neural activity that produced the original experience can be replicated later in time. This process gives rise to recall, or memory, which enables us to use past experiences as a guide to how to behave in the present.

LANGUAGE
Language involves both producing speech and analyzing what others say to understand the meaning. It depends on the brain's ability to link objects with abstract symbols and then to convey the symbols—and thus the ideas they represent—to others via words. In addition to facilitating communication between people, language enables individuals to reflect on their own ideas.

EMOTIONS

Certain stimuli (including some thoughts and imaginings) cause changes in the body by activating areas in the limbic system, especially the amygdala. Conscious "feelings" occur when signals from the limbic system are sent on to "association areas" in the prefrontal cortex that support consciousness. During adolescence, the amygdala is relied heavily upon for processing emotional information, because the prefrontal cortex only matures when a person reaches their late 20s.

BRAIN FACTS

FEATURE	FACT
Structure	The brain is highly compact. If you smoothed out all the wrinkles in the cortex, the brain would cover an area of about 2½ square ft (2,300 square cm).
Connectivity	The brain has around 100 billion neurons. There are more potential connections between the neurons than there are atoms in the universe.
Growth	A fetus grows neurons at the rate of 250,000 a minute. A person is born with nearly all the neurons of an adult, but the neural networks are not mature yet.
Signaling speed	Information travels at different speeds within different types of neurons. Transmission speeds range from 3 to 330 feet/sec (1 to 100 meters/sec).
Utilizing the whole brain	The claim that we only use 10 percent of our brains is false—we use all of it. Some complex functions, such as memory, involve many areas at once.
Regeneration	You do not "lose" brain cells as you age, although some functions may decline. You can maintain the networks or even form new ones by exercising your brain.
Pain-free zone	Brain tissue has no pain receptors, so despite the fact it registers pain from all parts of the body, it does not actually feel pain itself.

SENSATIONS

Information from the environment enters the brain via the different sense organs and is transmitted to specific areas of the cerebral cortex called the primary sensory areas. This information includes some input from the body itself. In the absence of external stimuli, the sensory areas continue to be active and are thought to generate the experiences that we know as dreams, hallucinations, and imagination.

THOUGHTS

The brain uses sensations, perceptions, and emotions to generate action plans. Some of the plans give rise to internalized brain activity, or thoughts. "Inner speech," for example, is actually generated by the motor areas, but has no visible sign. Some activity occurs in the hippocampus, which we experience as recollection.

PERCEPTIONS

Most of the time we are receiving information from many sensory areas at once, as with the combination of auditory and visual signals at a fireworks display. These signals may be communicated to association areas, which bind all of this information together. If these items of "bound" information become conscious, they form what is known as a multisensory perception. There is a great deal of current neuroscientific research on how the binding process forms a unified perception, because it is still not fully understood.

THE NERVOUS SYSTEM

THE NERVOUS SYSTEM IS THE BODY'S MAJOR COMMUNICATION AND CONTROL NETWORK. DATA, IN THE FORM OF ELECTRICAL SIGNALS, IS RELAYED CONSTANTLY FROM THE SENSE ORGANS TO AND FROM THE BRAIN, THROUGH COMPLEX NETWORKS OF NEURONS AND ON A TIMESCALE MEASURED IN MILLISECONDS.

Although it is a single, unified communications network, the nervous system consists of three anatomical and functional subdivisions. The central nervous system (CNS) is the coordinating system for the body. It comprises the brain and spinal cord, which are surrounded and protected by the skull and vertebral column respectively. The peripheral nervous system (PNS) is a complex network of nerves extending across the body, branching out from 12 pairs of cranial nerves originating in the brain and 31 pairs of spinal nerves emanating from the spinal cord. It relays information between the body and the brain in the form of nerve impulses. It has an afferent division (through which messages are sent to the brain) and an efferent division (which carries messages from the brain to the body). Finally, there is the autonomic nervous system (ANS), which shares some nerve structures with both the CNS and PNS. It functions "automatically" without conscious awareness, controlling basic functions, such as body temperature, blood pressure, and heart rate.

Sensory input travels quickly from receptor points throughout the body via the afferent network of the PNS to the brain, which processes, coordinates, and interprets the data in just fractions of a second. The brain makes an executive decision that is conveyed via the efferent division of the PNS to muscles, which take the action needed to respond to environmental change rapidly.

Brain

Facial nerve

Supraclavicular nerve

Axillary nerve
Phrenic nerve

Brachial plexus

Vagus nerve

Lateral pectoral nerve

Deltoid nerve

Ulnar nerve

Musculocutaneous nerve

Lateral cutaneous branches of intercostal nerves

Intercostal nerves

Medial cutaneous branches of intercostal nerves

Dorsal branches of intercostal nerves

Subcostal nerve

Obturator nerve

Iliohypogastric nerve

Ilioinguinal nerve

Filum terminale

Femoral nerve

Spinal ganglion

Radial nerve

Spinal cord

Median nerve

Gluteal nerve

Common palmar digital nerve

Deep branch of ulnar nerve

Muscular branches of sciatic nerve

Anterior cutaneous branches of femoral nerve

Muscular branch of femoral nerve

Common peroneal nerve

Muscular branch of tibial nerve

Deep peroneal nerve

Superficial peroneal nerve

Medial dorsal cutaneous nerve

Medial plantar nerve

Pudendal nerve

Sciatic nerve

Tibial nerve

Infrapatellar branch of saphenous nerve

Cutaneous branch of saphenous nerve

Interosseous nerve

Saphenous nerve

Intermediate dorsal cutaneous nerve

Lateral plantar nerve

THE BRAIN AND THE BODY

Increasingly, the interaction between brain and body is being understood in much finer detail. The organization of the nervous system (and for that matter, all the other systems of the body, such as the cardiovascular and endocrine systems) can be considered at various different functional levels, from the entire system down to individual cells, the basic unit of all living things. The chart below shows six of these levels and their features. While it is possible to view organs with the naked eye, tissues, networks, cells, and molecules all have to be viewed with the aid of a microscope.

SYSTEM—THE CENTRAL NERVOUS SYSTEM
The brain and the spinal cord together make up the CNS.

ORGAN—THE BRAIN
The central organ of the CNS, the brain is a complex, integrated collection of tissues that controls the functions of the human body.

TISSUES—NUCLEI
These are groups of neurons (nuclei) that work together to perform specialized functions.

NETWORKS
Neural networks consist of thousands of neurons and the connections between them (synapses).

CELLS—NEURONS
Neurons are the basic units of the CNS. They transmit electrical signals, process the data, and communicate with each other via synapses.

MOLECULES
These are the smallest recognized unit, comprising two or more atoms. All the body's cells contain working parts made of millions of them.

41

THE BRAIN AND THE NERVOUS SYSTEM

THE BRAIN SITS AT THE TOP OF THE BODY, DIRECTING AND COORDINATING ALL ACTION AND ACTIVITY THROUGHOUT ITS ENTIRETY. IT DOES SO VIA THE SPINAL CORD, AND THE NERVES THAT STEM FROM IT AT VARIOUS POINTS ALONG ITS LENGTH AND BRANCH OUT INTO A NETWORK THAT SPANS THE WHOLE BODY.

cortex

brainstem

EXTENT OF THE SPINAL CORD
The spinal cord extends from the brainstem down to the first lumbar vertebra, where it forms a filament, known as the filum terminale, that extends to the coccyx.

spinal cord

filum terminale

coccyx

lumbar region

THE SPINAL CORD

The spinal cord carries information to and from the brain and all parts of the body except the head, which is served by the cranial nerves. The signals that travel along the spinal cord are known as nerve impulses. The cord itself comprises a bundle of nerve fibers, which are the long projections of nerve cells. They extend from the base of the brain to the lower region of the spine. The cord is roughly the width of a pencil, tapering at its base to a narrow bunch of fibers. Data from the sensory organs in different parts of the body is collected via the spinal nerves and transmitted along the spinal cord to the brain. The spinal cord also sends motor information, such as movement commands, from the brain out to the body, again transmitted via the spinal nerve network.

SPINAL CORD ANATOMY
The core of the spinal cord is gray matter, which is composed of nerve cells (neurons). The outer layer of white matter insulates the long fibers (axons) that extend from the nerve cells.

Nerve fibers
Bundles of nerve fibers carry signals to and from spinal cord and specific areas of the brain

White matter

Gray matter

Central canal
Filled with cerebrospinal fluid, which provides nourishment

Spinal nerve
Carries both sensory and motor information between brain and body

Anterior fissure
Deep groove along front of spinal cord

Motor nerve rootlet
Individual nerve fiber that emerges from front of spinal cord; carries signals to muscles

Spinal nerve root

Spinal nerve

Spinal nerve

Spinal cord

HOW SPINAL NERVES ATTACH
There are gaps in the vertebrae of the backbone through which spinal nerves enter the spinal cord. The nerves divide into spinal nerve roots, each made up of tiny rootlets that enter the back and front parts of the cord.

REAR OF BODY

Vertebra

Sensory root ganglion
Cluster of nerve cell bodies on each spinal nerve; partially processes incoming signals

Sensory nerve root
Nerve splits into rootlets that enter spinal cord at rear, carrying incoming signals about touch sensations to brain

Subarachnoid space

Pia mater

Arachnoid

Dura mater

Meninges
Three layers of connective tissues that protect spinal cord; cerebrospinal fluid fills space under middle layer

FRONT OF BODY

SPINAL NERVES

There are 31 pairs of spinal nerves. These branch out from the spinal cord, dividing and subdividing to form a network connecting the spinal cord to every part of the body. The spinal nerves carry information from receptors around the body to the spinal cord. From here the information passes to the brain for processing. Spinal nerves also transmit motor information from the brain to the body's muscles and glands so that the brain's instructions can be carried out swiftly.

SPINAL REGIONS
Each of the 31 pairs of nerves belong to one of four spinal regions—cervical, thoracic, lumbar, or sacral.

Cervical region
Eight pairs of cervical nerves serve chest, head, neck, shoulders, arms, and hands

Thoracic region
12 pairs of thoracic nerves connect to back and abdominal muscles and intercostal muscles

Lumbar region
Five pairs of lumbar nerves form network to serve lower abdomen, thighs, and legs

Sacral region
Six pairs of sacral nerves connect to legs, feet, and anal and genital areas

DERMATOMES

Spinal nerves contain a special fiber, the dorsal root, that sends sensory information from the skin to the brain. All but one pair of spinal nerves serves a specific area of the body, or dermatome. Nerve fibers in contact with skin receptors join up along the network of fibers in one dermatome to form the relevant dorsal root, which enters the spinal cord and conveys sensory impulses from that dermatome to the brain.

MAP OF DERMATOMES
This map shows the 30 dermatomes of the body. Each zone is served by a corresponding pair of spinal nerves.

CRANIAL NERVES

There are 12 pairs of cranial nerves that are linked directly to the brain and do not enter the spinal cord. They allow sensory information to pass from the organs of the head, such as the eyes and ears, to the brain and also convey motor information from the brain to these organs–for example, directions for moving the mouth and lips in speech. The cranial nerves are named for the body part they serve, such as the optic nerve for the eyes, and are also assigned Roman numerals, following anatomical convention.

Optic nerve (II, sensory)
Visual information from retina is conveyed to brain by optic nerve at back of eye; optic nerves from both eyes meet at point known as optic chiasm, then signals from both visual fields are sent to opposite sides of brain

Oculomotor, trochlear, and abducens nerves (III, IV, VI, motor)
Three nerves regulating voluntary movements of eye muscles, allowing movement of eyeball and eyelids; oculomotor nerve also allows for pupil constriction

Olfactory nerve (I, sensory)
Smell molecules in nasal cavity trigger nerve impulses that pass along this nerve to olfactory bulb, then on to limbic areas (see pp.64–65) of brain

Trigeminal nerve (V, two sensory and one mixed branch)
Ophthalmic and maxillary branches of this nerve convey signals from eyes, teeth, and face, and other sensory fibers carry impulses from lower jaw; motor fibers control muscles involved with chewing

Vestibulocochlear nerve (VIII, sensory)
Vestibular branch of this nerve collects information from inner ear about head orientation and balance; cochlear branch is concerned with sound and hearing signals from ear

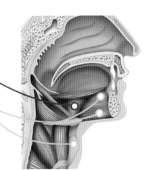

Glossopharyngeal and hypoglossal nerves (IX, XII, both mixed)
Motor fibers of these nerves control most of the muscles involved with tongue movement and swallowing; sensory fibers convey information on taste, touch, and temperature from tongue and pharynx and can trigger gag reflex if stimulated

Facial nerve (VII, mixed)
Sensory fibers collect information from taste buds at front two-thirds of tongue; motor fibers are predominantly responsible for muscle movements controlling facial expression and also function of salivary gland and lacrimal gland, which secretes tears and lubricates the surface of the eye and conjunctiva of the eyelid

CRANIAL NERVE CONNECTIONS

The cranial nerves I and II connect to the cerebrum, while cranial nerves III to XII connect to the brainstem. The fibers of sensory cranial nerves each project from a cell body that is located outside the brain itself, in sensory ganglia or elsewhere along the trunks of sensory nerves.

Spinal accessory nerve (XI, mixed)
Motor functions responsible for muscles and movements of head, neck, and shoulders; also stimulates muscles of larynx and pharynx, which are involved in swallowing; sensory functions unknown

Vagus nerve (X, mixed)
Longest and most branched of all cranial nerves, with autonomic, sensory, and motor fibers; serves lower part of head, throat, neck, chest, and abdomen, and plays role in many functions, including swallowing, breathing, heartbeat, and production of stomach acid

BRAIN SIZE, ENERGY USE, AND PROTECTION

THE BRAIN ACCOUNTS FOR AROUND 2 PERCENT OF TOTAL BODY WEIGHT, BUT CONSUMES A DISPROPORTIONATE AMOUNT OF FUEL TO SUPPORT ITS MANY ACTIVITIES. IT HAS SEVERAL FORMS OF PROTECTION—THE LAYERS OF MEMBRANE SURROUNDING IT, A BONY SKULL, AND FLUID PRODUCED IN ITS CHAMBERS (VENTRICLES) TO ABSORB THE IMPACT OF SHOCKS.

WEIGHT AND VOLUME

The average adult human brain weighs about 3¼lb (1.5kg). Its volume and shape are similar to those of an average-sized cauliflower, and the consistency of its tissues is similar to stiff jelly. The size of a person's brain bears little relation to his or her intelligence, and every brain, whatever its weight and volume, has roughly the same number of neurons and synapses. After the age of 20 or so, brain mass decreases by about 1/32oz (1g) per year. New neurons are made throughout life, but not enough to replace those that die off with age. This is generally no cause for concern, as there are plenty of neurons left to carry out the brain's functions.

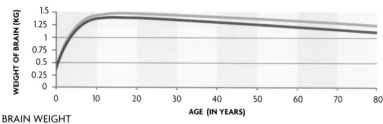

BRAIN WEIGHT
The brain's weight increases from birth and reaches its maximum during adolescence. The number of neurons is fixed in infancy but, as the body grows, they grow in size and form new connections. The male brain is consistently heavier than the female brain from birth.

BRAIN WEIGHT AND BODY WEIGHT
This graph shows brain weight as a percentage of total body weight over the course of a lifetime. Proportionally, a baby's brain is around six times larger than an adult's. Despite being lighter than the male brain overall, the female brain after the age of 13 is actually heavier than the male brain as a proportion of the entire body's weight.

KEY

▬▬▬ FEMALE
▬▬▬ MALE

80% brain tissue
10% blood
10% CSF

INTRACRANAL CONTENT
Brain tissue comprises gray and white matter, which consist of neurons and supporting glial cells respectively. A series of ventricles is filled with cerebrospinal fluid (CSF) and the brain is also richly supplied with blood vessels.

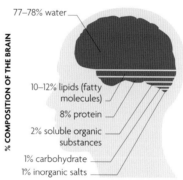

77–78% water
10–12% lipids (fatty molecules)
8% protein
2% soluble organic substances
1% carbohydrate
1% inorganic salts

COMPOSITION OF THE BRAIN
The brain consists mainly of water, which occurs in the cytoplasm of neurons and glial cells, as well as being a major constituent of blood. The brain is also rich in lipids—fatty molecules that make up cell membranes.

LENGTH, WIDTH, AND HEIGHT

The brain is housed within the intracranial cavity, so measurements of the skull effectively relate to the size of the brain. The actual length, width, and height of an individual human brain can be measured using MRI scanning. There is considerable variation in the size of the adult human brain, but the average dimensions are given against the diagrams below. Bear in mind that, because of the numerous complex folds within the cerebrum, the brain has a much larger surface area than is apparent from its overall shape.

6½ IN (167MM)

LEFT HEMISPHERE

5½ IN (140MM)

3½ IN (93MM)

FRONT

BRAIN VOLUME AND LIFESTYLE

A recent study linked alcohol consumption to brain shrinkage. Participants disclosed their drinking habits and MRI scanning was used to measure each person's ratio of brain volume to skull size. It was found that abstainers had greater brain volumes than former drinkers, light drinkers, moderate drinkers, or heavy drinkers. On average, abstainers had 1.6 percent greater brain volume than heavy drinkers. Interestingly, the effects were most marked among elderly women. In another study, participants between the ages of 60 and 79 took up either regular aerobic exercise or toning and stretching exercises for six months. MRI scans of each participant taken both before and after the six-month period showed an increase in the brain volumes of those doing aerobic exercise, suggesting that aerobic exercise can help maintain the health of the brain in older adults.

BRAIN OF A NORMAL MALE

BRAIN OF AN ALCOHOLIC
cerebellar degeneration

ALCOHOLISM AND BRAIN ATROPHY
Alcoholism can lead to cerebellar degeneration as shown above. The low quality of the scan was due to the man's withdrawal symptoms, preventing him from sitting still.

OXYGEN AND GLUCOSE SUPPLY

Glucose is the brain's sole fuel, except under conditions of starvation, when it breaks down protein. The brain is by far the body's hungriest organ. Although it accounts for just 2 percent of the body's weight, it requires a staggering 20 percent of its total glucose supplies. This is obtained from dietary carbohydrate, which is transported to the brain via the bloodstream. It consumes roughly 4oz (120g) of glucose (about 420kcal) per day. Because the brain cannot store glucose, it must be readily available at all times via the blood supply. Without oxygen or glucose, the brain can last for only about 10 minutes before irreparable damage occurs. This is why prompt resuscitation is needed in cases of cardiac arrest.

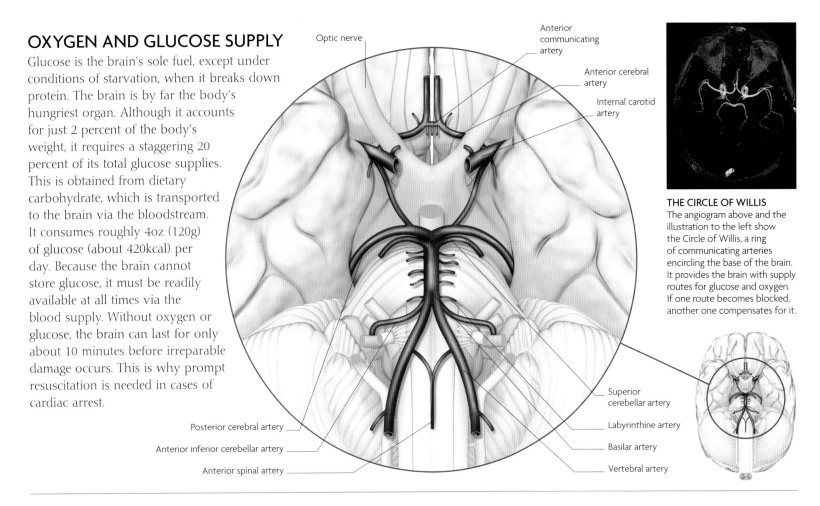

Optic nerve
Anterior communicating artery
Anterior cerebral artery
Internal carotid artery
Superior cerebellar artery
Labyrinthine artery
Basilar artery
Vertebral artery
Posterior cerebral artery
Anterior inferior cerebellar artery
Anterior spinal artery

THE CIRCLE OF WILLIS
The angiogram above and the illustration to the left show the Circle of Willis, a ring of communicating arteries encircling the base of the brain. It provides the brain with supply routes for glucose and oxygen. If one route becomes blocked, another one compensates for it.

PROTECTING THE BRAIN

The brain has several defense mechanisms to protect it from damage. The bony skull acts as a box, containing the brain and buffering it against blows. The meninges are three layers of membranes that line the skull, enclosing the brain and providing extra layers of protection between the skull and the brain. Cerebrospinal fluid circulates within the brain, nourishing brain tissue and working as a shock absorber to reduce the impact of knocks.

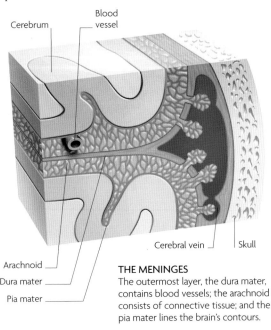

Cerebrum
Blood vessel
Arachnoid
Dura mater
Pia mater
Cerebral vein
Skull

THE MENINGES
The outermost layer, the dura mater, contains blood vessels; the arachnoid consists of connective tissue; and the pia mater lines the brain's contours.

CEREBROSPINAL FLUID FLOW

Brain tissue floats in cerebrospinal fluid (CSF) within the skull. CSF absorbs shocks from blows to the brain. It is produced in a series of connected chambers within the brain known as the ventricles, and is renewed four to five times per day. It contains proteins and glucose to nourish brain cells, as well as white blood cells to protect against infection. It moves through the ventricles, propelled by the pulsation of the cerebral arteries.

1 Site of fluid production (choroid plexus)
CSF is produced in the clusters of thin-walled capillaries (the choroid plexus) that line the walls of the ventricles.

2 Direction of flow
CSF flows from the lateral ventricles into the third and fourth ventricles. It then continues up the back of the brain, down around the spinal cord, and to the front of the brain, as indicated by the arrows.

3 Circulation around spinal cord
Helped by vertebral movement, fluid travels downward along the back of the spinal cord, into the central canal, and upward along the front of the cord.

4 Site of reabsorption (arachnoid granulations)
After traveling around the brain, the fluid is finally reabsorbed into the bloodstream through tiny arachnoid granulations (projections from the arachnoid layer of the meninges into the sagittal sinus).

Sagittal sinus
Lateral ventricle
Dura matter
Third ventricle
Fourth ventricle
Cerebellum
Skull
Spinal cord
Central canal

CIRCLE OF WILLIS
The major arteries of the brain can be seen in this MRI scan. They include the Circle of Willis (below center) at the base of the brain, where arteries from the neck meet before branching.

OXYGEN SUPPLY
This arteriograph shows arteries carrying oxygen-rich blood to the brain. The arrangement of the arteries allows blood to be supplied by another route if one of the pathways is blocked.

BRAINS EVOLVED TO ENABLE ANIMALS TO RESPOND TO ENVIRONMENTAL CHANGES. THE
HUMAN BRAIN HAS EVOLVED TO ITS PRESENT COMPLEXITY THROUGH SEVERAL STAGES,
MANY OF WHICH ARE COMMON TO ALL ANIMALS. ITS ORIGINS CAN BE SEEN IN THE
BRAINS OF OTHER SPECIES, IN WHICH MORE PRIMITIVE STRUCTURES REMAIN.

Brain

Oesophagus

Ventral nerve cord

EVOLUTION OF THE INVERTEBRATE BRAIN

All animals have to respond to changes in their internal and external environment in
order to survive. To do this, they have evolved cells that are sensitive to stimuli such as
light and to vibrations. The sensory cells are, in turn, connected to other cells that can
move the organism or change its state in response to the stimulus. This system of
interconnected nervous tissue is a crude form of brain. In invertebrates, such as worms,
the nervous system is distributed throughout the creature's
body, as a loose network of reactive fibers. Some of these
networks contain small masses of nerves, known as ganglia.
These are the forerunners of the structures that, in some
species, have become the central nervous system or brain.

Ganglia

PRIMITIVE NERVOUS SYSTEM
The simplest system, as seen in this
hydra (a tiny aquatic invertebrate),
consists of a loose network of
sensory cells with clumps of
interconnected cells called ganglia.

EARTHWORM BRAIN
The earthworm has a crude brain,
cerebral ganglion, which is connec
to a cord of nervous tissue (the
ventral nerve cord) that runs the
length of its body. Nerve fibers fro
the cord extend into each segmen
so muscle contraction along the b
can be coordinated to produce
movement in response to stimuli.

EVOLUTION OF THE VERTEBRATE BRAIN

Through the course of evolution, the brain has undergone
considerable changes. Compared to the primitive nervous
systems of invertebrates, the brain of vertebrates is a
well-developed, highly interconnected organ. The central
nervous system is connected to the rest of the body by a
peripheral nervous system that includes the fibers running
to and from the sensory organs. The basic vertebrate
brain–also sometimes referred to as the "reptilian brain"–

consists of the cluster of nuclei that lies just above the
brainstem in humans. They include the modules that
produce arousal, sensation, and reaction to stimuli. It is
unlikely, however, that these nuclei alone are sufficient to
produce consciousness. This basic vertebrate brain does
not include more advanced features, such as the limbic
system or cerebral cortex, which exist only in the brains
of mammals.

KEY TO VERTEBRAT
BRAIN AREAS
- Cerebellum
- Optic lobe
- Cerebrum
- Pituitary gland
- Medulla
- Olfactory bulb

FISH
A fish's cerebrum receives sensory signals from the
sense organs and combines them with information
from the internal organs and nerves to guide action.
Fish have a large cerebellum in order to coordinate
movement and gauge pressure.

FISH

AMPHIBIANS
The amphibian brain resembles the fish brain except
that the cerebrum is roofed over with nervous
tissue. The main function of this region is to perceive
smell, as reflected by the large olfactory bulb. The
forebrain is much larger than the cerebellum.

FROG

REPTILES
Modern reptiles show greater development in the
basal parts of the forebrain, and the cerebrum is
much larger than the optic lobe. The olfactory bulb
is large in comparison with the other structures of
the brain and is well developed.

TURTLE

MAMMAL BRAINS

The mammalian brain comprises a cluster of structures that evolved on top of the basic vertebrate brain, known as the limbic system, and a wrinkled covering called the cortex, which interconnects with the limbic structures beneath.
The limbic system is the part of the brain that produces emotions. These are responses to stimuli that go beyond the basic "grab" or "avoid" reactions in the vertebrate brain, and produce subtle and complex actions that are not always predictable. The limbic system also contains structures that encode experiences as memories, to be recalled for use in guiding future actions. The emotional and memory faculties greatly increase the range and complexity of behavior that a mammal displays, because it is not governed purely by instinct.

ELEPHANT

HUMAN

DOLPHIN

WOLF

CAT

BRAIN SIZE AND SHAPE
One striking aspect of mammalian brain evolution is the development of the cortex. This outer layer has evolved to serve the particular needs of each species, and therefore varies dramatically between one animal and another. A few mammals, such as humans, elephants, and dolphins, have a disproportionately large cortex compared to most mammals.

HOMINID BRAINS

The brains of hominids (modern humans and their ancestors) underwent a surge of evolutionary changes that left them, in some ways, distinctly different even from their near relatives, such as chimpanzees and gorillas. The main distinction between human and other mammalian brains is the size and density of the cortex, and particularly of the frontal lobe, which is responsible for complex thought, conscious judgement, and self-reflection. No one knows why the human brain evolved as it did–it may have been due to some change in diet forced by the environment, or the product of living in groups (see p.138) that depended on close interdependence for survival.

Bar chart showing brain volume (cubic centimeters):
- MODERN HUMANS
- HOMO NEANDERTHALENSIS
- HOMO ERECTUS
- HOMO HABILIS
- GORILLA
- CHIMPANZEE

Axis: 0, 200, 400, 600, 800, 1000, 1200, 1400, 1600

BRAIN VOLUME (CUBIC CENTIMETERS)

DOES SIZE MATTER?
The growth of the human brain over the course of evolution is thought to be the reason why we are so dominant. However, size is not the only factor that matters for intelligence or survival—the way brains are wired up may be more important. Neanderthals had bigger brains than humans, but were less innovative and were finally superseded by other hominids.

NEANDERTHAL SKULL

▶ BIRDS
Birds' brains are similar to those of reptiles except that the cerebellum is highly developed to control balance and position in flight. Despite the size of the olfactory bulb, most birds have a poor sense of smell, with some exceptions, such as the kiwi.

THRUSH

▶ MAMMALS
In mammals, the cerebellum is relatively small compared to the forebrain. The cerebrum is covered in wrinkled cortex; these wrinkles allow a greater volume of cortex to fit into the skull, compared to the smooth surface of the reptilian brain.

CAT

▶ MAN
The human brain is completely dominated by the cerebrum, and the cortex is intricately folded to allow the maximum amount to be contained in the skull. The cerebellum remains large and active, however, to enable complex motor activity.

HUMAN

BRAIN ANATOMY IS HIDDEN, SECRET, AND MORE COMPLEX
THAN ANY OTHER PART OF THE BODY. THE BASIC BUILDING
BLOCK OF THE BRAIN IS THE CELL. SIGNALING CELLS KNOWN
AS NEURONS FORM LARGER STRUCTURES CALLED NUCLEI
THAT CARRY OUT PARTICULAR FUNCTIONS. THEY ALSO
CLUSTER TOGETHER TO FORM THE THICK, LAMINATED SHEET
OF GRAY MATTER FORMING THE COVERING OF THE BRAIN
CALLED THE CORTEX. DEEP FISSURES IN ITS SURFACE DIVIDE
THE BRAIN INTO TWO HALVES (THE HEMISPHERES), EACH
WITH FIVE LOBES. THESE MAJOR DIVISIONS "SPECIALIZE" IN

BRAIN ANATOMY

BRAIN STRUCTURES

THE BRAIN HAS A COMPLEX AND MANY-LAYERED ANATOMY. PEELING BACK THE DOMINANT CEREBRAL HEMISPHERES REVEALS A FURTHER SET OF STRUCTURES WITHIN. SOME ARE DISCRETE MASSES, SUCH AS THE CEREBELLUM AND THALAMUS, WHILE OTHERS ARE ZONES OF NERVE FIBERS OR NERVE CELLS WITHIN LARGER STRUCTURES, DISCERNIBLE ONLY BY MICROSCOPIC EXAMINATION.

Corpus callosum

Putamen

Caudate nucleus

Right hemisphere

Cerebellum

Amygdala

Hippocampus

EXPLODED HEAD

A whole head "exploded" sideways reveals the main brain regions or divisions. The central brainstem stands up like a fist on an arm, and the cerebrum wraps over and around it, dominating it both physically and mentally. The next largest structure after the cerebrum is the cerebellum at the lower rear, comprising about ten percent of the brain's total volume. In common with standard anatomical terminology, right and left refer to the owner rather than the viewer. So here the right hemisphere of the cerebrum is on the left of the picture.

THE BRAIN HIERARCHY

The brain's major parts can be classified or categorized in several ways. In all of these systems, the dominant part is the cerebrum, the large pinky-gray wrinkled structure that forms more than three-quarters of the brain's total volume. The cerebrum is divided into left and right hemispheres, which are linked by a "bridge" of nerve fibers, the corpus callosum. The cerebrum, which includes the hippocampus and amygdala, is also known as the telencephalon. Together with the parts it wraps around—the thalamus, hypothalamus, and associated parts, collectively known as the diencephalon—it comprises the major brain "division" known as the forebrain (prosencephalon). Below the forebrain is the midbrain (mesencephalon), a small division that includes groups of nerve-cell bodies known as nuclei, such as the basal ganglia. Below the midbrain is the hindbrain (rhombencephalon), with the pons as its uppermost part, and beneath it the cerebellum and the medulla, which tapers to merge with the spinal cord.

Left hemisphere

Fornix

Thalamus

Hypothalamus

Interior globus pallidus

Subthalamic nucleus

Exterior globus pallidus

Superior colliculus

Geniculate nucleus

Midbrain

Trigeminal nerve

Optic chiasm

Pituitary gland

Pons

Olive (rounded protrusion that contains the olivary nuclei)

Pyramid (anterior medulla)

Medulla

Cervical spinal cord (in neck)

Thoracic spinal cord (in chest)

Occipital bone of skull

Foramen magnum (hole for spinal cord)

Sphenoid bone of skull

Nasal cavity

Cervical vertebra (neck backbone)

Maxilla (upper jaw bone of skull)

Spinal nerve

SCALP SKIN
The skin of the scalp has only a thin underlying layer of subcutaneous fat and the hard skull is just beneath, so it wounds relatively easily and bleeds copiously.

SCALP NERVES
Many small peripheral nerves branch through and under the scalp skin from cranial nerves II, III, and V. Even faint contact registers, allowing us to react quickly and avoid injury.

SKULL
The upper domed part of the skull, called the neurocranium, forms a "braincase" to shield against knocks and jolts. This function is aided by the meninges (see p.56).

Gyrus

Sulcus

Right thalamus

Internal globus pallidus

External globus pallidus

Putamen

Caudate nucleus

Right cerebral hemisphere

FRONTAL BONE
The neurocranium is composed of eight bones. Most prominent is the frontal bone under the forehead. The left and right parietals are behind it, the occipital below them at the lower rear, and the two temporals on the lower sides. The sphenoid and ethmoid bones are at the lower front, behind the nose area.

FACIAL BONES
Complicated in shape, the facial bones have gaps (foramina) in them. Some allow cranial nerves to pass from the brain within the neurocranium, out to the nasal epithelium in the nose cavity, the eyes in their sockets, the inner ear, and other sensory parts. Blood vessels have similar sets of skull foramina.

CEREBELLUM
This name means "little brain," referring to the pattern of grooves and bulges on the cerebellar surface, which reflects the external appearance of the cerebrum. The cerebellum is connected to the brainstem immediately in front of it by three pairs of thick, short, stalklike extensions, called the cerebellar peduncles.

CEREBRAL CORTEX
The thin grayish covering of each cerebral hemisphere is called the cerebral cortex. It has a characteristic pattern of bulges (gyri), shallower grooves (sulci), and deeper ones (fissures).

Fornix

Pineal gland

Subthalamic nucleus

Left thalamus

Midbrain

Mamillary body

Hypothalamus

Left olfactory tract
(cranial nerve I)

LEFT AND RIGHT HEMISPHERES

An overhead view of the "exploded" brain shows how the two cerebral hemispheres can be neatly separated by cutting through the corpus callosum. Many other brain structures are symmetrically paired in this way, such as the thalamus, which is sometimes described as "two hen's eggs sitting side by side." The cerebellum at the lower rear of the brain is accommodated within a bowl-like cavity of the skull known as the posterior cranial fossa. The cranial nerves (numbered I to XII, see p.43) enter the brain directly rather than connecting to the spinal cord.

Scalp

Skull

Dura mater and arachnoid
The outer two meninges are the tough, strong dura mater attached to the inside of the skull, and the blood-rich arachnoid

Superior sagittal sinus
Around the brain's midline is a shallow groove containing blood, which is part of the venous return to heart

Subarachnoid space
This gap between the arachnoid and pia mater is filled with cushioning cerebrospinal fluid

Pia mater
Innermost meninx

Corpus callosum
Main link between left and right cerebral hemispheres is a highway of more than 200 million nerve fibers

Hypothalamus
Situated under the thalamus, as its name implies ("hypo" means "under"), the sugar-cube-sized hypothalamus has many important functions, including temperature control and basic behavioral drives

Pituitary gland
"Master gland" of hormonal or endocrine system hangs by a stalk from hypothalamus above

Cerebellum
Responsible for balance and posture

Neck vertebra

Thalamus
Processes and sends on sensory information to higher brain areas

Pons
"Crossroads" area consisting mainly of nerve fibers

Medulla
Regulates vital functions such as heartbeat and respiration

SLICED DOWN THE MIDDLE
A medial sagittal section (a cut through the brain from front to rear, exactly in the middle or center line between the eyes) shows the sliced corpus callosum and brainstem. The left cerebral hemisphere and thalamus are off-center, so they remain unsectioned.

Spinal cord

SECTIONING THE BRAIN

HORIZONTAL　　**CORONAL**　　**SAGITTAL**　　**MEDIAL**

Specific names are given to various sections or slices of the brain, which show different views of the internal parts. For example, a sagittal section that is not medial (down the middle), misses the corpus callosum and cuts down through a cerebral hemisphere to reveal its intricate pattern of surface folds and grooves.

BRAIN ZONES AND PARTITIONS

THE BRAIN'S PHYSICAL STRUCTURE BROADLY REFLECTS ITS MENTAL ORGANIZATION. IN GENERAL, HIGHER MENTAL PROCESSES OCCUR IN THE UPPER REGIONS, WHILE THE BRAIN'S LOWER REGIONS TAKE CARE OF BASIC LIFE SUPPORT.

VERTICAL ORGANIZATION

The uppermost brain region, the cerebral cortex, is mostly involved in conscious sensations, abstract thought processes, reasoning, planning, working memory, and similar higher mental processes. The limbic areas (see pp.64–65) on the brain's innermost sides, around the brainstem, deal largely with more emotional and instinctive behaviors and reactions, as well as long-term memory. The thalamus is a preprocessing and relay center, primarily for sensory information coming from lower in the brainstem, bound for the cerebral hemispheres above. Moving down the brainstem into the medulla are the so-called "vegetative" centers of the brain, which sustain life even if the person has lost consciousness.

LESS CONSCIOUS, MORE AUTOMATIC
The brain's vertical zonation moves from high-level mental activity in the cerebral cortex gradually through to more basic or "primitive" lower functions, especially the autonomic centers of the medulla in the lower brainstem that deal with vital body functions, such as breathing and heartbeat.

CORTICAL → LIMBIC → MIDBRAIN → BRAINSTEM

LEFT AND RIGHT

Structurally, the left and right cerebral hemispheres look broadly similar. Functionally, however, speech and language, stepwise reasoning and analysis, and certain communicating actions are based mainly on the left side in most people. Since nerve fibers cross from left to right at the base of the brain, this dominant left side receives sensory information from, and sends messages to, muscles in the right side of the body–including the right hand. Meanwhile, the right hemisphere is more concerned with sensory inputs, auditory and visual awareness, creative abilities, and spatial–temporal awareness (what happens in our surroundings, second by second).

LEFT-HANDED PERSON
In a PET brain scan where yellow and red show increasing activity, a left-handed person involved in word recognition has busy areas at the right front cerebral cortex.

RIGHT-HANDED PERSON
On the same test in a right-handed subject, the left side of the cortex shows a similar pattern, with activity largely in the frontal region and the temporal and parietal areas.

ANARCHIC HAND SYNDROME

In anarchic hand syndrome (AHS), a person has one hand that is no longer under conscious control and seems to move on its own, almost as if possessed by another intelligence. The problem is usually due to an abnormality in the motor center of the cortex on the opposite side of the brain to the hand. Nerve signals sent from here to control the hand do not register any conscious intention for the action.

DR. STRANGELOVE
In this 1964 film the "hero" struggled with AHS as his leather-gloved right hand even tried to kill him.

THE ASYMMETRICAL BRAIN

In recent years, new and more accurate scanning techniques, especially MRI (see p.13), have shown that on average, brains are not as symmetrical in their left–right structure as was once believed. The scanning computer can be programmed to exaggerate any subtle departures from an exact mirror image. For example, near the lateral sulcus (Sylvian fissure), the part of the temporal lobe for understanding speech is slightly larger on the left than on the right. The lateral sulcus itself is also usually different in shape, being longer and less curved on the left than the right. This is partly due to a twisting effect known as Yakovlevian torque, which warps the right side of the brain forward.

Right lateral sulcus · FRONT · RIGHT HEMISPHERE · LEFT HEMISPHERE · Left occipital lobe · BACK

SEEN FROM BELOW
An asymmetry-enhanced MRI scan of the brain's underside reveals left–right differences, including a right frontal lobe that protrudes more than its counterpart, and a longer left occipital lobe that twists across the midline.

THE HOLLOW BRAIN

The brain has an internal system of chambers (ventricles), which are filled with a liquid–cerebrospinal fluid (CSF)–produced by the ventricle linings. The upper two chambers are the left and right lateral ventricles, one in each cerebral hemisphere, with hornlike forward- and side-facing projections. Small openings connect them to the third ventricle in the midbrain, which in turn links to the fourth ventricle in the pons and medulla. CSF flows slowly and continuously through the ventricles, then out via small openings into the subarachnoid space around the brain and the spinal cord.

VENTRICLES
Two large lateral ventricles communicate along ducts with the third ventricle (yellow, upper center), which lies between and below them.

CEREBROSPINAL FLUID
CSF is made by the ventricle lining (green). It physically cushions the brain, distributes nutrients, and collects wastes.

THE NUCLEI OF THE BRAIN

IN THE BRAIN, NUCLEI ARE DISCRETE COLLECTIONS OF THE CELL BODIES OF NEURONS (NERVE CELLS). THEIR NERVE FIBERS OR AXONS SPREAD OUTWARD TO PROJECT, OR LINK, TO VARIOUS OTHER BRAIN PARTS. THE BRAIN HAS MORE THAN 30 SETS OF NUCLEI, MOSTLY PAIRED LEFT AND RIGHT.

GENERAL STRUCTURE

To the naked eye, most brain nuclei resemble "islands" of gray matter (nerve-cell bodies) within the white matter of nerve fibers. Many nuclei are unencapsulated–not contained within a membrane or covering–so they may lack sharp delineation from surrounding tissues. An older term for some of these nuclei is "ganglia." However, this term is now usually reserved for similar structures in the peripheral nervous system, where groups of nerve-cell bodies are generally encapsulated into a discrete structure.

MAIN NUCLEI AND THEIR FUNCTIONS	
Basal	A system of nuclei (including some listed here) involved in motor control and learning.
Caudate	Involved in motor control and learning, especially processing feedback.
Subthalamic	Implicated in impulsive actions, including obsession–compulsion.
Thalamus	A major processing and relay area for inputs to the cerebral cortex (see pp.66–67).
Amygdala	Part of the limbic system, the amygdala is involved in learning, memory, and emotions.
Facial nucleus	One of several paired brainstem nuclei for cranial nerves, in this case nerve VII (facial).

CORPUS STRIATUM
This micrograph shows the nerve cell bodies (dark) and nerve fibers (pale) that make this brain region look striped or striated.

THE BASAL NUCLEI

The basal nuclei (also known as the basal ganglia) is the collective name for several pairs of nuclei at the "base" of the cerebral hemispheres–adjacent to their inner surfaces, around and below the thalamus. They include the putamen, caudate nuclei, globus pallidus, subthalamic nuclei, and substantia nigra. The putamen and caudate nuclei are together called the dorsal striatum because of the striped or striated appearance of their tissues. Together with the globus pallidus, or "pale sphere," the putamen and caudate nuclei are known as the corpus striatum.

THE SUBTHALAMIC NUCLEI AND GLOBUS PALLIDUS

As the name implies, each one of the paired subthalamic nuclei is situated beneath the thalamus. They are also immediately above the substantia nigra. Each nucleus is about the size and shape of a partly squashed pea and is almost surrounded by nerve fibers passing to, from, or around it. Most of the incoming (afferent) nerve fibers are from the globus pallidus, along with some from the cerebral cortex and the substantia nigra. The majority of the outgoing (efferent) nerve fibers carry signals to the globus pallidus and the substantia nigra. The globus pallidus and the putamen are sometimes termed the lentiform or lenticular nucleus.

SUBSTANTIA NIGRA

The substantia nigra or "black substance" paired nuclei are among the lowest, or most basal, of the basal nuclei. Each is situated just beneath a subthalamic nucleus. The dark color that is characteristic of these nuclei is caused by the body pigment melanin (also found in the skin) that is part of the biochemical pathways involving the neurotransmitter dopamine. Degeneration of substantia nigra neurons is seen in Parkinson's disease (see p.234).

Electrode

STIMULATION
Deep brain stimulation of basal nuclei, such as the substantia nigra, using electrodes is part of research into and treatment for Parkinson's.

CONNECTIONS AND FUNCTIONS

Most brain nuclei have multiple nerve connections, both inputs and outputs, and carry out wide-ranging functions. The C-shaped caudate nuclei above and to the side of the thalamus, and next to the lateral ventricle, have a head part, main body, and tapering tail. They are involved in motor (muscle) control and also in learning and memory. The rounded putamen, the outermost of the main basal ganglia, partly follows the shape of the caudate nucleus and is intricately linked anatomically to it. It, too, is heavily involved in motor control and movements, and in learning. The putamen has major nerve connections with the globus pallidus and substantia nigra. All of the basal ganglia work together as an integrated brain system to help ensure that physical movements are smooth and coordinated. Problems with one or more of the nuclei can lead to movement disorders such as tremors, tics, Parkinson's disease (see p.234), Tourette syndrome (see p.243), and Huntington's disease (see p.234). The subthalamic nuclei also have roles in impulsive actions and movement intentions.

LOCATION OF BASAL NUCLEI

Fornix

Caudate nucleus head

Thalamus

Putamen

Substantia nigra
Plays central roles in planning and monitoring of movements

MOTOR CONTROL

External globus pallidus

Internal globus pallidus

Subthalamic nucleus

Caudate nucleus tail

BASAL CIRCUITS
Incoming motor messages (indicated with red arrows) from the cortex pass via the caudate nucleus and putamen, then the globus pallidus, to the thalamus and back to the cortex (right side of diagram). Outgoing connections are shown in blue. Feedback loops within the basal nuclei "automatically" monitor and adjust ongoing movements (left side).

Mamillary body
Relay station between amygdala, hippocampus, and thalamus

MONITORING MOVEMENT

THE HIPPOCAMPUS
A micrograph of stained hippocampal tissue shows cellular organization that is similar to that in various brain nuclei. The neuron bodies are red, the axons (fibers) and other projections are blue. The glial cells, which provide support and nourishment, are green.

THE THALAMUS, HYPOTHALAMUS, AND PITUITARY GLAND

THE THALAMUS IS SITUATED AT THE ANATOMICAL CORE OF THE BRAIN. ITS POSITION MAKES IT PERFECTLY SITUATED TO ACT AS A RELAY STATION BETWEEN THE SENSE ORGANS AND THE BRAIN. SITTING BENEATH THE THALAMUS, THE HYPOTHALAMUS AND THE PITUITARY GLAND LINK THE CENTRAL NERVOUS SYSTEM AND THE ENDOCRINE SYSTEM.

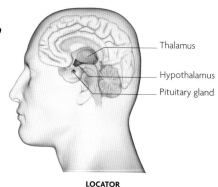

Thalamus

Hypothalamus

Pituitary gland

LOCATOR

THE THALAMUS

Paired, egg-shaped masses that sit side by side make up the thalamus. In a typical brain, each mass is about 1¼in (3cm) long and ½in (1.5cm) across. There are no direct nerve connections from one mass to the other–in fact, the fluid-filled chamber of the third ventricle lies between them. The thalamus is the major relay station for nerve signals coming from all the senses except smell. It screens, sorts, and preprocesses this continuing torrent of sensory information and sends it on to the cerebral cortex.

INSIDE THE THALAMUS

Each side (one of which is shown here) contains more than 20 nuclei consisting of "gray matter"—that is, collections of nerve-cell bodies. These nuclei, sometimes called thalamic bodies, are in groups separated by sheets of white matter (myelinated nerve fibers) known as laminae. The whole thalamus is enveloped in a similar white-matter wrapping.

FRONT OF THALAMUS

Nuclei of midline

Intralaminar nuclei

Anterior nucleus

Lateral dorsal nucleus

Medial dorsal nucleus

Centromedian nucleus

Medial ventral posterior nucleus

Lateral anterior nucleus

Internal lamina

Lateral ventral nucleus

Reticular nucleus

Lateral ventral posterior nucleus

Lateral posterior nucleus

THALAMIC NEURONS
Densely interconnected neuron bodies and nerve fibers (green) receive physical and nutritional support from glial cells (red).

Lateral nuclei (pulvinars)

Medial geniculate nucleus

Lateral geniculate nucleus

REAR OF THALAMUS

INNER EAR
Nerve impulses from the cochleas of the inner ears go mostly to the medial geniculate nuclei, which forward them on to the auditory cerebral cortex (Brodmann areas 41 and 42, see p.67).

RETINA
Information from the retinas, about what the eyes see, arrives at the lateral geniculate nuclei. After processing, it passes to the primary visual cortex (area 17) and visual association cortex.

VISUAL CORTEX
Working with the lateral geniculate nuclei, each much larger lateral nucleus (or pulvinar) sends accessory sensory information to several parts of the visual cortex (see pp.82–83).

FACE AND MOUTH
Sensory information from the facial skin and interior of the mouth travels along the trigeminal nerve and the trigeminothalamic tract to the medial ventral posterior nuclei.

PREMOTOR CORTEX
The thalamus has both incoming (afferent) and outgoing (efferent) nerve fibers. Many nerve fibers to the lateral anterior nuclei are afferent, from the premotor area of the cerebral cortex.

PREFRONTAL CORTEX
Most of the incoming signals for the medial dorsal nuclei are from the cerebral prefrontal cortex, and also from the hypothalamus when concerning emotions.

Fornix

Paraventricular nucleus
Contains neurosecretory cells; also involved in control of blood pressure, body temperature, and appetite

Dorsomedial nucleus
Important in eating, drinking, and regulation and conscious awareness of body weight

Mamillothalamic tract
This bundle of nerve fibers conveys messages between parts of the limbic system

THE HYPOTHALAMUS

Not much larger than the end segment of the little finger, weighing just ⁵/₃₂oz (4g), and comprising only 0.4 percent of total brain volume, the hypothalamus has many and varied vital roles–in conscious behavior, emotions and instincts, and automatic control of body systems and processes. It consists of more than a dozen paired nuclei (regions of interlinked nerve-cell bodies) clustered into the floor of the diencephalon and separated by the lateral ventricle. Its secretory cells make hormones (called releasing factors) that enter the bloodstream, and its neurosecretory cells produce hormonelike substances that travel along nerve axons down to the pituitary gland (see below).

Optic chiasm

Suprachiasmatic nucleus ("body clock")

Supraoptic nucleus
Two hormones, antidiuretic (ADH or vasopressin) and oxytocin, are produced by neurosecretory cells in the supraoptic nucleus

Posterior nucleus
Increases heart rate and blood pressure, dilates pupils, and other autonomic responses as part of "fight or flight" reaction

OXYTOCIN CRYSTALS
This birth and breastfeeding hormone is manufactured by neurosecretory cells in the paraventricular and supraoptic nuclei of the hypothalamus.

THE PITUITARY GLAND

The hypothalamus integrates the body's two systems for coordination and control: the nervous system around and above it; and the endocrine system (see p.114-15) via the pituitary just below it. The pea-sized pituitary (hypophysis), often called the body's "master hormone gland," has two distinct lobes. The anterior lobe (adenohypophysis) makes several hormones that release into the bloodstream to regulate other endocrine glands around the body, such as the thyroid. The posterior lobe (neurohypophysis) receives two hormones along axons from the hypothalamus.

Neurosecretory cell axons

Hypophyseal portal system
These blood vessels carry releasing factors to the anterior lobe

Pituitary stalk

Artery

SKIN

ADRENAL GLANDS

KIDNEYS

ENDOCRINE CELL
This micrograph shows somatotroph cells in the anterior pituitary. These cells store their growth hormone as granules (red dots) ready for export.

THYROID GLAND

Anterior lobe
Forming two-thirds of the pituitary bulk, the anterior lobe manufactures about eight major hormones; it is under the control of nerve messages and regulatory substances, called releasing factors, made in the hypothalamus

SEX GLANDS

Vein

BONES AND GENERAL BODY GROWTH

BREASTS

UTERUS AND BREASTS

Posterior lobe
Hypothalamic ADH and oxytocin are stored here and released as instructed

KEY TO PITUITARY HORMONES
- Melanocyte-stimulating hormone (MSH)
- Adrenocoricotropic hormone (ATCH)
- Thyroid-stimulating hormone (TSH)
- Follicle-stimulating hormone (FSH), Luteinizing hormone (LH)
- Growth hormone (GH)
- Oxytocin
- Antidiuretic hormone (ADH)
- Prolactin

THE BRAINSTEM AND CEREBELLUM

THE BRAINSTEM IS PERHAPS MISNAMED. IT IS NOT A STEM LEADING TO THE SEPARATE BRAIN ABOVE, BUT AN INTEGRAL PART OF THE BRAIN ITSELF. IT IS SHAPED RATHER LIKE A WIDENING UPRIGHT STALK, ON TOP OF WHICH ARE THE THALAMUS AND THE DOME OF THE CEREBRAL HEMISPHERES. CURLED AROUND THE LOWER BRAINSTEM, AT THE REAR OF THE BRAIN, SITS THE CEREBELLUM.

BRAINSTEM ANATOMY

The brainstem includes almost all of the brain except for the highest parts, which make up the forebrain (cerebrum and diencephalon, see p.52). Its uppermost region is the midbrain comprising an upper "roof" or tectum incorporating the superior and inferior colliculi or bulges at the rear, and the tegmentum to the front. Below the midbrain is the hindbrain. At its front is the large bulge of the pons. Behind and below this is the medulla, which narrows to merge with the uppermost end of the body's main nerve, the spinal cord. The cerebellum joins to the rear of the medulla by three pairs of stalks, known as the cerebellar peduncles.

CONNECTING THE BRAIN
This MRI scan shows how the upper brainstem is at about level with the eyes, and its lower region joins the spinal cord at a gap through the base of the skull, the foramen magnum.

Thalamus

Pineal body

Superior colliculus

Inferior colliculus

Superior cerebellar peduncle

Middle cerebellar peduncle

Inferior cerebellar peduncle

Median sulcus

Lateral sulcus

Fasciculus gracilis

Fasciculus cuneatus

REAR   **FRONT**

Midbrain

❶

❷ Cranial nerve IV (trochlear)

Pons

Cranial nerve V (trigeminal)

❸

Floor of fourth ventricle (fluid-filled chamber)

Cranial nerve VII (facial)

Cranial nerve X (vagus)

❹

Medulla

❺

Cranial nerve XI (accessory)

❻

Spinal cord

THE BRAINSTEM
This view of the brainstem, with the cerebellum removed, reveals the medulla and bundles of axons called fascicles. The cranial nerves join various parts of the brainstem.

FRONT   **RIGHT**   **BACK**   **LEFT**

360-DEGREE VIEW

The brainstem consists of the structures shown here inferior to, or below, the thalamus (green). Major landmarks are the pons (blue), the cerebellum (pinkish brown), and the medulla (creamy beige). In some categorizations, the thalamus is included as part of the brainstem.

BRAINSTEM SECTIONS
The horizontal cross sections of the brainstem shown here match the numbers in the illustration above left. Nuclei are shown in green; the white matter of nerve fiber tracts is pale. In each section, the rear of the body is uppermost.

INTERNAL STRUCTURE

Within the brainstem are groupings of nerve-cell bodies known as nuclei (see pp.58–59) and numerous bundles of nerve fibers or axons, called nerve tracts. For example, the pontine nuclei of the front or ventral pons are involved in learning and remembering motor skills–they act as relay stations for nerve signals from the motor cortex, which are traveling to the cerebellum behind the pons (see panel, opposite).

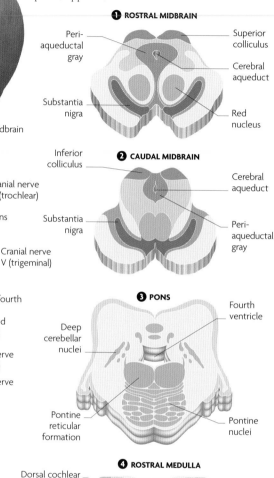

❶ ROSTRAL MIDBRAIN

Peri-aqueductal gray

Superior colliculus

Cerebral aqueduct

Substantia nigra

Red nucleus

❷ CAUDAL MIDBRAIN

Inferior colliculus

Cerebral aqueduct

Substantia nigra

Peri-aqueductal gray

❸ PONS

Deep cerebellar nuclei

Fourth ventricle

Pontine reticular formation

Pontine nuclei

❹ ROSTRAL MEDULLA

Dorsal cochlear nucleus

Raphe nucleus

Ventral cochlear nucleus

Inferior olive

Superior olive

Medullary pyramid

❺ MID-MEDULLA

Nucleus of the solitary tract

Vestibular nucleus

Inferior olive

Medullary reticular formation

Medullary pyramid

❻ MEDULLA-SPINAL CORD JUNCTION

Dorsal column nuclei

Spinal canal

Medial lemniscus

Medullary pyramid

BRAINSTEM FUNCTIONS

The brainstem is highly involved in mid- to low-order mental activities, for example, the almost "automatic" scanning movements of the eyes as we watch something pass by, rather than higher activities such as abstract thought. It is also the site of subconscious or autonomic control mechanisms, of which we are usually unaware. The medulla, in particular, houses groups of nuclei that are centers for respiratory (breathing), cardiac (heartbeat), and vasomotor (blood pressure) monitoring and control, as well as for vomiting, sneezing, swallowing, and coughing.

07:30 Melatonin secretion stops
START OF THE DAY
08:30 Bowel movement likely
04:30 Lowest body temperature
10:00 High alertness
06:45 Sharpest rise in blood pressure
09:00 Highest testosterone secretion
02:00 Deepest sleep
Noon
Midnight
14:30 Best coordination
22:30 Bowel movements suppressed
19:00 Highest body temperature
15:30 Fastest reaction time
21:00 Melatonin secretion starts
18:30 Highest blood pressure
17:00 Greatest cardiovascular efficiency and muscle strength

CIRCADIAN RHYTHM
Information from the "body clock" (see p.184) is passed to the brainstem so that basic body processes follow a 24-hour rhythm.

LOCKED-IN SYNDROME

Damage to certain parts of the brainstem, especially the forward-facing area of the pons, can produce a condition known as "locked-in" or ventral pontine syndrome. The sufferer is aware of his or her surroundings and able to see and hear, but cannot activate any voluntary muscles—those that are under conscious control—and so is unable to move or react. Damage may be due to injury or the lack of blood supply during a stroke. In some cases, the eye muscles continue to function, allowing communication by eye movements.

THE CEREBELLUM

The "little brain" is the lower, rearmost part of the entire brain. It resembles the wrinkled appearance of the cerebrum above, but its grooves and bulges are finer and organized into more regular patterns. Major anatomical parts of the cerebellum include: the long, slim vermis ("worm") in the center; two flocculonodular lobes beneath, one on each side; and outside these, two much larger lateral lobes, each of which is divided into several lobules. The two lateral lobes are reminiscent of the two hemispheres of the cerebrum and are sometimes termed cerebellar hemispheres. The cerebellum's main functions are to coordinate body movements through integrated control of muscles, including balance and posture, and equilibrium.

INTERNAL STRUCTURE

The cerebellum has a similar layered microstructure to the cerebrum. The outer layer, or cerebellar cortex, is gray matter composed of nerve-cell bodies and their dendrite projections. Beneath this is a medullary area of white matter consisting largely of nerve fibers. Toward the center are collections of more nerve-cell bodies known as deep cerebellar nuclei. Nerve fibers run from these nuclei to the cerebral cortex high above. In a cross section at almost any angle through the cerebellum, the white matter between the cortex and deep nuclei forms a complex branching pattern known as the arbor vitae.

CEREBELLUM CELLS
The main types of nerve cells in the cerebellar cortex are known as Purkinje cells (red), supported by glial cells (green).

THE CEREBELLUM
The grooves in the cerebellar surface are termed fissures, and the bulges are known as folia. In each image, the front is uppermost.

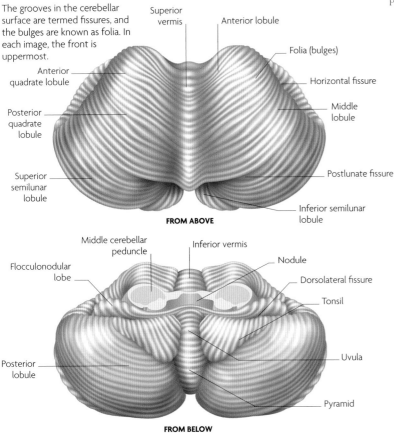

Superior vermis
Anterior lobule
Folia (bulges)
Anterior quadrate lobule
Horizontal fissure
Middle lobule
Posterior quadrate lobule
Superior semilunar lobule
Postlunate fissure
Inferior semilunar lobule

FROM ABOVE

Middle cerebellar peduncle
Inferior vermis
Flocculonodular lobe
Nodule
Dorsolateral fissure
Tonsil
Uvula
Posterior lobule
Pyramid

FROM BELOW

CROSS SECTION OF CEREBELLUM

Stellate interneuron

Purkinje cell
Has many branching dendrites

Golgi cells
One of various inhibitory interneurons including basket and stellate cells

CEREBELLAR CORTEX
Several types of cortical cells occupy the three distinct layers of the cortex, which are from the outside inward, the molecular, Purkinje, and granule layers.

Folium
Bulge in cerebellar surface

Horizontal axon
Long fiber extends from granule cell

White matter
Chiefly nerve fibers (axons)

Climbing fibers

Granule cell
Has long axons

THE LIMBIC SYSTEM

THE LIMBIC SYSTEM IS INVOLVED IN INSTINCTIVE BEHAVIORS, DEEP-SEATED EMOTIONS, AND BASIC IMPULSES SUCH AS SEX, ANGER, PLEASURE, AND GENERAL SURVIVAL. IT ALSO FORMS A LINK BETWEEN CENTERS OF HIGHER CONSCIOUSNESS, IN THE CEREBRAL CORTEX, AND THE BRAINSTEM, WHICH REGULATES THE BODY'S SYSTEMS.

COMPONENTS OF THE LIMBIC SYSTEM

The limbic system includes the areas of the cortex and adjacent parts known as the limbic lobe (see opposite page), along with the amygdala, hypothalamus, thalamus, mamillary bodies, and other deeper, more central brain structures. The system is also "hard-wired" into parts of the sensory system, especially the sense of smell. Nerve fibers link all of these parts intimately and also connect them to other areas of the brain, particularly the lower frontal cortex, with its roles in expectation, reward, and decision-making.

Fornix
Corpus callosum
Mamillary bodies

AT THE BRAIN'S CORE
Situated approximately in the anatomical center or core of the brain, the limbic system is a varied collection of structures extending from the cerebrum inward and down to the brainstem.

Fornix
This tract of nerve fibers connects the mamillary bodies and hippocampus

Cingulate gyrus
Part of limbic cortex just above corpus callosum

Column of fornix

Mamillary bodies
Small lumps of nerve cells, these relay signals to thalamus, contributing to alertness and memory formation

Olfactory bulbs
Tracts of sensory nerve cells extend from nasal cavity into the brain; they part-process smell information before it enters conscious awareness

LIMBIC STRUCTURES
The name of this system is derived from the Latin *limbus*, meaning "border" or "edge." Its major structures form a circular, beltlike transition zone between the relatively plain-looking main cerebral cortex and the more distinctive bodies, tracts, and nuclei of the inner, lower brain.

Hypothalamus
Chief link and mediator between nervous system and hormonal or endocrine system (see p.61)

Pons

Hippocampus
Named after its vague S-shaped resemblance to a seahorse, this part is involved in memory and spatial awareness

Midbrain
The limbic system extends nerve fibers from thalamus and other higher parts into this uppermost part of the brainstem and also to the basal nuclei

Amygdala
Almond-shaped neuron clusters that are heavily involved in memory and emotional responses

Parahippocampal gyrus
This area of cortex flanking the hippocampus is active when viewing scenes and places

360-DEGREE VIEW

FRONT

RIGHT SIDE

BACK

LEFT SIDE

These views of the limbic system show how it is situated in the center of the brain and occupies parts of the inner or medial surfaces of the cerebral cortex. The cingulate gyrus, the hippocampus, and the parahippocampal gyrus—all part of the cerebral cortex—arch around and down below the corpus callosum.

Cingulate gyrus
Ridge above the corpus callosum

Parahippocampal gyrus
Limbic lobe ridge below corpus callosum

Cingulate sulcus
Groove or valley with cingulate gyrus extending on either side of it

Corpus callosum

Hippocampus and amygdala

WRAP-AROUND SHAPE
The cortical areas known as the limbic lobe (highlighted here in brown) comprise inner or medial surfaces of the cerebral cortex, which wrap around the innermost, central portions of the brain—the brainstem.

THE LIMBIC LOBE

The structures of the limbic system are surrounded by an area of the cortex referred to as the limbic lobe. The lobe forms a collarlike or ringlike shape on the inner surfaces of the cerebral hemispheres, both above and below the corpus callosum. The upper part is the cingulate gyrus, on either side of the cingulate sulcus. The lower part is the parahippocampal gyrus, delineated below by the collateral fissure and rhinal sulcus. The cingulate and parahippocampal gyri are together known as the fornicate gyrus. As such, the limbic lobe comprises the inward-facing parts of other cortical lobes, including the temporal, parietal, and frontal, where the left and right lobes curve around to face each other. The hippocampus and amygdala are not integral to this split-ring shape, but are considered as anatomically part of the limbic lobe as well as components of the limbic system.

THE HIPPOCAMPUS

The hippocampus is strung along the upper edge of the parahippocampal gyrus. The hippocampus interlocks with another ridge, known as the dentate gyrus–together the two form the hippocampal–dentate complex. It is part of the cerebral cortex, but it has only one, two, or three layers of cells, rather than the usual six layers found in most of the more "advanced" regions of the cortex.

The main functions of the hippocampus include spatial awareness, and memory formation and recall. In particular, the hippocampus helps select transient information for memorizing and then pass it through to longer-term memory areas. Damage to it can prevent a person from forming new memories, even though memories from before the damage are intact.

NEURONS
A light micrograph of a section through the hippocampus reveals neurons that have been labeled with green fluorescent protein. Also seen are ion channels (colored gold) that allow the exchange of sodium and calcium ions across the cell membrane. This exchange propagates nerve impulses.

Inferior horn of lateral ventricle

Fimbria

CA3

CA2

CA4

CA1

Subicular cortex

Dentate gyrus

Enthorhinal cortex

Parahippocampal gyrus

White matter

SECTION OF HIPPOCAMPUS

LOCATION OF HIPPOCAMPUS

HIPPOCAMPAL STRUCTURES
This cross section shows a coronal slice through the hippocampus. The detailed structures of the cell layers in the hippocampus change around its curve, from the region known as CA1 (cornis ammonis 1) to CA4. The main nerve-signal inputs are from the parahippocampal gyrus, the fornix, and the hippocampus in the opposite hemisphere.

THE CEREBRAL CORTEX

THE CEREBRAL CORTEX IS THE OUTER LAYER OF THE BRAIN'S MOST DOMINANT PART, THE CEREBRUM. IT IS THE BULGING WRINKLED SURFACE WE SEE WHEN LOOKING AT THE BRAIN FROM ANY ANGLE. IT IS COMMONLY KNOWN AS GRAY MATTER FROM ITS COLOR, WHICH CONTRASTS WITH THE WHITE MATTER IN THE LAYER BELOW.

THE CEREBRAL LOBES

Bulges and grooves help divide the cortex into four to six paired lobes, according to the anatomical system used. The main and deepest groove is the longitudinal fissure that separates the cerebral hemispheres. Both the extent and the names of the lobes are also partly related to the overlying bones of the skull, known as the neurocranium. For example, the two frontal lobes are approximately beneath the frontal bone, and likewise for the occipital lobes under the occipital bone. In some naming systems, the limbic lobe (see p.65) and the insula, or central lobe, are distinguished as separate from other lobes.

MEDIAL VIEW OF THE CORTEX

Frontal lobe
Parietal lobe
Temporal lobe
Occipital lobe

Frontal lobe
Parietal lobe
Temporal lobe
Occipital lobe

LATERAL VIEW OF THE CORTEX

LOBE DIVISIONS
The cortex can be divided into four areas called lobes (shown here). In some classifications, the forward part of the frontal lobe is separated as the prefrontal lobe, but the term prefrontal cortex is more generally accepted.

CORTICAL LANDMARKS

Rounded bulges of the cortex are known as gyri; grooves are termed sulci when relatively shallow and fissures when deeper. The overall patterns of gyri and sulci are similar but rarely identical among normal brains—individual variations occur. They are also similar for the left and right of an individual's brain, although there are minor asymmetries (see p.57).

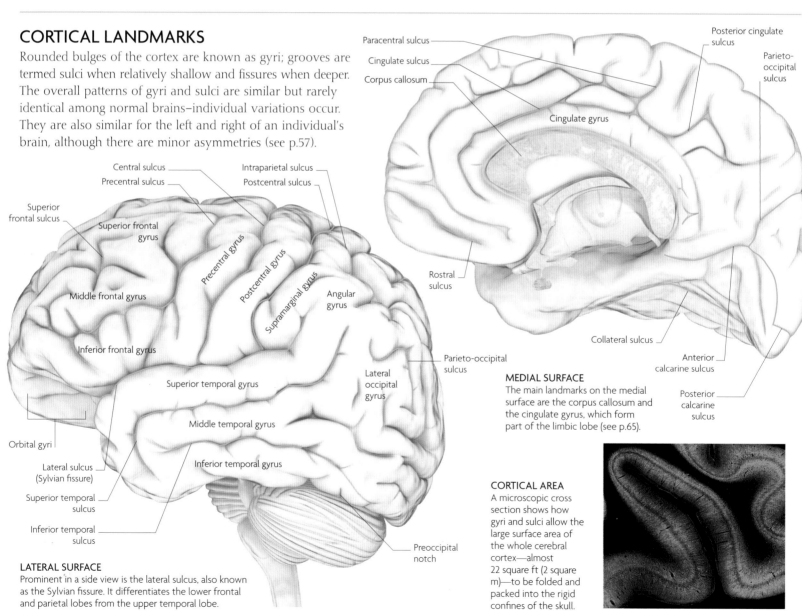

Paracentral sulcus
Cingulate sulcus
Corpus callosum
Cingulate gyrus
Posterior cingulate sulcus
Parieto-occipital sulcus
Rostral sulcus
Collateral sulcus
Anterior calcarine sulcus
Posterior calcarine sulcus

MEDIAL SURFACE
The main landmarks on the medial surface are the corpus callosum and the cingulate gyrus, which form part of the limbic lobe (see p.65).

Central sulcus
Precentral sulcus
Intraparietal sulcus
Postcentral sulcus
Superior frontal sulcus
Superior frontal gyrus
Precentral gyrus
Postcentral gyrus
Supramarginal gyrus
Angular gyrus
Middle frontal gyrus
Inferior frontal gyrus
Superior temporal gyrus
Lateral occipital gyrus
Middle temporal gyrus
Orbital gyri
Lateral sulcus (Sylvian fissure)
Superior temporal sulcus
Inferior temporal sulcus
Inferior temporal gyrus
Parieto-occipital sulcus
Preoccipital notch

LATERAL SURFACE
Prominent in a side view is the lateral sulcus, also known as the Sylvian fissure. It differentiates the lower frontal and parietal lobes from the upper temporal lobe.

CORTICAL AREA
A microscopic cross section shows how gyri and sulci allow the large surface area of the whole cerebral cortex—almost 22 square ft (2 square m)—to be folded and packed into the rigid confines of the skull.

FUNCTIONAL AREAS

The cortex can be "mapped" in three ways. One is by gross anatomy, as defined by sulci and gyri (see opposite page). A second is by microscopic anatomy—the shapes and types of cells and their connections, as pioneered by Korbinian Brodmann (see panel, below). The map of areas shown here is named after him. The third method is by neurological function, when small areas are stimulated to study the sensations or movements this produces. The three "maps" only partially coincide.

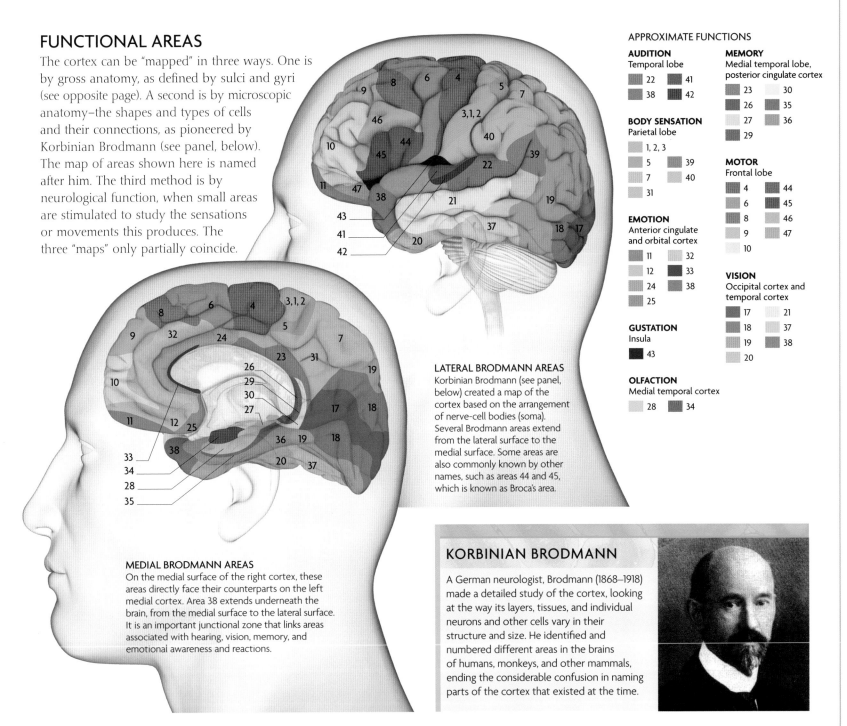

APPROXIMATE FUNCTIONS

AUDITION
Temporal lobe

22		41	
38		42	

BODY SENSATION
Parietal lobe

1, 2, 3	
5	39
7	40
31	

EMOTION
Anterior cingulate and orbital cortex

11	32
12	33
24	38
25	

GUSTATION
Insula

43

OLFACTION
Medial temporal cortex

28	34

MEMORY
Medial temporal lobe, posterior cingulate cortex

23	30
26	35
27	36
29	

MOTOR
Frontal lobe

4	44
6	45
8	46
9	47
10	

VISION
Occipital cortex and temporal cortex

17	21
18	37
19	38
20	

LATERAL BRODMANN AREAS
Korbinian Brodmann (see panel, below) created a map of the cortex based on the arrangement of nerve-cell bodies (soma). Several Brodmann areas extend from the lateral surface to the medial surface. Some areas are also commonly known by other names, such as areas 44 and 45, which is known as Broca's area.

MEDIAL BRODMANN AREAS
On the medial surface of the right cortex, these areas directly face their counterparts on the left medial cortex. Area 38 extends underneath the brain, from the medial surface to the lateral surface. It is an important junctional zone that links areas associated with hearing, vision, memory, and emotional awareness and reactions.

KORBINIAN BRODMANN

A German neurologist, Brodmann (1868–1918) made a detailed study of the cortex, looking at the way its layers, tissues, and individual neurons and other cells vary in their structure and size. He identified and numbered different areas in the brains of humans, monkeys, and other mammals, ending the considerable confusion in naming parts of the cortex that existed at the time.

STRUCTURE OF THE CORTEX

The highly convoluted "sheet" of gray matter that constitutes the cerebral cortex varies in thickness from about 1/16 to 3/16 in (2 to 5mm). Estimates of its cell numbers vary from 10 billion to more than 50 billion neurons and about five to ten times this number of glial (supporting) and other cells. The neurons are organized into six layers, known generally from the outside inward as the molecular, external granular, external pyramidal, internal granular, internal pyramidal and multiform layers. Each Brodmann area has its characteristic types and shapes of neurons. For example, primary motor area 4 is rich in pyramidal cells.

CORTEX COMPONENTS
Relatively low magnification of cortical tissue shows neurons (far left, blue-gray) packed among supporting glial cells (red). Higher magnification reveals an individual axon at the cortex base (second from left). Different laboratory stains show four of the six cortical layers (third from left) and fatty myelin wrapped around an axon (below).

CORTEX TISSUE

NERVE FIBER

CEREBRAL LAYERS

OLIGODENDROCYTE CELL

MICROANATOMY OF A NEURON
The cell body of a neuron is about 10–100 micrometers across, that is, $\frac{1}{100}$ th to $\frac{1}{10}$ th of one millimeter. The axon is 0.2–20 micrometers in diameter; dendrites are usually slimmer. In the central nervous system, dendrites are typically 10–50 micrometers long, and axons can be up to a few centimeters (inches) in length.

Axon (nerve fiber)
Most neurons have just one main axon or sending neurite, also called an axonal process or nerve fiber; it is usually much longer and thicker than the dendrites

Myelin sheath
Spiral wrapping of myelin around certain axons helps speed and insulate the nerve impulses they carry

Oligodendrocyte
Manufactures myelin sheaths for axons of brain neurons

Neuron cell body

Axon end bulb

Synapse
Communication point between neurons

Dendrite

Microtubules
Flexible, rod-like assemblies form the structural "scaffolding" of the cell

Golgi complex
Stores and processes proteins made by the ribosomes, ready for export from the cell

BRAIN CELLS

THERE ARE OVER A THOUSAND TYPES OF BRAIN CELL, WHICH FALL INTO TWO BROAD GROUPS: NEURONS AND GLIAL CELLS. NEURONS SEND ELECTRICAL SIGNALS, OR "FIRE," IN RESPONSE TO STIMULI. THERE ARE ABOUT 86 BILLION NEURONS IN AN AVERAGE HUMAN BRAIN AND TEN TIMES AS MANY GLIAL CELLS.

NEURONS

Like hepatocyte cells in the liver, osteoctyes in bone, or erythrocytes (red cells) in blood, each neuron is a self-contained functioning unit. Its internal components, the organelles, include a nucleus harboring the genetic material (DNA), energy-providing mitochondria, and protein-making ribosomes. As in most other types of cells, the organelles are concentrated in the main cell body. In addition, characteristic features of neurons are neurites–long, thin, fingerlike or threadlike extensions from the cell body (soma). The two main types are dendrites and axons. Usually dendrites receive nerve signals, while axons send them onward.

Vacuoles
Baglike containers inside the cell that store various substances such as wastes or excess water

Cell membrane
Outer covering or "skin" of the cell; in neurons, it is specialized to convey or propagate nerve impulses (see p.72)

Cytoplasm
The cell's individual organelles are suspended in this jellylike, solute-packed fluid

Rough endoplasmic reticulum
Sheets of membrane are folded, stacked into piles, and studded with tiny, spherical ribosomes

Mitochondrion
Cellular "power station" that splits apart sugar and fat molecules to release their chemical energy

Ribosomes
Ball-like structures that assemble proteins

Smooth endoplasmic reticulum
Tubes and layers that help transport and store materials

Nucleus
Contains DNA that instructs how the cell develops and functions

TYPES OF NEURON

Neurons can be categorized structurally according to the location of the cell body in relation to the axon and dendrites, and also the number of dendrites and axon branches (see illustration, below). In some regions of the brain, peripheral nervous system, and sense organs, neuron types are organized and easily recognized. For example, the retina of the eye contains ranks of bipolar neurons (see p.80). However, in many other regions, the neurons are mixed in shape and form a complex, interconnected web. In the cortex, one neuron may receive signals from many thousands of other neurons via its multitudinous branching dendrites. Signals are conducted to the soma, around this, and then away along the axon–always by the cell membrane, not through the cytoplasm.

UNIPOLAR NEURON
One axon extends from the cell body and divides into two or more branches.

Cell body
Axon
Axon terminals
Axon branch
Axon branch
Dendrites

BIPOLAR NEURON
The cell body has one set of dendritic extensions and one axonal extension or process.

Cell body
Dendrites
Axon
Axon terminals

MULTIPOLAR NEURON
Many sets of dendrites and one main axon is the design for most of the brain's neurons.

Axon
Cell body
Dendrites
Axon terminals

NEURON REGENERATION

Each neuron has its own immensely complex, highly individual shape and sets of connections, via synapses, to other neurons. Its links are shaped by its history and how it is used over time, as some of its connections weaken and fade while others strengthen. This uniqueness makes any disease or damage very serious. The neuron is unlikely to reform all of its extensions and their links. Even if regrowth occurs, it is slow and at first random, as the dendrites and axon "feel" their way according to the nerve signals being received and sent.

Cell body
Myelin sheath
Degenerating fiber terminal
Damaged nerve fiber (axon)
INJURED NERVE

Nerve fiber sprouts new endings
Empty section of myelin sheath
Fiber has degenerated
EARLY STAGE OF REPAIR

Regrown fiber
Regenerated terminals
NERVE FUNCTION RESTORED

NEUROGENESIS
The brain can form new nerve cells. Neural progenitor cells (shown in this micrograph) are a stage in specialization between stem cells and fully formed nerve cells. At this stage they can specialize into neurons or support cells.

REPAIRING NERVE FIBERS
Nerve cell repair is a very slow process, if it occurs at all. The damaged or severed end of the axon (fiber) can be encouraged to send out new sprout growths by treating it with substances called nerve growth factors. A sprout that finds an empty myelin sheath may then grow through it.

GLIAL CELLS

Glial cells give physical support to neurons (glia means "glue" in Greek) but they are also thought to influence neurons' electrical activity. They provide physical support for the thin dendrites and axons that wind their way around the neural network, and supply nutrition for neurons in the form of sugars and raw materials for growth and repair. There are several types of glial cells. Oligodendrocytes make myelin sheathing, a task performed in peripheral nerves by Schwann cells. Microglia destroy invading microbes and clear up debris from degenerating neurons. Astrocytes are thought to affect neuronal behavior and play a role in memory and sleep.

OLIGODENDROCYTES UNDER ATTACK
In multiple sclerosis (MS) oligodendrocytes (purple), which normally make insulating myelin sheaths around nerve axons in the brain and spinal cord, are attacked and destroyed by microglia (yellow).

SYNAPSES

Synapses are communication sites where neurons pass nerve impulses among themselves. Many neurons do not actually touch one another, but pass their signals via chemicals (neurotransmitters) across an incredibly thin gap, called the synaptic cleft (see pp.72–73). Microanatomically, synapses are divided into types according to the sites where the neurons almost touch. These sites include the soma, the dendrites, the axons, and tiny narrow projections called dendritic spines found on certain kinds of dendrites (see illustration, right). Axospinodendritic synapses form more than 50 percent of all synapses in the brain; axodendritic synapses constitute about 30 percent.

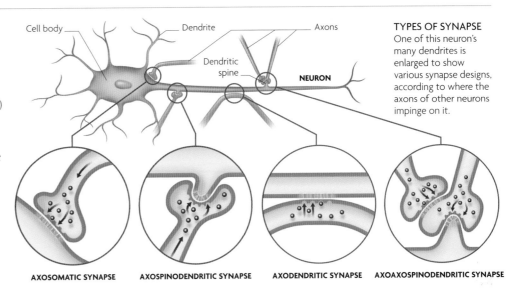

Cell body
Dendrite
Axons
Dendritic spine
NEURON

TYPES OF SYNAPSE
One of this neuron's many dendrites is enlarged to show various synapse designs, according to where the axons of other neurons impinge on it.

AXOSOMATIC SYNAPSE
AXOSPINODENDRITIC SYNAPSE
AXODENDRITIC SYNAPSE
AXOAXOSPINODENDRITIC SYNAPSE

GLIAL CELLS
In this light micrograph, star-shaped astrocytes (lighter green) can be seen along with other support cells, or neuroglia. Together, they make up the brain's connective tissue and provide protection to neurons. The cell nuclei are colored blue. Astrocytes modulate the activity of neurons and play a part in memory formation and sleep.

NERVE IMPULSES

A NERVE IMPULSE OR SIGNAL CAN BE THOUGHT OF AS A TINY, BRIEF "SPIKE" OF ELECTRICITY TRAVELING THROUGH A NEURON. AT A MORE FUNDAMENTAL LEVEL, IT CONSISTS OF CHEMICAL PARTICLES MOVING ACROSS THE CELL'S OUTER MEMBRANE, FROM ONE SIDE TO THE OTHER.

Neurofibral node

Myelin-coated internode

ANATOMY OF AN IMPULSE

Nerve signals are composed of series of discrete impulses, also known as action potentials. A single impulse is caused by a traveling "wave" of chemical particles called ions, which have electrical charges and are mainly the minerals sodium, potassium, and chloride. In the brain, and throughout the body, most impulses in most neurons are of the same strength–about 100 millivolts (0.1 volt). They are also of the same duration–around one millisecond ($1/1,000$ of a second)–but travel at varying speeds. The information they convey depends on how frequently they pass in terms of impulses per second, where they came from, and where they are heading.

SPEED OF CONDUCTION

Impulses travel at widely differing rates, from 3 to more than 330ft/s (1–100m/s), depending on the type of nerve carrying them. They are fastest in myelinated axons. Here the impulse "jumps" rapidly between the myelin-coated sections from one gap (neurofibral node), to the next node.

IMPULSE HEADS TOWARD SYNAPSE

AXON IS POLARIZED AT REST

AXON DEPOLARIZES AS IMPULSE PASSES

IMPULSE ARRIVES AT SYNAPSE

CHANGING FORM

A nerve impulse is always based on chemical particles. As it passes along a dendrite or axon, it consists of moving electrically charged ions, but at a synapse, it relies more on the structural shape of the chemical neurotransmitter.

Positive ions pumped out across membrane, restoring resting potential

Excess of positive ions inside produces a positive charge and the potential across the membrane changes from -70mV to peak at +30mV relative to the outside

Direction of nerve impulse

Positive ions pumped in

Excess of positive ions on outside of cell membrane

Region outside the axon consists of extracellular fluid

Cell's axon membrane

Axon of nerve cell contains intracellular fluid

Neuron membranes have the ability to actively pump charged ions through gatelike channels

"Action potential" across membrane

ELECTRICAL WAVE

The nerve impulse is based chiefly on the movement of positively charged sodium and potassium ions through a neuron's cell membrane. The nerve signal moves along the membrane as a wave of depolarization and repolarization.

3 Repolarization
To restore the balance of electrical charges, positive potassium ions flow in the opposite direction to the sodium ions. This stimulates adjacent areas of the membrane behind the depolarized area, disrupting their resting potentials.

2 Depolarization
The arrival of an impulse is known as depolarization. Sodium ions, which are positive, flow quickly through sodium ion channels in the neuron's axon membrane, from outside to inside. The inside is now positive compared to the outside.

1 Resting potential
When no impulse is passing, there are more potassium and negative ions inside the neuron's axon membrane, and more sodium and other positive ions outside. This causes a polarization or difference in electrical potential across the membrane, with the outside positive.

1 Synaptic vesicles
The neurotransmitter molecules are manufactured in the neuron's cell body (called the soma), which could be some distance from the end of the axon. To provide a continuing supply of these molecules at the synapse, they are transported along the axon by neurotubules that work like ultramicroscopic conveyor belts, and then packaged into membrane-covered, ball-like containers called synaptic vesicles.

Axon
Neurotubule
Microfilament
Axon membrane
Axon end bulb
Neurotransmitter molecules
Receptor site
Emptying vesicle
Mitochondrion
Presynaptic membrane
Synaptic cleft
Positive ions
Postsynaptic membrane

AT THE SYNAPSE

The synaptic cleft separating the membranes of the sending pre-synaptic) cell and the receiving (postsynaptic) cell has a width of some 20nm (20 billionths of a meter). This is so narrow that the neurotransmitter molecules can pass across it extremely quickly by simple diffusion—moving from a region of higher concentration to one of lower concentration. Depending on the neurotransmitter, the time taken for the impulse to pass from the pre- to the postsynaptic membranes is typically less than 2ms ($^1/_{500}$ of a second). There is then a recovery delay or clearance time, as the concentrations of neurotransmitter subside, before the next impulse can be sent across. This may last several tenths of a second.

2 Discharge of neurotransmitter
When the nerve impulse or action potential reaches the presynaptic membrane of the axon end bulb, it causes synaptic vesicles to fuse or merge with the membrane. This releases the neurotransmitter molecules to pass or diffuse across the synaptic cleft to the post-synaptic membrane and slot into receptor sites.

Membrane channel opens
Ions pass through channel

3 Post-synaptic excitation
Neurotransmitter molecules slot into the same-shaped receptor sites of gatelike membrane channels in the postsynaptic membrane (such as the dendrite of the next nerve cell). When this happens, the channel opens and allows positive ions to flow from the outside to the inside of the post-synaptic cell. This triggers a new wave of depolarization, which continues the impulse if it is strong enough.

NEUROTRANSMITTERS

Neurotransmitters are chemicals that allow signals to pass between a neuron and another cell. There are several groups of neurotransmitter molecules. One contains only acetylcholine. A second is known as biogenic amines, or monoamines, and includes dopamine, histamine, norepinephrine, and serotonin. The third group is composed of amino acids, such as GABA, glutamic acid, aspartic acid, and glycine. Many of these substances have other roles in the body. For example, histamine is involved in the inflammatory response. Amino acids (apart from GABA) are also very common, being the building blocks for hundreds of kinds of protein molecules.

Oxygen
Carbon
Hydrogen
Nitrogen

GABA MOLECULE
GABA is the chief inhibitory neurotransmitter throughout much of the human brain and nervous system.

SMALL MOLECULE NEUROTRANSMITTER	
Several common examples of neurotransmitters are listed together with their typical effects at synapses.	
NEUROTRANSMITTER CHEMICAL NAME	**USUAL POST-SYNAPTIC EFFECT**
Acetylcholine	Mostly excitatory
Gamma aminobutyric acid (GABA)	Inhibitory
Glycine	Inhibitory
Glutamate	Excitatory
Aspartate	Excitatory
Dopamine	Excitatory and inhibitory
Noradrenaline	Mostly excitatory
Serotonin	Inhibitory
Histamine	Excitatory

EXCITATION AND INHIBITION
A particular neurotransmitter can either excite a receiving nerve cell, helping depolarize the axon hillock (where the soma and axon meet) and continue a nerve impulse, or inhibit it by preventing depolarization from taking place. Which of these occurs depends on the type of membrane channel on the receiving cell.

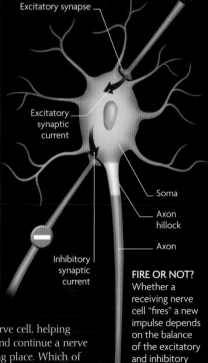

Excitatory synapse
Excitatory synaptic current
Inhibitory synaptic current
Soma
Axon hillock
Axon

FIRE OR NOT?
Whether a receiving nerve cell "fires" a new impulse depends on the balance of the excitatory and inhibitory currents.

BRAIN MAPPING AND SIMULATION

CREATING AN ARTIFICAL BRAIN IS A LONG-HELD DREAM THAT IS FINALLY BEING MADE POSSIBLE THANKS TO ADVANCES IN COMPUTER POWER. TWO GLOBAL PROJECTS ARE NOW UNDERWAY TO REPRODUCE A DIGITAL SIMULATION OF THE HUMAN ORGAN. IF THIS IS ACHIEVED IT WILL EFFECTIVELY BE A BRAIN, ALTHOUGH WHETHER IT WILL BE CONSCIOUS AND WHAT SORT OF EXPERIENCE IT MIGHT HAVE ARE UNKNOWN.

THE CONNECTOME

The connections between neurons form the "wiring" of the brain, and in order to recreate a working simulation it is essential to know in detail the route taken by information passing from one neuron to another. A global initiative called the Connectome project charts these pathways using a form of MRI scanning called diffusion tensor imaging. The connecting fibers of the brain are skeins of myelin-coated axons, which snake out from one cell to contact another. The overall pattern of neural pathways is similar in all of us, but differs in detail from person to person. It is these differences that make each of us unique. For instance, people with relatively few pathways from their amygdala, the area deep in the brain that generates fear, to their prefrontal cortex are likely to be less nervous than people whose neural wiring allows their forebrain to be deluged by doom alerts from the amygdala.

INPUT

OUTPUT

NEAT THEORY
Neural networks provide a neat theoretical model of how the brain works. The virtual neurons form a mini-brain. When data is fed into the system, it changes in a way believed to be similar to that of the physical human brain. Connections form between all neurons in the network.

Neuron recieves input from first-level "sensory" neurons and passes data on

Each neuron is connected to all other neurons in the network

COMPLEX WEB
This image of cells in a minute section of neocortex reveals that the network of fibers in the brain is incredibly complex. To produce a model of a brain that really behaves like a human one involves tracing each and every fiber.

Fibers travel through the limbic system and up to the cortex

Thick skein of fibers forms the corpus callosum, which carries signals from one hemisphere to the other

Fibers narrow at base of brain to form spinal cord and peripheral nervous system

KEY

	FIBERS RUN LEFT TO RIGHT
	FIBERS RUN FRONT TO BACK
	FIBERS RUN UP AND DOWN

ARCHITECTURE OF THE BRAIN
This 3D reconstruction of connecting nerve fibers is based on data gathered by polarized light imaging of a postmortem brain. Myelin-coated nerve fibers reflect light in distinct ways, allowing scientists to map the orientation of axons.

SLICING THE BRAIN

Scientists already have highly detailed visual models of the human brain available to them on computers. The one shown below was built up by slicing a dead woman's brain into 7,400 slices, staining the sections to show the details, and then building the information into a 3D model. Many slices were slightly damaged in the process, so scientists had to "fill in" the missing connections. Although the model does not function, researchers can deduce a great deal about how the brain works from examining its structure in light of what is already known about which parts of the brain do what.

BIGBRAIN VIEWER
The BigBrain is a free, publicly available online tool that gives access to a detailed view of human brain anatomy. It allows researchers to study connections between cortical regions and redefines the traditional map of the brain.

DIGITAL MODELING

The biggest challenge facing neuroscientists is to simulate an entire human brain. The current approach is to identify every neuron in a normal brain and then trace all the connections between them. Bit by bit, the entire organ and its wiring will be determined and the information converted to a digital model, which will be stored on one or more supercomputers. The system could then be run on demand, fed by digital input that mimics sensations triggered by the environment. This should, in theory, function like a real brain. In Europe, this mammoth task is being undertaken by the European Union flagship Human Brain Project (HBP), and a similar endeavor, Brain Research through Advancing Innovative Neurotechnologies (BRAIN), is underway in the US.

PATCH CLAMP
The electrical output of neurons is recorded using a 12-patch clamp instrument (below). The patch clamp allows 12 living neurons to be studied at the same time.

BLUE BRAIN PROJECT
Neurons in the cortex are so dense it is almost impossible to visualize them. The Swiss Blue Brain Project has produced the digital equivalent of around one million neurons and their billion interconnections, as seen here.

THE SELF-BUILD BRAIN

Another approach to brain simulation is to let a virtual brain grow digitally. The idea is to create a neural network, a system of computer-based information nodes organized to communicate with one another, that will restructure itself as it receives new data. NeuraBASE, for example, is a computer-based artificial-intelligence system that starts with virtual motor and sensory neurons, each of which responds to an element of information. Real-life stimuli are fed into the system, much as the brain is fed with experiences through the senses. The neurons in NeuraBASE form associations as neurons in the brain do. The virtual links form networks that become denser as more stimuli is fed in, just as biological brains learn through experience. Given enough computer resources, NeuraBASE could in theory grow itself to function like a brain.

LEARNING PROGRAM
NeuraBASE learns to recognize hand-drawn figures and reproduce them. It does not just copy the input but, like a human brain, it recognizes the idea encapsulated in the input even when—like the 5 here—it is incomplete.

SUBMITTED INPUT

RECOGNIZED AND RECALLED

AUTOMATA

Attempts to replicate brainlike systems go back a long way. Automata—apparently driven by internal intelligence—were popular entertainments in the 18th century and are the forerunners of today's robots. Lifelike figures had hidden clockwork mechanisms. These moved their limbs and allowed them to carry out seemingly intelligent actions like writing. Although the workings of such mechanical "brains" seem crude today, the idea—to make an artificial system that functions like a human being—is the same as that driving today's huge projects.

THERE ARE NO SIGHTS, SOUNDS, TASTES, OR SMELLS IN THE WORLD—JUST VARIOUS TYPES OF WAVES AND MOLECULES. SENSATIONS, THEREFORE, ARE "VIRTUAL" CONSTRUCTS CREATED BY THE BRAIN. THE SENSE ORGANS BEGIN THIS EXTRAORDINARY ACT OF TRANSFORMATION BY TURNING STIMULI, SUCH AS LIGHT WAVES OR THE TOUCH OF CERTAIN MOLECULES, INTO ELECTRICAL SIGNALS THAT ARE CARRIED TO BRAIN AREAS DEDICATED TO DEALING WITH THAT TYPE OF INPUT. SOME STIMULI ALSO ORIGINATE FROM WITHIN THE REST OF THE BODY. ALTHOUGH SOME SENSATIONS ARE CONSCIOUSLY EXPERIENCED, MANY REMAIN UNCONSCIOUS.

THE SENSES

HOW WE SENSE THE WORLD

THE BRAIN REACHES OUT TO THE ENVIRONMENT VIA OUR SENSE ORGANS, WHICH RESPOND TO VARIOUS STIMULI SUCH AS LIGHT, SOUND WAVES, AND PRESSURE. THE INFORMATION IS TRANSMITTED AS ELECTRICAL SIGNALS TO SPECIALIZED AREAS OF THE CEREBRAL CORTEX (THE OUTER LAYER OF THE CEREBRUM) TO BE PROCESSED INTO SENSATIONS SUCH AS VISION, HEARING, AND TOUCH.

Touch area

Auditory area

Visual area

MIXED SENSES

Sensory neurons respond to data from specific sense organs. Visual cortical neurons, for example, are most sensitive to signals from the eyes. But this specialization is not rigid. Visual neurons have been found to respond more strongly to weak light signals if accompanied by sound, suggesting that they are activated by data from the ears as well as the eyes. What you see also influences what you hear. In a phenomenon known as the McGurk effect, if someone says "ba," while you watch someone mouthing "ga," you hear a third sound, "da." This is the brain's attempt to make sense of conflicting inputs. Other studies show that in people who are blind or deaf, some neurons that would normally process visual or auditory stimuli are "hijacked" by the other senses. Hence, blind people hear better and deaf people see better.

HEARING PERSON PROCESSES SPEECH	DEAF PERSON PROCESSES SIGNING
LEFT SIDE OF BRAIN	LEFT SIDE OF BRAIN
RIGHT SIDE OF BRAIN	RIGHT SIDE OF BRAIN

"HEARING" WITHOUT SOUND
These fMRI scans of human brains show some sensory neurons that are activated by speech in hearing people being used in deaf people to process sign language.

SYNESTHESIA

Most people are aware of only a single sensation in response to one type of stimulus. For example, sound waves make noise. But some people experience more than one sensation in response to a single stimulus. They may "see" sounds as well as hear them, or "taste" images. Called synesthesia, this sensory duplication occurs when the neural pathway from a sense organ diverges and carries data on one type of stimulus to a part of the brain that normally processes another type.

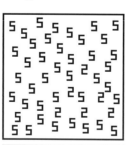

NUMBER TEST
Some synesthetes see numbers as having different colors. Variations in shape "pop out" (bottom) for them.

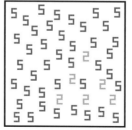

CONTROL GROUP	SYNESTHETES

Larger area responds to sounds

Increased activity

RICHER EXPERIENCE
These fMRI scans show brain activity in people listening to sounds. In response, those with synesthesia generate more sensations than others, suggesting that the condition enriches everyday experiences by increasing sensation.

ROUTES TO SENSATION
Sense organs detect stimuli, turn the information into electrical signals, and transmit these to areas of the brain that are specialized to process specific types of sensory information into sensations such as sound, vision, taste, smell, touch, and pain. Some of this data is then "forwarded" to areas of the brain that make it conscious.

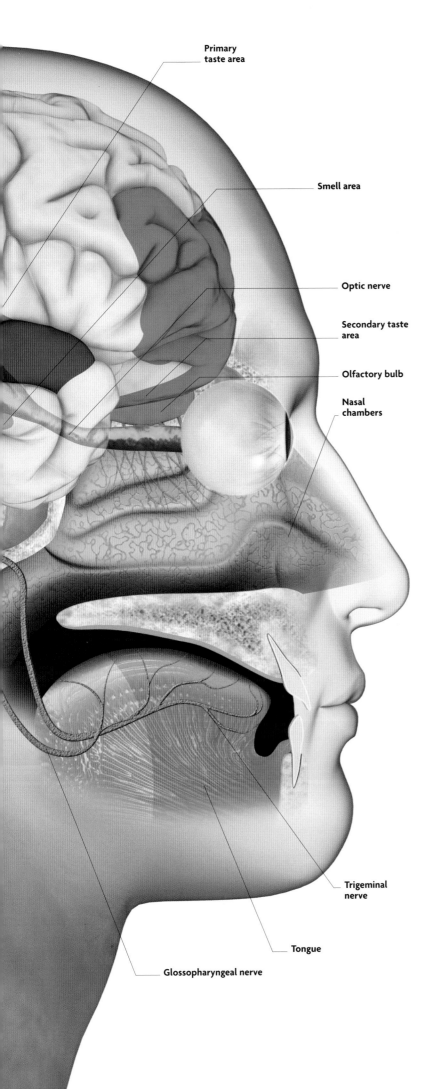

Primary
taste area

Smell area

Optic nerve

Secondary taste
area

Olfactory bulb

Nasal
chambers

Trigeminal
nerve

Tongue

Glossopharyngeal nerve

CONSCIOUS AND UNCONSCIOUS SENSATION

Our brains are bombarded with sensory information, but only a fraction of it reaches consciousness. Most sensory signals fizzle out unnoticed. Especially "loud" or important data grabs our attention (see pp.182–83), and we become conscious of it. Sensations we are not conscious of may still guide our actions. For example, unconscious sensations relating to our body position allow us to move without thinking about it. Also, sights and sounds that we fail to notice may nevertheless influence our behavior.

BLINDSIGHT

Blindsight gives visual knowledge without conscious vision. It is likely that we all have it, but it is most easily measured in people who are blind due to cortical damage. Such people cannot knowingly see, but if something is put in front of them they can correctly "guess" what it looks like, without knowing how. Most blindsight studies use moving objects. The subjects say they can't see the objects, but can usually "guess" the direction of movement correctly.

"GUESSING" MOVEMENT
Blindsight for movement is probably due to information from the eyes stimulating the visual movement area directly via an unconscious route. Conscious vision depends on activation in the primary visual cortex, stimulated via another pathway.

Moving object

Visual input

Optic nerve

Optic chiasm

Thalamus

Visual
movement area

Visual
cortex

BOTTOM-UP AND TOP-DOWN PROCESSING

Sensations are triggered externally, by an occurrence that impacts on a sense organ, and internally, by memory or imagination. The former is known as "bottom-up," and the latter as "top-down" processing (see p.87). The two combine to create our experience of reality. Each person's experience of a given event is different. Physiological differences affect bottom-up processing. One person's color-processing area in the brain may be highly sensitive, for example, so that colors are more vibrant than average. Also, an individual's own memories, knowledge, and expectations affect top-down processing.

BOTTOM-UP VISION
Bottom-up processing alone presents the viewer with a meaningless array of seemingly random blobs and shapes.

TOP-DOWN VISION
Top-down processing imposes a pattern on the image that helps the viewer understand it.

THE EYE

THE EYE IS AN EXTENSION OF THE BRAIN. IT CONTAINS
ABOUT 125 MILLION LIGHT-SENSITIVE NERVE CELLS, KNOWN
AS PHOTORECEPTORS, WHICH GENERATE ELECTRICAL SIGNALS
THAT ALLOW THE BRAIN TO FORM VISUAL IMAGES.

THE STRUCTURE OF THE EYE

The eyeball is a fluid-filled orb with a hole in the front (the pupil);
a sheet of nerve cells (the retina), some of which are light-sensitive,
at the back; and a lens in between. The pupil is surrounded by
pigmented fibers (the iris) and covered by a sheet of clear tissue
(the cornea) that merges with the tough outer surface or the
"white" of the eye (the sclera). The optic nerve passes through
a hole in the back of the eye (the optic disk) to enter the brain.

Optic nerve

OPTIC NERVE
This colored MRI scan shows the thick
bundle of fibers, the optic nerve, that
connects each eye to the brain.

SEQUENCE OF VISION

Light passes through the cornea and enters the eye through the pupil.
The iris controls how much enters by changing shape, so the pupil
appears smaller in bright light and expands in shade. Light rays then
pass through the lens, which bends (refracts) the light so it converges
on the retina. If focusing on a near object, the lens thickens to increase
refraction, but if the object is distant, the lens needs to flatten. The
light then hits the photoreceptors in the retina, some of which fire,
sending electrical signals to the brain via the optic nerve.

Object

Cornea

Light rays
Cross inside eye

Retina

Inverted image
Crossed rays produce
an upside-down
image on retina

EYE MECHANISM
The workings of the
eye transform images
made from light into
electrical impulses to
send to the brain.

Iris

Lens
Bends incoming
light rays

**Optic
nerve**

Iris
Muscular ring that
alters size of pupil

Pupil
Hole in iris that
narrows in bright
light or widens in
dim light

Cornea
Transparent layer
covering front
of eye

Lens
Transparent disk
that adjusts to
focus light rays

Conjunctiva
Covering of cornea
and eyelid lining

VISUAL PATHWAYS

Information from the eyes has to travel right to the
back of the brain before it starts to be turned into
conscious vision. En route, it passes through two
major junctions, and half of it crosses from one
side of the brain to the other. Signals from the
two optic nerves first converge at a crossover
junction called the optic chiasm. Fibers carrying
information from the left side of each retina join
up and proceed as the left optic tract, while fibers
carrying information from the right side form the
right optic tract. Each tract ends at the lateral
geniculate nucleus, which is part of the thalamus,
but their signals continue to the visual cortex via
bands of nerve fibers, called the optic radiation.

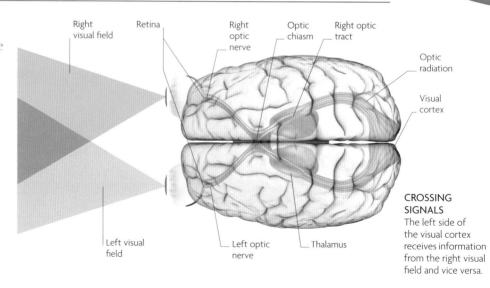

Right
visual field

Retina

Right
optic
nerve

Optic
chiasm

Right optic
tract

Optic
radiation

Visual
cortex

Left visual
field

Left optic
nerve

Thalamus

**CROSSING
SIGNALS**
The left side of
the visual cortex
receives information
from the right visual
field and vice versa.

Sclera
Protective outer sheath of eyeball

Choroid
Blood-rich layer

Retina
Layers of light-sensitive rod and cone cells

Fovea
Area of densely packed rods and cones

Optic disk
Point at which nerve fibers exit

Optic nerve
Carries signals to visual cortex

Inner surface of retina

Blood vessel

Bundle of axons extending from ganglion cells

Cell nucleus

Eye muscle
Eye held in socket by strong bands of muscle

RETINAL NERVE CELL
This light micrograph shows, in yellow, a nerve cell (neuron) from the retina. Its lightninglike extensions pass signals from light-sensitive cells to the brain.

THE RETINA

The retina contains three layers of cells, each one connecting to the next via junctions between neurons (synapses), through which information (electrical impulses) can pass. The first two layers send signals to the visual cortex in the brain, but these cells do not respond directly to the light. The third layer, at the very back of the retina, bears light-sensitive (photoreceptive) cells–the rods and cones. Light must pass over the first two layers to these cells to trigger any neural activity. Rods, which make up 90 percent of photoreceptors, are responsible for vision in dim light. Cones detect fine detail and color.

RODS AND CONES
Cell type and number can differ. Some people have more red-sensing cones (left) than others (top).

Amacrine cell Bipolar cell

Ganglion cell

BACK OF RETINA

Rod cell

Cone cell

Horizontal cell

EYE ANATOMY
The eye comprises three main outer layers and an inner chamber, which is filled with a thick, clear fluid, known as vitreous humor.

LAYERS OF RETINAL CELLS
The first two layers of cells, containing the ganglion, amacrine, and bipolar cells, connect directly with the optic nerve to send signals to the brain. Horizontal cells receive and regulate input from the light-sensitive rods and cones in the third layer.

THE FOVEA

The central part of the retina allows for far sharper vision than the periphery because it contains more cones (which pick up detail and color) than rods. Right in the center of the retina is the fovea, a tiny pitted area where cones are most densely packed. In addition to being more numerous, foveal cones can also pass on more detail, because almost every one has a dedicated signal-sending pathway to the brain. Light-sensitive cells elsewhere on the retina must share these means of output.

FOVEAL MAGNIFICATION
This electron micrograph shows the part of the retina that gives sharpest vision, the foveal pit.

BLIND SPOT

Signal-carrying nerve fibers bundle together at the optic disk in the back of the eye to form the optic nerve. Consequently, this area has no light-sensitive cells, so it forms a "blind spot." We are unaware of this gap in our vision because the brain "fills in" the area we can't see.

OPTIC DISK
This opthalmoscope image of a retina shows the optic disk, the site of the blind spot.

THE VISUAL CORTEX

THE VISUAL AREAS OF THE BRAIN ARE AT THE BACK OF THE BRAIN; THEREFORE, INFORMATION FROM THE EYES HAS TO TRAVEL THE FULL DEPTH OF THE SKULL BEFORE IT BEGINS TO BE PROCESSED INTO SIGHT. VISUAL INFORMATION CAN GUIDE ACTIONS WITHIN ONE-FIFTH OF A SECOND, BUT IT TAKES ABOUT HALF A SECOND FOR US TO SEE AN OBJECT CONSCIOUSLY.

VISUAL AREAS

The visual cortex is divided into several functional areas, each of which specializes in a particular aspect of vision (see table, right). The process is similar to assembly-line production: raw material is checked in by V1, then sent on to other vision areas, which contribute shape, color, depth, and motion. These components are then combined to form a whole image. Because of the modular nature of vision, if one of the sight areas is damaged, a particular visual component may be lost while the others remain intact. Cell death in the motion-detecting area, for example, may cause the world to be seen as a series of still snapshots.

AREAS OF THE VISUAL CORTEX	
AREA	**FUNCTION**
V1	Responds to visual stimuli
V2	Passes on information and responds to complex shapes
V3A, V3D, VP	Registers angles and symmetry, and combines motion and direction
V4D, V4V	Responds to color, orientation, form, and movement
V5	Responds to movement
V6	Detects motion in periphery of visual field
V7	Involved in perception of symmetry
V8	Probably involved in processing of color

VERTICAL SECTION

Spiny stellate cells communicate with neighboring layers

Pyramidal cells send messages to other areas of the visual cortex

I
II
III
IVA
IVB
IVC
V
VI

CORTICAL LAYERS
The primary visual cortex consists of several cell layers, numbered I to VI, each of which contains a special mix of cells. Each layer sends and receives signals to and from different parts of the brain.

THE MIND'S MIRROR
The crisscrossed layout of the visual pathways (see p.80) causes the view seen by the eyes to be reversed, so it registers on the primary visual cortex (V1) as a mirror image. Signals from the left field of vision end up in the right hemisphere and vice versa. The information is passed between the two sides to give a shared view. In certain rare conditions, each side of the brain sees something different–the person appears to be in "two minds" (see p.11, p.199).

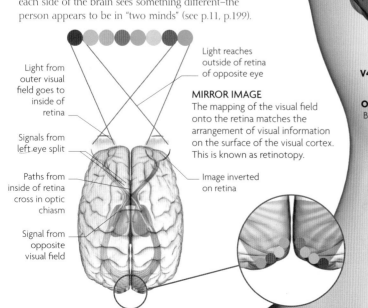

Light from outer visual field goes to inside of retina

Signals from left eye split

Paths from inside of retina cross in optic chiasm

Signal from opposite visual field

Light reaches outside of retina of opposite eye

MIRROR IMAGE
The mapping of the visual field onto the retina matches the arrangement of visual information on the surface of the visual cortex. This is known as retinotopy.

Image inverted on retina

V6
V3A
V3D
V2
V1
V2
V4V
V8
VP

INTERIOR CORTEX
Some, but not all, of the visual processing areas curve around the back of the brain and into the groove between the hemispheres.

Occipital lobe
Location of visual cortex areas

Thalamus

V7

V3a

V3

V2

V1

V4D

Optic radiation
Bundle of axons running from thalamus to visual cortex

V5

Lateral geniculate nucleus
Area of thalamus that sends signals on to visual cortex

Optic nerve

Temporal lobe
Location of object-recognition pathway

THE SEEING BRAIN
Signals from the eyes arrive at V1, which passes them to other visual areas for further processing (see also pp.84–85). Activation in V1 is not sufficient for conscious sight, but is necessary for it. As long as we are consciously seeing something, V1 is kept activated.

DISTINGUISHING COLORS

In theory the human visual system can distinguish millions of colors, but in practice the number of colors we see depends on whether we have learned to see them. Presented with a globe showing all possible colors, people can easily distinguish those for which they have distinct names. But if a range of hues is lumped together under a single name, they often find it hard to see the differences.

ENGLISH HUES
This globe shows the spectrum of color, which is divided into eight basic categories (red, orange, green, blue, purple, yellow, and brown) in the English language.

OTHER HUES
Studies suggest that language affects how people see the globe. For example, the Berinmo tribe of Papua New Guinea split colors into five categories, each of which relates to a different hue from those above.

RECOGNIZING OBJECTS

Conscious sight requires the brain to recognize what it is seeing. To achieve this, the image is forwarded from the occipital lobe to other brain areas concerned with emotion and memory. Here it gains information relating to its function, its identity, and its emotional significance. One of the first stops is in the object-recognition area, which runs along the bottom rim of the temporal lobe. Human faces are dealt with in a particular subregion that has evolved to make fine distinctions. Its ability to distinguish tiny differences between individual faces makes nearly all of us "experts" at recognizing one another.

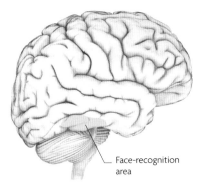
Face-recognition area

FACE-RECOGNITION AREA
Part of the brain's object-recognition path scrutinizes things of importance. This area processes objects that call for fine discrimination, such as faces.

GREEBLES

Greebles are organic-looking objects used in studies that, like faces, are each slightly different from one another. At first sight the differences are easily overlooked, but as people become familiar with Greebles their brains start processing the sight of them in the face-recognition area. This allows them to see the tiny differences very clearly and they become Greeble "experts."

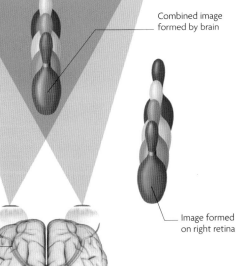

DEPTH AND DIMENSION

The brain uses two types of cues to produce our three-dimensional view of the world. One is the slightly different image recorded by each eye (spatial binocular disparity), and the other is the way the perceived shape of an object shifts as it moves. Both cues come together in an area of the brain called the anterior intraparietal area (AIP), which lies between the visual processing areas and the part of the brain devoted to monitoring our position in space.

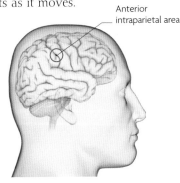
Anterior intraparietal area

DEPTH AREA
The AIP combines two types of visual cue to calculate distance and depth. This information guides the movements involved in reaching out and grasping objects.

Central visual field

Combined image formed by brain

Image formed on left retina

Image formed on right retina

Optic nerve

Optic chiasm

Thalamus

Lateral geniculate nucleus

Left cerebral hemisphere

Right cerebral hemisphere

Visual cortex

STEREOGRAM

Stereoscopic images make use of the way the brain processes visual information to trick it into seeing a three-dimensional image when in fact there is only a flat plane. One way to do this is to present, side by side, two minutely differing images of the same scene. The difference between them is that which would normally be perceived by each eye—a tiny shift of perspective equal to the distance between the eyes. These illusions were popular in Victorian times.

PHANTOM IMAGE
If you can force your eyes to cross or to diverge, so that each eye sees just one picture, a ghostly third image appears in the center in three dimensions.

3-D VISION
The slightly differing views provided by each eye, combined with information about how shapes change as they move across the visual field, produce a three-dimensional view of the world.

VISUAL PATHWAYS

CONSCIOUS VISION IS THE FAMILIAR PROCESS OF SEEING SOMETHING, WHILE UNCONSCIOUS VISION USES INFORMATION FROM THE EYES TO GUIDE BEHAVIOR WITHOUT OUR KNOWING IT IS HAPPENING. THE TWO TYPES OF VISION ARE PROCESSED ALONG SEPARATE PATHWAYS IN THE BRAIN. THE UPPER (DORSAL) ROUTE, IS UNCONSCIOUS AND GUIDES ACTION, WHILE THE LOWER (VENTRAL) PATH IS CONSCIOUS AND RECOGNIZES OBJECTS.

DORSAL AND VENTRAL ROUTES
Electrical signals from the eyes travel to the primary visual cortex, where the brain begins to process them into vision. The signals are then sent on to other brain regions via the two separate dorsal and ventral pathways.

DORSAL

THE "WHERE" PATHWAY

The dorsal, or "where," pathway carries signals triggered by a visual stimulus–for example, the light bouncing off a nearby object–from the visual cortex to the parietal cortex. Along the way, it passes through areas that calculate the object's location in relation to the viewer and creates an action plan in relation to it. The dorsal path gathers information about motion and timing that is integrated into the action plan. All the information needed to, say, duck a flying object, is gathered along this path with no need for conscious thought.

Parietal lobes
Depth and position of object in relation to observer are gauged

V7
Contributes to perception of symmetry

V3a
Information on motion and direction is collated here

VENTRAL

THE "WHAT" PATHWAY

The ventral, or "what," pathway follows a route that takes it first through a series of visual processing areas, each of which adds a specific aspect of perception, such as shape, color, depth, and so on (see pp.88–89). The loosely formed representation then passes into the bottom edge of the temporal lobe, where it is matched or compared to visual memories in order to achieve recognition. Some information continues along this pathway to the frontal lobes, where it is assessed for meaning and significance. At this stage, it becomes a conscious perception.

V3
Angles and orientation analyzed—paths split here

V2
Information passed on through secondary visual cortex—complex shapes are registered here

V1
Signals from eyes received in primary visual cortex

V4D
Involved in perception of color, orientation, form, and movement

V5
Direction of movement detected here

RECOGNIZING FACES

Different types of visual stimuli are processed in different parts of the brain. Faces, which are recognized by the pattern of human facial features, activate the face-recognition area. This extracts information about facial expression and forwards it to relevant brain areas. When a face matches a memory, the information is sent to the frontal lobes for further processing.

FAMILIAR PERSON
Emotional recognition is near-instant. The pathway runs from the visual cortex via the face area to the amygdala.

Face-recognition area · Amygdala

Primary visual cortex

SEEING SOMEONE FAMILIAR

EMOTIONAL

Primary visual cortex

Face-recognition area

SEEING SOMEONE FAMOUS

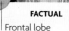

FACTUAL
Frontal lobe

FAMOUS PERSON
When a face matches a memory of a famous person, such as Marilyn Monroe, the information is shunted to the frontal lobes for processing.

DAMAGE TO THE DORSAL PATHWAY

Damage to the dorsal visual pathway causes a number of disorders, all of which affect the ability to deal with objects in space. A person may, for example, be unable to see that two objects are in different places or to correctly see their spatial relationship, one to the other. They may find it impossible to reach out and grasp an object accurately or to know where it lies in relation to themselves. For example, a person may say something like, "I know there is a banana there but I don't know where it is." Patients may also suffer visual attention defects (see pp.182–83).

Frontal lobe
Some information from dorsal route arrives in frontal lobes, where it is consciously perceived

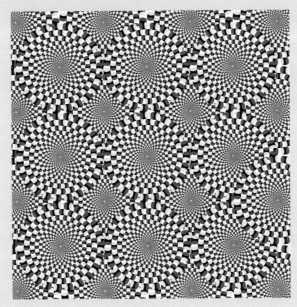

STILL LIFE

The ability to see movement is vital for survival. Many animals, such as frogs, can only see things in motion. The motion area of the human brain is tiny and more than 90 percent of neurons here are specialized to detect direction of movement. It is generally well protected from injury but, very rarely, a person may lose motion vision due to a stroke. The effect is profoundly disturbing, reducing the world to a series of snapshots. Day-to-day life becomes difficult—crossing the road, for example, is perilous as approaching traffic appears first to be distant and then suddenly close. Pouring a cup of tea is difficult because the column of liquid seems to be frozen and then overflowing.

ILLUSORY MOTION
The brain frequently detects motion where there is actually none. Many different types of illusions can do this. Most of them depend on exciting motion-detecting neurons, causing them to fire and thus create the effect of movement.

PROSOPAGNOSIA

If the face-recognition area is damaged, or fails for some reason to develop normally, people may be unable to recognize people they know—even their closest friends and members of their own family. Prosopagnosia is severely socially disabling. Affected people may get quite good at identifying people by features other than their face (by voice or clothing) but these techniques are slower and less reliable than normal face recognition. Face recognition relies on detailed information about distances between features. In the faces above, the shape of the features or the distance between them have been manipulated. People with prosopagnosia are unable to spot the differences.

EYES CLOSE   **EYES ENLARGED**   **EYES APART**   **MOUTH ENLARGED**

ALTERED IMAGES
These photographs have had features, such as mouth or eye size, altered or have been changed configurally—the eyes moved together or further apart.

Inferior temporal lobe
Fusiform gyrus involved in recognizing objects, especially faces

MONA LISA ILLUSION
The face-recognition area only processes stimuli that have the pattern of facial features. So a picture of an upturned face is not processed here but is dealt with by an area that is not sensitive to facial expression. The upturned image of Mona Lisa seems at first to be normal. Turn it the right way up, though, and the face area alerts you to something very wrong!

DAMAGE TO THE VENTRAL PATHWAY

Damage to the ventral pathway results in one or another form of visual agnosia–the inability to recognize what one is seeing. Prosopagnosia, the inability to recognize faces (see panel, above), is one type of agnosia, but there are many others. Visual agnosia is generally divided into two categories: apperceptive and associative. The first type results from damage to the parts of the pathway in the occipital lobe and manifests itself as an inability to form a properly constructed perception. Hence a person with apperceptive agnosia cannot copy or draw an object, even though they may be able to see the parts of it quite clearly. Associative agnosia is an inability to identify objects. The person sees the object and may be able to mime an appropriate action in relation to it–for example, using a fork to raise food to the mouth–yet be unable to say what it is.

 LETTER   **FANTASY OBJECT**

AGNOSIA TESTS
Tests for agnosia include recognizing objects from their silhouettes, telling fantasy objects from real ones, or identifying an incomplete letter.

 SILHOUETTE

So strong is the attraction of faces that even the portraits within the picture get close and repeated study

Eye gaze and mouth are scrutinized for clues to the intentions and inner states of the characters in the picture

The viewer's gaze lingers here to scrutinize the interplay between the "main" characters

The eye passes straight across the floor, pausing briefly when the pathway is obstructed, but not stopping long enough to see it

VISUAL PERCEPTION

WE DO NOT SEE WHAT WE THINK WE SEE. WHEN WE LOOK AT A SCENE WE HAVE THE IMPRESSION OF SEEING ALL OF IT IN ONE GLANCE, BUT IN PRACTICE WE TYPICALLY PICK OUT JUST A FEW TINY DETAILS.

TOP-DOWN AND BOTTOM-UP PROCESSING

Visual perception is momentary, partial, and fragmentary. "Bottom-up" visual processing presets the brain with information about the whole field of vision, but "top-down" processes select which parts of the scene to make conscious. When we look at a picture, our eyes typically alight on a few thumbnail-size areas that we scan in sequence repeatedly. The rest of the image remains a blur unless we deliberately turn our attention to it. Eye-tracking studies (see left) show that the parts of a scene that we look at most closely are those that relate to other people. Although this visual selection is determined by "higher" brain functions–those involved in social concerns rather than, say, ducking a low branch–people are often unaware of what they are looking at. When asked, they may say they are looking at one thing when in fact their eyes have been resting on another.

MAKING SENSE OF PICTURES

The brain works hard to make sense of visual information. Looking at a complex scene (see left) activates processes that distinguish target objects, such as people, from the background and then selects which bits of the target to focus on. These details are then scrutinized while the conscious brain pieces together the story. This interpretation begins unconsciously. Colors and shades are not recognized just by the type and amount of light reflected from them. The unconscious brain works out an object's most likely color or shade from its context.

CYLINDER ILLUSION
The squares A and B are identical shades but B looks lighter because we assume that the cylinder is casting a shadow over it.

COLOR ILLUSION
The color you see depends on those around it. Pink next to white looks paler than pink next to green. This is due to "lateral inhibition," which defines objects from their surroundings.

LAUGHTER PLAYS TRICKS ON THE EYES

Laughing literally changes the way you see the world. Normally, when you look at a Necker cube the image switches between two competing 3-D images, a situation known as binocular rivalry. This rivalry occurs because each eye sends a slightly different image to each side of the brain (see p.83), and the brain switches conscious awareness of one to the other. One theory on why switching stops during laughter is that amusement is a state in which information from both halves of the brain merges more than usual.

NECKER CUBE

---

the possibility of others intruding on the scene and altering the human dynamics within it

Pointing to an object increases its significance and makes it worthy of a look

TUNING IN TO DETAIL
The white lines on this image track the viewer's eyes as they navigate around the scene. The circles represent where the gaze rests—the larger the circle, the longer the eye lingers.

SEEING SEEMS TO BE INSTANTANEOUS AND EFFORTLESS, AND VISUAL
IMAGES ALWAYS APPEAR FULLY FORMED. UNCONSCIOUSLY, HOWEVER, THE
BRAIN IS CONSTANTLY UNDERTAKING A MAJOR FEAT OF CONSTRUCTION
TO PRESENT US WITH OUR VIEW OF THE WORLD.

VISUAL PERCEPTION

One way of thinking about visual perception is to
see it as the end product that emerges from a long
and complicated assembly line. The construction
process begins in earnest when information from
the eyes–the raw material–reaches the primary
visual cortex at the back of the brain. This is then
sent along two main pathways (see pp.84–85),
through a number of cortical and subcortical areas.
Each of these responds by creating neural activity
that generates various aspects of vision such as
color, form, location, and movement. Eventually,
the various elements are bound together and we
become conscious of a meaningful sight.

2 Retinal cells
The light passes through the lens and
then through two layers of retinal cells
before hitting the light-sensitive
rods and cones at the back.

1 Light enters the eye
Light waves enter the eye through the pupil,
a hole in the center of the iris. The pupil expands
to let in more light in shady conditions, and
contracts when the light is bright, so a relatively
constant amount of light is allowed in.

3 The optic nerve
The light-sensitive retinal cells fire and send
signals along their axons, which are bundled
together to form the optic nerve. The
nerve crosses at the optic chiasm, and
the nerve fibers connect with a
specialized part of the
thalamus.

4 The optic radiation
The signals are then sent from the
thalamus on to the visual cortex via a
thick band of tissue known as the
optic radiation.

**8 Perception
(frontal lobes)**
Once all the visual
elements of a sight
have been brought
together and the
object has been
recognized, it
is presented to
consciousness as
a full "perception."

HOW WE SEE
Although we are beginning to understand how
information from the eye is used to recognize
objects and guide behavior, no one knows
how vision becomes conscious and why it
feels the way it does (see pp.178–79).

5 THE DORSAL ROUTE

Information from the eyes is registered by the primary visual cortex and then sent forward along two pathways for further processing. The dorsal route takes it up through areas that are concerned with charting the location of the target object in relation to the viewer. Along this route, neuronal activity encodes the object's position, movement, and some aspects of its size and shape. The dorsal route ends in the parietal areas, which construct action plans relative to the viewed object. This process occurs unconsciously.

DORSAL

Motion
Movement is processed along the dorsal pathway. It is an essential component of any "action plan" (see p.121), and the brain not only notes current motion, but also predicts where an object will be in a split second. This ensures that any action plan is well timed.

Depth
In order to calculate the depth of an object, the brain combines visual signals from both eyes—each of which has a slightly different view (see p.83)—along with information about how the shape of the image alters as the eyes move.

6 THE VENTRAL ROUTE

The ventral route carries information from the primary visual cortex down through the temporal lobes, where the neural activity identifies the sights and "clothes" them with meaning. A face, for example, is distinguished and recognized here (see p.84), and information about it such as the name of the person is recalled from memory (see p.163). Information traveling along the ventral path is brought together with that from the dorsal path in the frontal lobes—resulting in conscious perception rather than action.

VENTRAL

Form
The brain has many different ways of "seeing" form. These include registering the orientation of light waves hitting an object and processing information about the way the waves reflect from its surfaces or outlines.

Color
Color discrimination begins in the retinal cells, some of which are tuned to fire in response to specific light wavelengths. Color processing continues in the brain, especially in an area known as V4 (see pp.82–83), which contains the majority of color-sensing neurons.

7 Recognition path

In order to see something properly, a person needs to have some idea of what is being seen. If an image is not recognized, it is less likely to be consciously registered and may be overlooked altogether. Recognition is not purely visual, but involves clothing the perception with knowledge—such as who or what it is, what its intention is (if it is sentient), why it is there, and what it is called. Some of these elements may be missing—you may see someone you know but fail to recall his or her name, for example. By contrast, the purely visual elements of a perception are nearly always intact.

SEEING WITH SOUND?

A device that turns visual information into sound has been reported to create visual experience in at least one user, who is otherwise blind. The device involves mounting a small camera on a person's head, which captures a moment-by-moment view of what would normally be the person's visual field. This information is then turned into a "soundscape" that is played into the user's ears. As the person learns to recognize the physical qualities matching the sounds—for example, that a single high-pitched tone signifies a vertical surface—they seem to cease to hear it as a noise and instead experience it much like normal vision. One woman claims that her experience of "hearing" the environment is sometimes indistinguishable from seeing it.

SOUNDSCAPE
This image is a computer reconstruction of one second of sound, as "seen" by the system that builds soundscapes from camera images.

THE EAR

THE EAR PICKS UP SOUND WAVES IN THE ENVIRONMENT AND TRANSLATES THIS INFORMATION INTO NERVE IMPULSES, WHICH ARE SENT TO THE BRAIN FOR PROCESSING. THE EAR ALSO SENSES THE MOTION AND POSITION OF THE BODY, WHICH ALLOWS THE BRAIN TO REGULATE BALANCE.

THE ANATOMY OF HEARING

The ear is divided into three sections: the outer ear, middle ear, and inner ear. The outer ear funnels sound waves along the ear canal to the eardrum (tympanic membrane)–the start of the middle ear. The sound waves cause the eardrum to vibrate, which in turn causes a chain of bones, known as the ear ossicles, to vibrate. One of these, the stapes, is attached to a membrane known as the oval window– the start of the inner ear. Beyond this is the maze of fluid-filled chambers of the spiral-shaped cochlea. The vibrations of the stapes on the oval window are converted into pressure waves, which travel in the fluid within the cochlea to the organ of Corti. Sensory hair cells on this organ transform the pressure waves into electrical impulses, which travel through the auditory nerve (specifically, the cochlear branch of the vestibulocochlear nerve) to the brain.

Scalp muscle

Auricular cartilage
Gives pinna distinctive C shape and flexibility

Temporal bone

Outer ear canal (exterior auditory canal)

Pinna (ear flap)
Skin-covered flap made of subcutaneous fat, connective tissue, and cartilage

OUTER EAR
The visible part of the outer ear is called the pinna. Its funnel shape helps collect sound waves and channel them into the ear canal (which extends roughly 1in/2.5cm) toward the middle ear.

Suspensory ligament
Holds bones in place but allows them to vibrate

Tympanum (eardrum)

Malleus (hammer)

Incus (anvil)

Stapes (stirrup)

Ear ossicles

Oval window
Membrane receives vibrations from stapes

Round window
Membrane relieves pressure by allowing cochlear fluid to bulge

Semicircular canals
Contain sensory organs involved in balance

Cochlear nerve
Carries nerve signals from inner ear to brain

Vestibulocochlear (auditory) nerve
Carries signals from semicircular canals and cochlea to brain

Cochlea
Contains sensory organ involved in hearing

Vestibular canal

Cochlear duct

Tympanic canal

Eustachian tube
Runs to upper throat

MIDDLE AND INNER EAR
The eardrum is the gateway to the middle ear, an air-filled cavity that houses the ear ossicles—the smallest bones in the body. The innermost of these, the stapes, is attached to the oval window, which leads into the cochlea. The cochlea and the semicircular canals comprise the inner ear.

ORGAN OF CORTI
Tiny hairs on this organ, found in the cochlea, transform sound waves into electrical impulses. Low-frequency sounds are picked up at the center of the cochlea's spiral and high-frequency sounds at the base, near the oval window.

Reissner's membrane
Divides cochlear duct and vestibular canal

Cochlear duct

Outer spiral sulcus

Hensen's cells

Outer hair cells

Basilar membrane
Membrane along which the organ of Corti is located

Tunnel of Corti

Vestibular canal
Conveys vibrations to basilar membrane

Tectorial membrane
Receives signals from hair cells

Stereocilia
Protrude from tip of hair cells and bend in response to vibrations

Modiolus

Inner spiral sulcus

Reticular lamina

Inner hair cell

Pillar cell

Auditory nerve

Tympanic canal

HAIRS ON THE ORGAN OF CORTI
This colored electron micrograph shows sound-sensing hairs. There are 20,000 or so outer hairs (yellow). Around 3,500 inner hairs (red) lead to the auditory nerve.

THE AUDITORY CORTEX

Sound information, in the form of electrical impulses, travels from the ear along the auditory nerve to the auditory cortex (situated in the temporal lobe, beneath the temples) for processing. In one of its three areas, the primary auditory cortex, different auditory neurons respond to specific sound frequencies. Also, some respond to the intensity of a sound rather than to its frequency, while others respond to more complex sounds, such as clicks, animal noises, and bursts of noise. It is thought that the secondary auditory cortex plays a part in processing harmony, rhythm, and melody, while the tertiary auditory cortex is involved in integrating the variety of sounds into a whole impression.

PERCEIVING SOUND FREQUENCIES
In the primary auditory cortex, neurons are sited according to the frequency each responds to, as are the sensory cells in the cochlea.

Corresponds to apex of cochlea

Corresponds to base of cochlea

AUDITORY RANGES

AUDITORY RANGES	
SPECIES	**FREQUENCY (HERTZ)**
Elephant	16–12,000
Goldfish	20–3,000
Human	64–23,000
Dog	67–45,000
Porpoise	75–150,000
Bullfrog	100–3,000
Owl	200–12,000
Bat	2,000–110,000

Many animals can hear sounds that humans cannot, both at higher and lower frequencies. Some animals pick up frequencies significantly higher than those humans can detect. For example, bats using echolocation can detect reflected sounds in the 14,000–100,000 Hertz range. The lower limit of the human auditory frequency range is fixed throughout life, but the upper limit begins to fall from adolescence. The maximum frequency heard by a normal middle-aged adult is between 14,000 and 16,000 Hertz.

HAIR CELLS AND FREQUENCY
This colored electron micrograph shows V-shaped sensory hair cells on the organ of Corti (see opposite page), each with multiple strands (yellow) or stereocilia. Cells are arranged within the cochlea according to the frequency of the sound each is able to detect.

THE COCHLEAR IMPLANT

Rather than restore hearing, this device helps the wearer have a perception of sound with no time lag, which can help with lip-reading. A microphone picks up sounds and passes them to a sound processor, which turns them into digital electrical signals. The transmitter conveys the signals, in the form of radio waves, to the implanted receiver, located beneath the skin. This receiver communicates via electrodes with the sensory hair cells in the cochlea, which pass the information on to the brain.

EXTERNAL APPARATUS
A transmitter, microphone, and sound processor convert environmental sounds into digital signals.

Receiver

Transmitter

Cochlear (auditory) nerve

Cochlea

Electrode

Microphone worn behind ear

Wire connected to sound processor

INTERNAL APPARATUS
Surgery is required to insert the receiver and electrodes that convey the sound information to the inner ear.

AUDITORY DISORDERS

Hearing loss is common but total deafness is rare and usually results from a congenital problem. Mild or severe hearing loss can result from ear disease, injury, or degeneration of the hearing system with age. Hearing loss is either conductive (a fault in the transferral of sound from the outer to inner ear) or sensorineural (sometimes known as nerve deafness, involving damage to the auditory nerves, or to the sensory parts of the inner ear). Common hearing disorders include otitis media and otosclerosis. Otitis media mainly affects young children and is an inflammation of the middle ear caused by a bacterial infection. Otosclerosis occurs when there is abnormal bone growth on the stapes bone of the middle ear, which stops it from vibrating and conducting sound waves on to the inner ear.

PERFORATED EARDRUM
The eardrum may become perforated due to infection, injury, or sudden exposure to an explosive noise that causes excessive vibration. Perforations can heal naturally.

NORMAL EARDRUM
The eardrum consists of a thin layer of fibrous tissue continuous with the skin of the outer ear and the mucous membrane of the middle ear.

MAKING SENSE OF SOUND

SOUND VIBRATIONS ARE TURNED INTO ELECTRICAL IMPULSES IN THE COCHLEA. FROM THERE, THEY TRAVEL TO THE AUDITORY CORTEX AND ITS ASSOCIATION AREAS VIA THE MEDULLA AND THE THALAMUS.

PERCEPTION OF SOUND

Sounds start as vibrations entering the ears. In the inner ear, receptor cells in the cochlea transform these vibrations into electrical signals, which pass along the cochlear nerve to the medulla in the brainstem, and then to the inferior colliculus. The cochlear nerve fibers divide so that most of the input from each ear can go to both hemispheres. At this stage, the source of the sound is determined by areas of the brainstem that compare input from both ears and analyze the delay (of about $1/1,500$ of a second) between the receipt of the signal by the ear nearest to the source and the ear farther away. The signals reach the auditory cortex via the thalamus, where frequency, quality, intensity, and meaning are perceived. The left auditory cortex is more concerned with the meaning and identification of sound; the right, with quality.

THE COCKTAIL-PARTY EFFECT

The brain not only receives signals from the ears, it also sends signals to them, creating a circuit that modulates input. Background noise is dimmed, and the longer a person concentrates on a single strand of conversation, the greater the effect of filtering. This makes it easy to hear words you are interested in but may reduce the background so much that important messages fail to get through. If your brain registers an important sound, such as your name, it will instantly identify the source of that sound and upgrade it from heard to listened to. This is known as the cocktail-party effect.

HEAR OR LISTEN
When in a noisy environment, such as at a party, the brain can tune in to listen to a particular conversation while still hearing the noise of background speech. Green areas in the scan above register the sound of speech while red areas process speech to the level of understanding —it is "listened to" as well as heard.

Sound crosses to right hemisphere
Most signals from left cochlea travel to right side of cortex

Right auditory cortex

Sound travels through ear along cochlear nerve

Corpus callosum

Medial geniculate body
Part of thalamus that receives signal

Left auditory cortex

Sound crosses to left hemisphere
Most sound signals received from right ear are processed here

Medulla in brainstem
Sound received in cochlear nucleus

THE HEARING BRAIN
Sound enters the ears and travels via the brainstem and thalamus to the auditory cortex. Here, it is processed by association areas, such as Wernicke's area, which is involved with interpreting speech.

NOISE OR MUSIC?

Sound consists of waves, or vibrations, whose characteristics are determined by the source of the sound. The main characteristics influencing our perception of sound are frequency (number of vibrations per second) and amplitude (the size of the waves' "peaks" and "troughs"). Frequency influences pitch, and amplitude governs loudness. Irregular sound-wave patterns tend to be experienced as noise; in contrast, music produces regular patterns.

Music is hard to define precisely, but the quality of musical notes depends upon their sound source–a musical instrument–and how it is being played. Another important factor in music is timbre, or the "quality" of a sound. Timbre depends upon how many different frequencies of the note are heard at once; multiple frequencies or overtones (harmony) make a richer timbre. The auditory cortex responds to different qualities in music. The primary region responds to frequencies and the secondary area to harmony and rhythm, while the tertiary area adds higher levels of appreciation and integration.

NOISE OR NOTE
Analysis of the wave forms of sounds reveals pure tones to be regular in frequency and amplitude, while noise is irregular.

AUDITORY CORTEX
The inner primary auditory cortex has areas associated with specific frequencies. The secondary and tertiary regions tune into more complex aspects of sound perception.

Primary cortex
Secondary cortex
Tertiary cortex

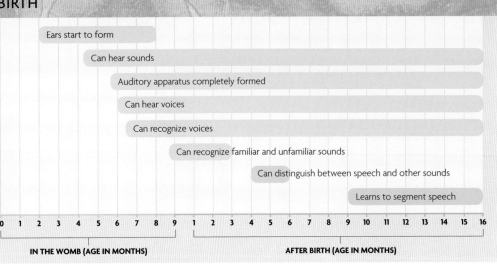

ACTIVITY DURING SPEECH
Speech tends to produce more intense activity in the left-hand side of the auditory cortex.

ACTIVITY DURING MUSIC
Music produces more pronounced activity on the right-hand side of the auditory cortex.

THE MOZART EFFECT

The French child-development expert Alfred Tomatis first described the "Mozart effect" in 1991. He claimed that listening to the music of the 18th-century classical composer Mozart could help the mental development of children under three. Researchers have also demonstrated that students listening to Mozart could improve their performance on tasks involving spatial reasoning and show a temporary increase in IQ. Recent research has given mixed results, but the idea has gained in popularity. The Mozart effect may, however, have more to do with changes in mood and arousal affecting mental performance than any direct impact on intelligence.

DEVELOPMENT OF HEARING

The development of hearing is a gradual process that begins in the womb and is complete by about the end of the first year of a baby's life. Research shows that the unborn child is capable of hearing by about the fourth month of gestation, but the auditory apparatus is not fully formed until about the sixth month. At birth, hearing is the most developed of the senses, so it is of prime importance to the baby in exploring its world. Studies have shown how the baby learns to recognize sounds in its first few months, gradually becomes able to distinguish between speech and non-speech sounds, and then begins to understand words. Children also lose the ability to hear differences between sounds that are not important in their native language. Many Japanese children, for example, can no longer hear the difference between "l" and "r," which they could distinguish at an earlier age.

DEVELOPMENT BEFORE AND AFTER BIRTH

The human fetus has some basic hearing capacity from the age of about 18 weeks. This ability matures and develops over the next few weeks, with low-frequency sounds outside the mother's body being heard better than those of high frequency. From birth up to four months, the baby starts to respond to loud or sudden sounds, beginning to localize them by turning the head. From three to six months, the baby begins to recognize and also make sounds. Between six and 12 months, he or she begins to babble, recognizes basic words like "mommy," and starts to recognize voices. The baby begins to form words from the age of about one year. Each child reaches these milestones in hearing and speech development at different times, but very slow development may indicate some problem with the hearing apparatus.

Ears start to form
Can hear sounds
Auditory apparatus completely formed
Can hear voices
Can recognize voices
Can recognize familiar and unfamiliar sounds
Can distinguish between speech and other sounds
Learns to segment speech

IN THE WOMB (AGE IN MONTHS) / AFTER BIRTH (AGE IN MONTHS)

HEARING

HEARING INVOLVES MECHANICAL VIBRATIONS FROM THE ENVIRONMENT—SPEECH, MUSIC, AND EVERYDAY NOISE—TRAVELING THROUGH THE OUTER, MIDDLE, AND INNER EAR. THE VIBRATIONS ARE TRANSFORMED TO ELECTRICAL SIGNALS, WHICH TRAVEL TO THE BRAIN TO BE INTERPRETED AS SOUND.

PATHWAY OF SOUND

The ear is a complex, exquisitely designed instrument for the capture of sound and its transport to the brain. Once mechanical vibrations from sound sources reach the inner ear, they are transformed into electrical impulses that shoot along the cochlear nerve to the brainstem. Here, they follow complex pathways up to the thalamus before arriving at the auditory cortex. Processing in the brain allows perception of the meaning, direction, and volume of a sound.

5 The cochlea
The cochlea contains three fluid-filled ducts. The vestibular canal transmits sound vibrations (blue) to the basilar membrane of the organ of Corti. Residual vibrations (red) travel back along the tympanic canal to the round window.

1 The outer ear
Sound waves are caught in the funnel-like curves of the outer ear that comprises the exterior "flap" of the pinna and the auditory canal.

2 The auditory canal
The sound waves continue along the 1in-(2.5cm)-long auditory canal, which extends from the concha (inner curve) of the outer ear to the eardrum and is lined with tiny hairs that protect it from the entry of foreign objects.

3 The eardrum
The eardrum, or tympanic membrane, vibrates as sound waves enter the auditory canal. It is a thin layer of fibrous tissue that forms a barrier between the outer ear and the middle ear.

4 Ossicles
Vibrations are passed on to a set of tiny bones called ossicles (see p.90), which act as a chain of levers. The stapes pushes and pulls on the oval window at the entrance to the cochlea, transmitting sound to the inner ear.

HEARING LIGHT

Hair cells turn sound vibrations into electrical signals that stimulate neurons in a healthy ear. Damage to the hair cells can lead to loss of hearing. However, research shows that infrared light is also capable of stimulating ear neurons. A team at Northwestern University in Chicago exposed inner-ear neurons in guinea pigs to infrared light. This resulted in electrical activity in the inferior colliculus suggesting that the light had caused soundlike input to be sent to the brain. This discovery could be turned into a new type of cochlear implant if fiberoptics targeting light to the inner ear are developed.

HAIR CELLS
Each hair cell is topped by about 100 projections called cilia. It is the movement of these in response to vibrations that generates electrical signals.

11 The thalamus
Nerve impulses are received and processed by specialized neurons in the medial geniculate nucleus of the thalamus. These signals are then sent to the primary auditory cortex, which also feeds information back to the thalamus.

12 The primary auditory cortex
The characteristics of a sound input are finally interpreted, after intermediate processing at the primary auditory cortex, which works with other cortical areas on sound perception.

6 The organ of Corti
Mechanical vibrations of sound are transformed into electrical signals by hair cells in the organ of Corti, which is the main organ of hearing and is located in the cochlea (see p.90).

7 The cochlear nerve
Sound impulses are transported from each hair cell in the organ of Corti via cochlear nerve endings that join together to form the nerve responsible for transmitting signals to specialized groups of neurons in the brainstem.

8 Cochlear nuclei
The cochlear nerve branches to connect to the two cochlear nuclei on the same side of the brain as the ear where the sound originally entered. After this, neural pathways branch and ascend in ways that are not yet fully understood.

10 The inferior colliculus
All the ascending auditory pathways—some of which bypass the superior olives—converge upon the inferior colliculi at the top of the brainstem and their input is then passed on toward the thalamus.

9 The superior olive
Cells in the ventral cochlear nucleus send signals up to the superior olives on both sides of the brainstem. Here the brain interprets the direction of sounds (see p.92). The superior olive then sends signals on to the midbrain.

HOW THE BRAIN HEARS
A sound begins as a wave of vibrations that is picked up by the trumpet-shaped outer ear. Vibrations travel through the middle ear before being converted into electrical signals by the organ of Corti. There are thought to be several nerve pathways that sound impulses take through the brainstem (see p.92) to reach the thalamus and primary auditory cortex for processing into the conscious perception of a sound.

SMELL

ALTHOUGH VISION HAS BECOME THE DOMINANT SENSE IN HUMANS, THE SENSE OF SMELL (OLFACTION) REMAINS IMPORTANT TO SURVIVAL BECAUSE IT CAN WARN US OF HAZARDOUS SUBSTANCES IN OUR ENVIRONMENT. THE SENSES OF SMELL AND TASTE ARE CLOSELY LINKED.

DETECTING SMELL

Like the sense of taste, smell is a chemical sense. Specialized receptors in the nasal cavity detect incoming molecules, which enter the nose on air currents and bind to receptor cells. Sniffing sucks up more odor molecules into the nose, allowing you to "sample" a smell. It is a reflex action that occurs when a smell attracts your attention, and can help warn of danger, such as smoke from a fire or rotting food. Olfactory receptors located high up in the nasal cavity send electrical impulses to the olfactory bulb, in the limbic area of the brain, for processing.

SMELL CENTERS IN THE BRAIN
The olfactory bulb is the smell gateway to the brain. Here, data about smells is processed in the forebrain (yellow), then sent to various areas of the brain, including the olfactory cortex adjacent to the hippocampus (red).

SMELL PATHWAYS

Odors are initially registered by receptor cells in the nasal cavity. These send electrical impulses along dedicated pathways to the olfactory bulb (each nostril connects to one olfactory bulb). The olfactory bulb is part of the brain's limbic system, the seat of our emotions, desires, and instincts, which is why smells can trigger strong emotional reactions. Once processed by the olfactory bulb, data is transmitted via three olfactory pathways to higher centers in the brain that process it in different ways. This process is called "orthonasal" smelling, in which smell data travels along pathways directly from the nose (see opposite). In "retronasal" smelling (see p.101), odors also have a flavor component that enters the olfactory pathways via the mouth.

SAME-SIDE PROCESSING
Unlike data gathered by the other sense organs, odors are processed on the same, not opposite, side of the brain as the nostril the sensory data was sent from.

RECEPTOR ARRAYS

There are around 1,000 types of receptor cell in the nasal cavity, but we can distinguish around 20,000 different smells so, clearly, there is more to smell reception than "one receptor, one smell." Research shows that each receptor has zones on it, each of which responds to a number of smell molecules. Also, multiple receptors respond to the same smell molecule—it may be that each receptor binds to a different part of it. A specific smell will activate a specific pattern or

"array" across the receptors, so that each smell has its own "signature." When the receptors forming a specific pattern are activated, this signature is sent to the brain for processing.

OLFACTORY RECEPTOR CELL
This colored electron micrograph shows tiny cilia projecting from a receptor cell. Odor molecules bind to the cilia and activate the receptor.

THE CHEMISTRY OF SMELL

There is still much to be learned about the relationship between chemical structure and smell. Scientists have identified eight primary odors (rather like the three primary colors): camphorous, fishy, malty, minty, musky, spermatic, sweaty, and urinous. Smells are often produced by a combination of many different smell molecules, often from different categories. Comparisons of the structures of smell molecules within each category have shown some similarities—for example, minty smelling compounds often share a similar molecular structure. However, tiny differences in molecular structure can produce very different smells. Octanol, a fatty alcohol, smells like oranges, while octanoic acid, a saturated fatty acid that differs from octanol by only one oxygen atom, smells like sweat.

SMELL AND MOLECULAR STRUCTURE
These two molecules differ significantly in their chemical structure, yet both of them conjure the same characteristic "mothball" smell of camphor. One theory is that it is not the shape of molecules that causes them to smell, but the frequency at which their atoms vibrate.

PRIMARY SMELLS
Scientists investigating the perception of smell have attempted to identify primary odors, which can be combined with one another to produce the much larger range of smells that we experience. To date, eight primary odors have been identified, including the distinctive smell of fish.

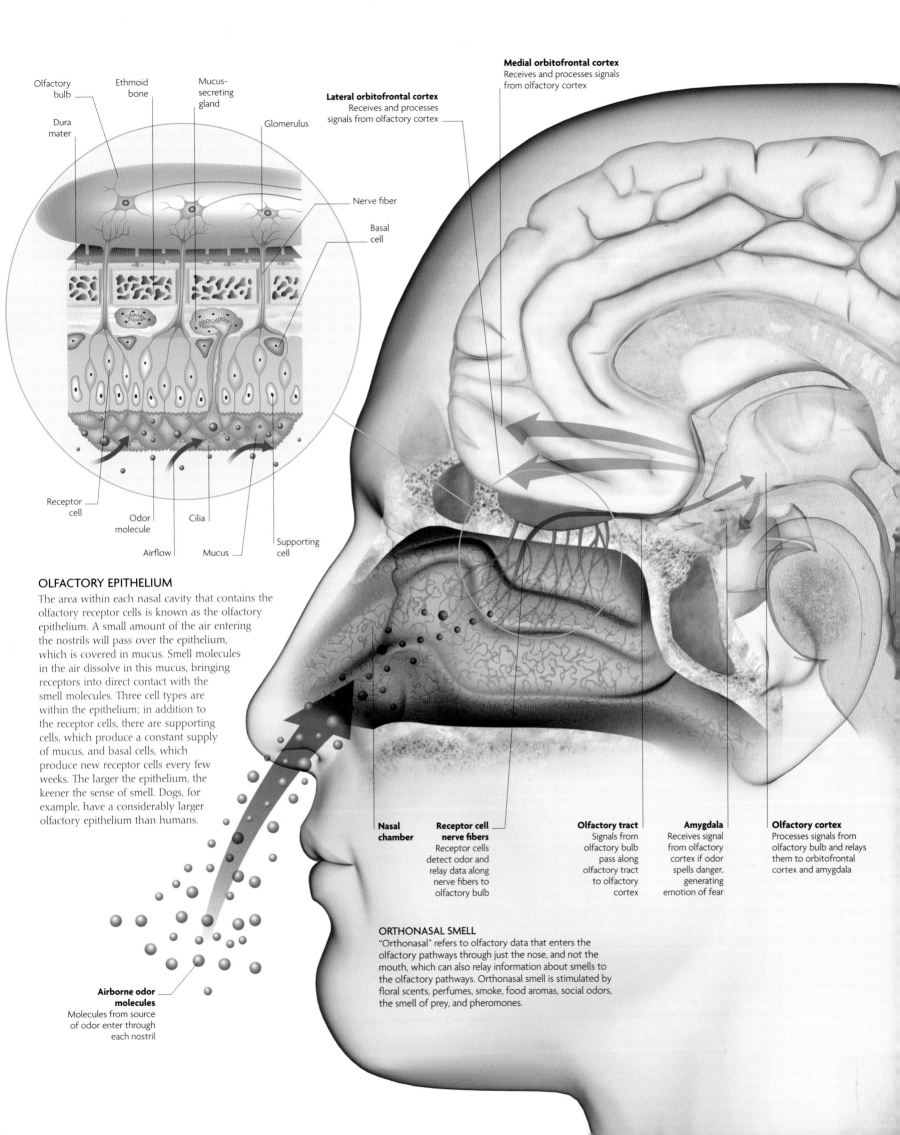

Olfactory
bulb

Dura
mater

Ethmoid
bone

Mucus-
secreting
gland

Glomerulus

Nerve fiber

Basal
cell

Receptor
cell

Odor
molecule

Cilia

Airflow

Mucus

Supporting
cell

OLFACTORY EPITHELIUM

The area within each nasal cavity that contains the olfactory receptor cells is known as the olfactory epithelium. A small amount of the air entering the nostrils will pass over the epithelium, which is covered in mucus. Smell molecules in the air dissolve in this mucus, bringing receptors into direct contact with the smell molecules. Three cell types are within the epithelium; in addition to the receptor cells, there are supporting cells, which produce a constant supply of mucus, and basal cells, which produce new receptor cells every few weeks. The larger the epithelium, the keener the sense of smell. Dogs, for example, have a considerably larger olfactory epithelium than humans.

**Airborne odor
molecules**
Molecules from source
of odor enter through
each nostril

Medial orbitofrontal cortex
Receives and processes signals
from olfactory cortex

Lateral orbitofrontal cortex
Receives and processes
signals from olfactory cortex

**Nasal
chamber**

**Receptor cell
nerve fibers**
Receptor cells
detect odor and
relay data along
nerve fibers to
olfactory bulb

Olfactory tract
Signals from
olfactory bulb
pass along
olfactory tract
to olfactory
cortex

Amygdala
Receives signal
from olfactory
cortex if odor
spells danger,
generating
emotion of fear

Olfactory cortex
Processes signals from
olfactory bulb and relays
them to orbitofrontal
cortex and amygdala

ORTHONASAL SMELL

"Orthonasal" refers to olfactory data that enters the olfactory pathways through just the nose, and not the mouth, which can also relay information about smells to the olfactory pathways. Orthonasal smell is stimulated by floral scents, perfumes, smoke, food aromas, social odors, the smell of prey, and pheromones.

PERCEIVING SMELL

SMELL IS MORE LIKELY TO EVOKE EMOTION AND MEMORY THAN THE OTHER SENSES. THE FACT THAT OLFACTORY AREAS OF THE BRAIN EVOLVED EARLY ON AND ARE WIRED INTO THE PRIMITIVE BRAIN SUGGESTS THAT SMELL IS VITAL FOR OUR SURVIVAL, AS WELL AS THE SURVIVAL OF OTHER ANIMALS.

THE EVOLUTION OF SMELL

The smell brain, centered around the olfactory bulb in the limbic system, is of ancient origin, having evolved about 50 million years ago in fish. The sense of smell was overtaken in importance by the sense of vision when humans began to walk on two legs, although it is still dominant for many animals. But smell is an important aspect of survival for humans, shown in the fact that we take prompt action if we smell gas or smoke, for example. It also plays an important role in sexual selection, emotional responses, and forming preferences for food and drink. All of these factors were probably of key importance in the lives of our ancestors.

DISGUST
When a bad odor is detected, such as that of rotting meat, it is natural to both feel and express disgust. Avoidance of the source of the odor follows, and it is almost impossible to eat food that smells bad.

OLFACTION IN ANIMALS

Although humans can smell some odors at a concentration as low as one part per trillion, our sense of smell is weak compared to that of other animals. The size of the surface area of the olfactory epithelium (see p.97) and the density of smell receptor cells indicate how sensitive an animal's sense of smell is. Dogs, for example, can identify a particular human from just a few odor molecules. Northern dogs, such as huskies and jackals, are renowned for their sense of smell. Hunting dogs and grayhounds have a weaker sense of smell—in the chase, they don't have time to distinguish prey from background smells.

SNIFFER DOG
A breed combining the behavioral characteristics of a domestic dog and a jackal's sense of smell makes an ideal sniffer dog for security work.

SMELL ACROSS SPECIES

SPECIES	NUMBER OF OLFACTORY RECEPTOR CELLS	AREA OF OLFACTORY EPITHELIUM
Human	12 million	1½ square in (10 square cm)
Cat	70 million	2¼ square in (21 square cm)
Rabbit	100 million	Data not available
Dog	1 billion	26½ square in (170 square cm)
Bloodhound	4 billion	59 square in (381 square cm)

SMELL PREFERENCES

Whether we find a smell nice, nasty, or neutral is very subjective and depends upon familiarity, intensity, and perception as pleasant or unpleasant. It is not clear if preferences are innate or learned, but much experimental evidence supports the latter possibility. Associative learning links pleasant smells to pleasant experiences, and vice versa. For example, people who fear the dentist do not like the clovelike smell of eugenol, which is used in dental cement; those without a fear of the dentist react positively or neutrally to this odor.

SUBJECTIVE RESPONSES
The distinctive smell of the durian fruit is perceived by some as revolting but others find it extremely tempting.

THE SIX WORST SMELLS IN THE WORLD

SMELL	DESCRIPTION
Decaying flesh	Repulsive to most people; may evoke thoughts of death
Skunk odor	Horrible to most, but a few people find it "interesting"
Vomit	Often associated with illness, which may heighten disgust
Feces or urine	Caused by gas released as bacteria break down food residue
Decaying food	Triggers an "adaptive" response to food that could cause illness
Isonitriles	Chemicals in nonlethal weapons described as "world's worst smell"

STEREOSCOPIC AND BLIND SMELL

It is generally believed that the human sense of smell has atrophied in relation to our other senses, but recent research shows that humans can still effectively track a scent. Using both nostrils to sample a smell, the human brain uses both sets of data to accurately pinpoint the location of the source of the odor. Therefore, as with vision and hearing, smell can be "stereoscopic," relying on both nostrils for a full understanding of a scent. "Blind" smell refers to the ability of the brain to detect a smell without being consciously aware of it, which has been demonstrated in experiments using fMRI scans showing how olfactory areas are activated without the participant's knowledge.

BLIND SMELL ACTIVATION
This fMRI scan shows widespread activity throughout the brain in areas including the thalamus (just above center), on exposure to an odor at concentrations that cannot be detected consciously.

Hippocampus
Only three synapses separate olfactory nerve from hippocampus

Amygdala
Only two synapses separate olfactory nerve from amygdala

Olfactory nerve
Carries signals from olfactory bulb; closely linked to hippocampus and amygdala

Olfactory bulb

Nasal chamber

SMELL AND MEMORY
The olfactory bulb is in the limbic system, close to the amygdala (associated with emotion) and the hippocampus (associated with memory). When you first encounter a smell, it becomes linked to the emotions you associate with the events of that time. Encountering the smell again may trigger this link, evoking the memory and associated emotion.

SMELL AND MEMORY

An event is associated with input from all the senses, co-ordinated by the hippocampus. Reexperiencing any of the sight, smell, or sound inputs may trigger a memory of the event, but smell seems most strongly associated with memory. This may be because olfactory regions are linked to all emotional areas in the limbic system. Research shows that a memory of a visual image is likely to fade within days, but the memory of a smell may persist for up to a year or even decades. The hippocampus may not even be crucial for the link, because people who sustain damage to this region can still recall scents from their childhood, even though suffering from general memory loss.

THE MADELEINE EFFECT

The madeleine effect is named after an episode in Marcel Proust's epic *Remembrance of Things Past*. As a mature adult, the novel's hero eats a madeleine soaked in lime-blossom tea and is mentally transported to his childhood and the house of his aunt, who used to serve madeleines before Sunday mass. Long before the effect was investigated scientifically, Proust recognized that taste and olfactory memories can take us further back than visual or auditory cues.

PROUST
French novelist Marcel Proust (1871–1922) wrote "the smell and taste of things remain poised a long time, ready to remind us...."

SMELL AND COMMUNICATION

Animals emit compounds called pheromones that are used as communication signals and detected by an accessory olfactory system in the brain. Humans recognize each other in a similar way–for example, infants prefer the smell of their mother's breast to that of other women. Research into the existence of pheromones in humans has found that women's menstrual cycles can synchronize when one woman is exposed to odorless compounds (supposing that these are pheromones) emitted from the underarms of another woman. In animals, the accessory olfactory system is linked to the vomeronasal region (VMO), an area in the nasal cavity that responds to pheromones. The VMO's existence in humans remains debatable.

MALE BODY SMELL
Male sweat contains androstenone, a musky compound. When sprayed on a waiting-room chair, most women choose that one. Androstadienone, another compound, affects men, making them more helpful. It is likely to stem from the need for men to hunt cooperatively.

USING SMELL COMMERCIALLY
Some estate agents claim that the smells of baking bread, cinnamon, and coffee can help sell a house by evoking a good feeling in potential purchasers. Equally, they advise banishing pets, so that animal smells do not put off buyers.

TASTE

LIKE SMELL, TASTE HAS A SURVIVAL VALUE—POISONOUS SUBSTANCES TEND TO TASTE BAD (USUALLY BITTER) WHILE THOSE THAT ARE NOURISHING TASTE PLEASURABLE (USUALLY SWEET OR SAVORY). TOGETHER, TASTE AND SMELL ALLOW ANIMALS TO EVALUATE AND RECOGNIZE WHAT THEY EAT AND DRINK.

THE EVOLUTION OF TASTE

The sense of taste enables animals, including humans, to make the most of the variety of foods available to them. Many plants that look tempting are toxic, so genes that enable us to detect (and therefore avoid) these toxins have an obvious survival value. One such gene that has been identified affords taste sensitivity to phenylthiocarbamide (PTC), an organic compound that resembles many toxic compounds found in plants.

EVOLVED TO REACT TO TASTES
Herbivores, such as deer, with fewer bitter-taste genes than omnivores, are less selective and therefore benefit from an increased food supply. They can tolerate more toxins because they have larger livers than omnivores, such as chimpanzees.

THE TONGUE

The tongue is the main sensory organ for taste detection. It is the body's most flexible muscular organ, as revealed by its work in both nutrition and communication. It has three interior muscles and three pairs of muscles connecting it to the mouth and throat. Its surface is dotted with tiny, pimplelike structures called papillae.

Other parts of the mouth, such as the palate, pharynx, and epiglottis can also detect taste stimuli.

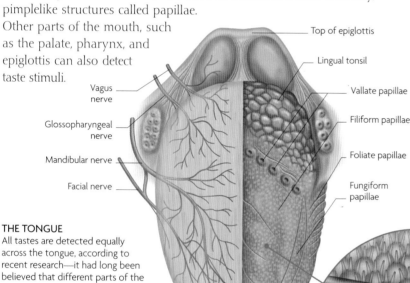

Top of epiglottis
Lingual tonsil
Vallate papillae
Filiform papillae
Foliate papillae
Fungiform papillae
Vagus nerve
Glossopharyngeal nerve
Mandibular nerve
Facial nerve

THE TONGUE
All tastes are detected equally across the tongue, according to recent research—it had long been believed that different parts of the tongue are dedicated to detecting specific tastes. The tongue is well supplied with nerves that carry taste-related data to the brain.

SUPERTASTERS

Around a quarter of the population are "supertasters," which means they have an overall higher level of tasting ability. They are very sensitive to a chemical called propylthiouracil (PROP), finding it incredibly bitter. Half the remaining population find PROP moderately bitter, and the final quarter cannot taste it at all. Supertasters find bitter compounds such as coffee too strong. They seem to have more fungiform papillae on the tongue, which may explain the increased sensitivity.

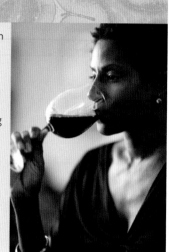

PAPILLAE
Papillae contain taste buds and are distributed across the tongue. Four types of papillae have been distinguished—vallate, filiform, foliate, and fungiform. Each type bears a different amount of taste buds. Fungiform and filiform are the smallest papillae, and vallate are the largest, and together form a V-shape across the rear of the tongue.

Tongue epithelium
Filiform papilla
Fungiform pailla
Vallate papilla
Mucus-secreting gland
Connective tissue
Taste pore
Taste hair
Gustatory receptor cell
Supporting cell
Nerve fibre
Epithelium of tongue

TASTE BUDS
A taste bud is composed of a group of about 25 receptor cells alongside supporting cells, layered together much like a bunch of bananas. The tips of the cells form a small pore, through which taste molecules enter and contact receptor molecules. These are borne on taste hairs (tiny projections called microvilli) that extend into the pore.

THE FIVE BASIC FLAVORS

Along with the basic tastes, people can detect other substances, such as fatty acids, through receptors in the upper airways. This suggests that taste is a part of smell, just as smell is a part of taste.

NAME	DESCRIPTION
Sweet	Often linked to energy-rich, high-calorie foods.
Sour	May be a danger sign, signaling unripe or "off" foods.
Salty	Most chemical salts, including sodium chloride, taste salty.
Bitter	May be linked to natural toxins, and is best avoided.
Umami	Savory ("umami" means "delicious" in Japanese).

TASTE AND SMELL BRAIN AREAS

Taste and smell are both chemical senses—receptors in the nose and mouth bind to incoming molecules, generating electrical signals to send to the brain. Both sets of signals pass along the cranial nerves. Smell-related (olfactory) signals travel from the nose to the olfactory bulb, then along the olfactory nerve to the olfactory cortex in the temporal lobe for processing (see also pp.96–97). The pathway of taste-related (gustatory) data travels from the mouth along branches of the trigeminal and glossopharyngeal nerves to the medulla, continues to the thalamus, then to primary gustatory areas of the cerebral cortex.

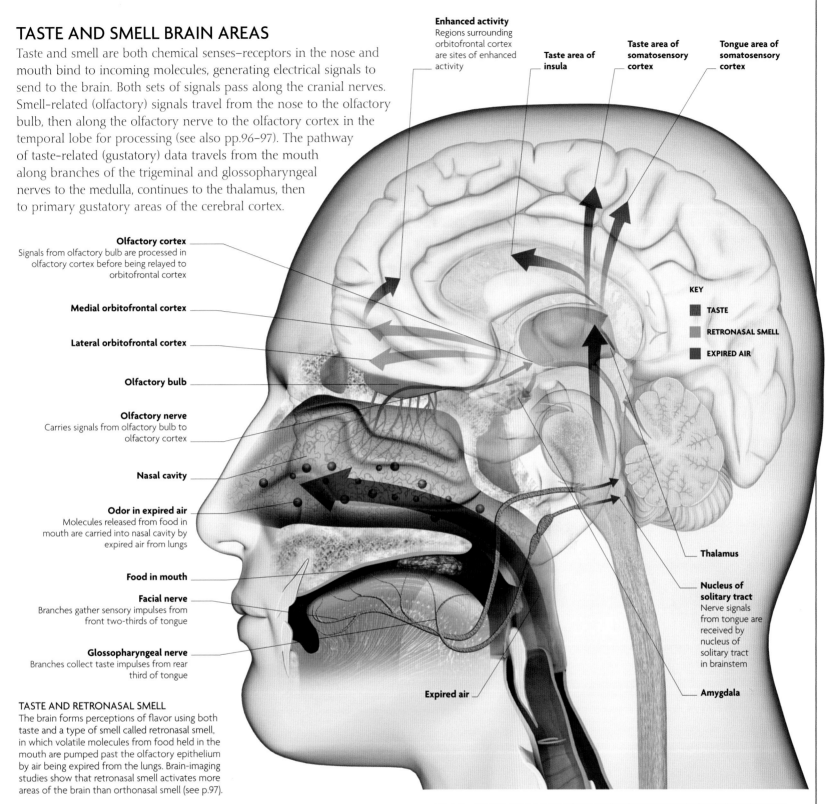

Enhanced activity
Regions surrounding orbitofrontal cortex are sites of enhanced activity

Taste area of insula

Taste area of somatosensory cortex

Tongue area of somatosensory cortex

Olfactory cortex
Signals from olfactory bulb are processed in olfactory cortex before being relayed to orbitofrontal cortex

Medial orbitofrontal cortex

Lateral orbitofrontal cortex

Olfactory bulb

Olfactory nerve
Carries signals from olfactory bulb to olfactory cortex

Nasal cavity

Odor in expired air
Molecules released from food in mouth are carried into nasal cavity by expired air from lungs

Food in mouth

Facial nerve
Branches gather sensory impulses from front two-thirds of tongue

Glossopharyngeal nerve
Branches collect taste impulses from rear third of tongue

Expired air

KEY
- TASTE
- RETRONASAL SMELL
- EXPIRED AIR

Thalamus

Nucleus of solitary tract
Nerve signals from tongue are received by nucleus of solitary tract in brainstem

Amygdala

TASTE AND RETRONASAL SMELL
The brain forms perceptions of flavor using both taste and a type of smell called retronasal smell, in which volatile molecules from food held in the mouth are pumped past the olfactory epithelium by air being expired from the lungs. Brain-imaging studies show that retronasal smell activates more areas of the brain than orthonasal smell (see p.97).

TASTE ASSOCIATIONS

When a food makes you ill (spoiled seafood, for example), the association can linger for a long time, making even the thought of that food repulsive. The phenomenon, known as flavor-aversion learning, has been demonstrated by researchers at Harvard Medical School who fed rats a sweet liquid with a substance that made them briefly ill. Thereafter, the rats avoided the liquid despite its tempting sweetness. When a food is paired with nausea, flavor-aversion learning has a survival value in teaching animals to avoid attractive-looking foods that may be toxic. It is a robust form of learning—occurring after one episode only, but lasting for many years.

TASTE AVERSION
As an alternative to killing coyotes that prey on domestic sheep, some farmers in the western US place lamb bait laced with an illness-inducing drug around their ranches. The coyotes learn to avoid lamb meat and therefore stop approaching sheep.

TOUCH

THERE ARE MANY KINDS OF TOUCH SENSATIONS. THESE INCLUDE
LIGHT TOUCH, PRESSURE, VIBRATION, AND TEMPERATURE AS WELL
AS PAIN (SEE PP.106–107), AND AWARENESS OF THE BODY'S POSITION
IN SPACE (PROPRIOCEPTIONS, SEE PP.104–105). THE SKIN IS THE
BODY'S MAIN SENSE ORGAN FOR TOUCH.

TOUCH RECEPTORS

There are around 20 types of touch receptor that respond to various
types of stimuli. For instance, light touch, a general category that
covers sensations ranging from a tap on the arm to stroking a cat's
fur, is detected by four different types of receptor cells: free nerve
endings, found in the epidermis; Merkel's disks, found in deeper
layers of the skin; Meissner's corpuscles, which are common in the
palms, soles of the feet, eyelids, genitals, and nipples; and, finally, the
root hair plexus, which responds when the hair moves. Pacinian and
Ruffini corpuscles respond to more intense pressure. The sensation
of itching is produced by
repetitive, low-level stimulation
of nerve fibers in the skin, while
feeling ticklish involves more
intense stimulation of the same
nerve endings when the stimulus
moves over the skin.

SKIN STRUCTURE

Skin is the largest sense organ and allows us
to interact fully with our surroundings. This
light micrograph reveals how the skin is
embedded with nerves, receptors, glands,
hair follicles, and a rich blood supply.

Merkel's disk
Mostly in lower
epidermis and
upper dermis

Sebaceous gland
Produces sebum
to protect hair
and lubricate skin

Hair
When body
is cold, hair
is pulled up
by dedicated
erector pili
muscle, which
is located
in dermis

**Meissner's
corpuscle**
Nerve endings
found in upper
dermis

Free nerve ending
Located at edge
of epidermis;
specialized to pick
up light touch

Epidermis
Outer layer of
skin; made up of
resilient, flat cells

Dermis
Contains
glands, blood
vessels, and
nerve endings

Hypodermis
Deepest layer
of skin, contains
fatty tissue

Pacinian corpuscle
Located deep in dermis

Adipose tissue
Fat storage; fat
supplies energy
and absorbs shocks

Bulbous corpuscle
Soft, capsulelike cells,
mostly located in
mucous membranes

Ruffini corpuscle
Mostly found in
middle and lower
layers of dermis

Sweat gland
Produces sweat
that passes to
skin's surface
via sweat duct

TYPES OF RECEPTORS

The variety of touch receptors gives rise to a wide range of
sensations. They are distributed throughout the body in the
skin, conjunctiva, bladder, and in muscles and joints.

TYPES OF TOUCH

The different types of touch sensation convey detailed,
complex information about the world around us and
can act as a warning signal. Touch is essential for
experiencing the texture and "feel" of objects. It also
plays a vital role in communicating with others.

SENSATION	RECEPTORS
Light touch	The skin is not deformed by light touch, for example a handshake or a kiss. Free nerve endings in the skin respond to light-touch stimuli.
Touch pressure	Pressure entailing short-lived skin deformation stimulates Pacinian corpuscles and Ruffini corpuscles, located deep in the skin.
Vibration	Pacinian corpuscles and Meissner's corpuscles (mechanoreceptors, detecting mechanical movements) respond to vibrations.
Heat and cold	Receptors are sensitive to either hot or cold, not temperature itself. Heat and cold receptors occur in specific spots on the skin.
Pain	Pain signals come from damaged tissue and stimulate nociceptors (see pp.106–107), which consist of free nerve endings.
Proprioception	Receptor cells located in muscles and joints send information to the brain about the position and movement of the body.

TOUCH PATHWAY

When a sense receptor is activated, it sends information
about touch stimuli as electrical impulses along a nerve
fiber of the sensory nerve network to the nerve root on the
spinal cord. The data enters the spinal cord and continues
upward to the brain. The processing of sensory data is
begun by nuclei in the upper (dorsal) column of the spinal
cord. From the brainstem, sensory data enters the thalamus,
where processing continues. The data then travels to the
postcentral gyrus of the cerebral cortex, the location of the
somatosensory cortex. Here, it is finally translated into a
touch perception.

1 FIRST ORDER TO SECOND ORDER
First-order neurons carry data from the
touch receptors of the upper thigh to the
spinal cord. Their cell bodies are found in
the dorsal root ganglia of the spinal cord.
On entering the spinal cord, they connect
with second-order neurons, most of which
are located in the gray matter of the spinal
cord, before traveling up the spinal cord
along the pathway known as the ascending
anterior spinothalamic tract.

White
matter

Gray
matter

**FRONT OF
SPINAL CORD**

Ventral horn

Signal passes
into spinal
cord

Sensory
information
from upper
thigh

Dorsal root
ganglion cell

Dorsal root
axon

Dorsal horn

BACK OF SPINAL CORD

Brain

Spinal cord

Somatosensory cortex

Thalamus

Cerebellum

Signal travels to cortex for interpretation

Ventral posterior nucleus

Signal travels to thalamus

Pons

Medulla

Signal continues from spinal cord to medulla

Dorsal column nuclei

Spinal cord

2 SECOND ORDER TO THIRD ORDER

From the spinal cord, the signal travels through the brainstem, crossing over to the other side of the brain. Here, the nerve fiber connects with a third-order neuron in the thalamus, and the signal is relayed to the somatosensory cortex to be processed. Nuclei in the dorsal spinal column and thalamus also process sensory impulses en route.

SOMATOSENSORY CORTEX

Touch sensations are turned into perceptions in the somatosensory cerebral cortex, which curls around the brain like a horseshoe. Data from the left side of the body ends on the right side of the brain, and vice versa. Each part of the cortex processes data from a different part of the body. It is possible to make a map of the cerebral cortex, dividing it into regions that correspond to distinct body parts. Such a map was first drawn by Wilder Penfield, a renowned Canadian neurosurgeon. Touch receptors are unevenly distributed across the body. For example, experiments show that the distance between touch receptors is far greater on the back than on the lips. The hands have the largest proportion of touch receptors in the body.

HOMUNCULUS
The size of the body parts with the most sensory and motor connections with the brain are proportionally enlarged on this distorted figure.

Dermatome
One of three regions of skin served by single pair of spinal nerves

SOMATOSENSORY CORTEX

Arm   Head   Trunk

Hand

Leg

Foot

Toes

Genitals

Fingers and thumb

Eye

Face

Lips

Tongue

TOUCH MAP
The touch pathway from a specific sense receptor ends in a region of the somatosensory cortex that corresponds to that part of the body.

Initial sensation
Touch receptors in the skin are activated by touch stimuli—they are linked to a nerve fiber within the body's sensory nerve network, along which they send signals to the brain

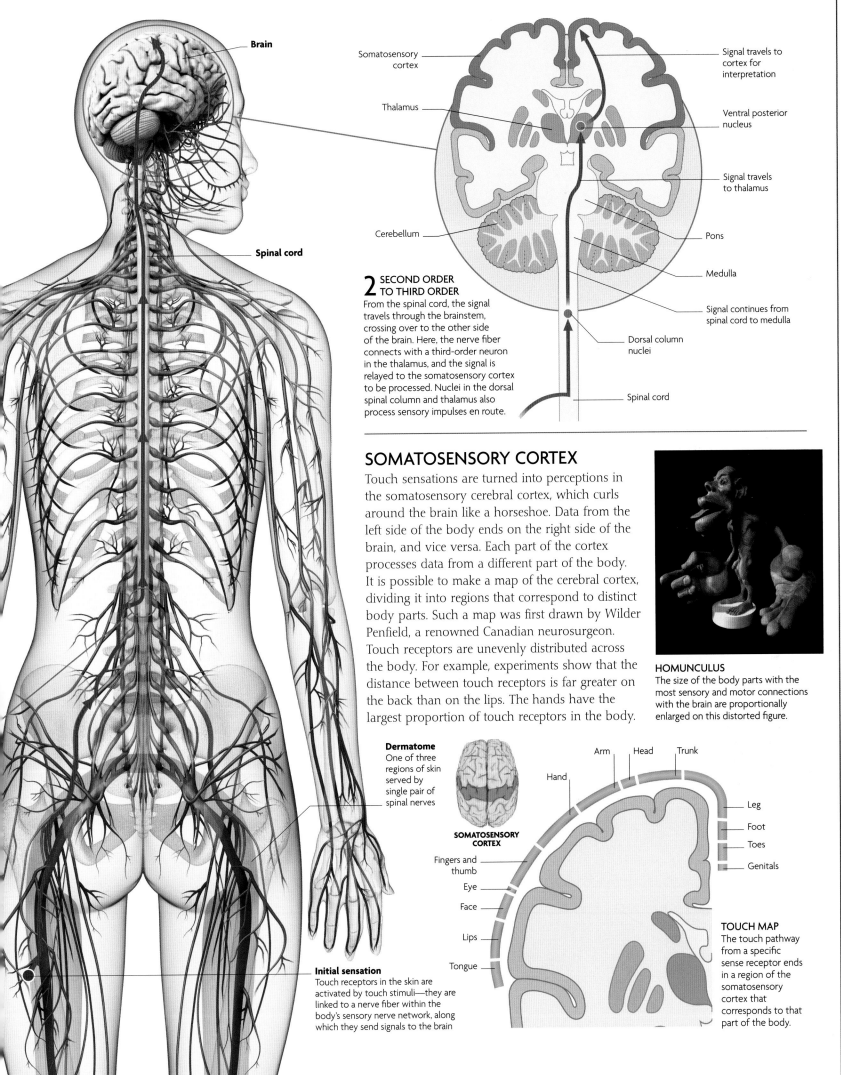

PROPRIOCEPTION—FROM *PROPRIO*, THE LATIN FOR "SELF"—IS SOMETIMES REFERRED TO AS THE SIXTH SENSE. IT IS THE SENSING OF BODY POSITION, MOVEMENT, AND POSTURE, INVOLVING FEEDBACK TO THE BRAIN FROM THE BODY. HOWEVER, THIS INFORMATION IS NOT ALWAYS MADE CONSCIOUS.

WHAT IS PROPRIOCEPTION?

Proprioception is our sense of how our bodies are positioned and moving in space. This "awareness" is produced by part of the somatic sensory system, and involves structures called proprioceptors in the muscles, tendons, joints, and ligaments that monitor changes in their length, tension, and pressure linked to changes in position. Proprioceptors send impulses to the brain. Upon processing this information, a decision can be made–to change position or to stop moving. The brain then sends signals back to the muscles based on the input from the proprioceptors–completing the feedback cycle.

Proprioceptive information is either made conscious or processed unconsciously. For example, keeping and adjusting balance is generally an unconscious process. Conscious proprioception usually involves some kind of cortical processing, resulting in decision-making. This normally ends in a command to the muscles to perform a movement. The sheer amount of proprioceptive input means that much is processed unconsciously.

Biceps muscle
Moves through arm elongation or contraction

Sensory cortex
Processes input from biceps

Sensory nerve

Sensory neuron
Carries sensory information to the brain

Muscle cell

Muscle spindle fiber
Detects changes in the length of the muscle

POSITIONAL SENSORS
Information from proprioceptors, such as muscle spindle-fibers, is sent to the brain for processing. There are also position sensors in the joints, load sensors within the tendons, and muscle-stretch detectors, all working together to create an image of the body's position.

Conscious pathway

Unconscious pathway

PROPRIOCEPTION PATHWAYS
Conscious proprioception uses the dorsal column–medial lemniscus pathway, which passes through the thalamus, and ends in the parietal lobe of the cortex. Unconscious proprioception involves spinocerebellar tracts, and ends in the cerebellum, the part of the brain at the back of the skull involved with the control of movement.

PHANTOM LIMBS

When someone has a part of the body amputated or removed–be it a limb, an extremity, or an organ, such as the appendix–they sometimes continue to have sensations, often including pain, in that area. Research has linked this to changes in the sensory cortex. Specifically, the somatosensory cortex undergoes a remapping process in which the areas near the "dead" area "take over", so that stimuli in these areas are felt as sensations in the area that has been lost. This reorganization of the cortex has been confirmed through imaging studies.

PHANTOM-LIMB-PAIN TREATMENT

Research has shown that the development of phantom-limb pain is linked to the plasticity of the sensory cortex. Trying to reverse the changes in the cortex can actually reduce the pain sensation for the patient. For instance, use of an electric prosthetic limb that is moved by signals from the patient's muscles was helpful. Brain scans revealed that this was linked with reversion of the cortex to its original state, maybe by replacing some of the original input.

NEURONS IN CORTEX

Toes and trunk | Arm and hand | Face

SENSORY INPUT

BEFORE AMPUTATION
Sensory inputs from the arm and hand are connected to the appropriate region of the sensory cortex. Other parts of the body are also connected to specific, neighbouring cortical regions.

Toes and trunk | Face

AFTER AMPUTATION
There is no sensory input from the amputated arm and hand, but the pathway to the cortex remains. Input from another part of the body takes over, reshaping the sensory map, which may produce sensations.

MIRROR TREATMENT
When a patient's remaining arm is shown as a mirror image and moved, it looks as though the missing arm is moving. Somehow, this illusion can relieve phantom-limb pain.

FINE BALANCE
Proprioceptors in the muscles, tendons, and skin work together with hair cells in the vestibule and semicircular canals of the inner ear to maintain balance. A gymnast will work on all aspects of strength, movement, and body coordination to achieve feats involving fine balance.

PAIN SIGNALS

PAIN IS PRIMARILY A WARNING SIGNAL. IT TELLS YOU THERE IS SOMETHING WRONG AND FORCES YOU TO TAKE ACTION. PAIN USUALLY OCCURS AS A RESULT OF STIMULATION OF SPECIALIZED NERVE FIBERS THAT EXTEND THROUGHOUT THE BODY.

PAIN PATHWAYS

Pain-transmitting nerve fibers permeate almost every part of the body. When stimulated by an injury, they send electrical signals from the site of the stimulus to the spinal cord. The signals then cross over the cord and continue up to the brain. This crossover means that pain from one side of the body activates the opposite side of the brain. As they pass through the medulla in the brainstem, pain signals trigger automatic bodily responses. The signals then arrive at the thalamus and are distributed to various regions of the brain to be processed.

FEELING PAIN
Pain is not felt until the brain has processed signals indicating injury.

1 INFLAMMATORY "SOUP"
Injury sets off the release of chemicals, such as bradykinin and ATP, which trigger the nerve impulses that are experienced as pain. Some chemicals—such as histamine, which is released by specialized white blood cells—also cause the injury site to become inflamed by making capillaries swell up.

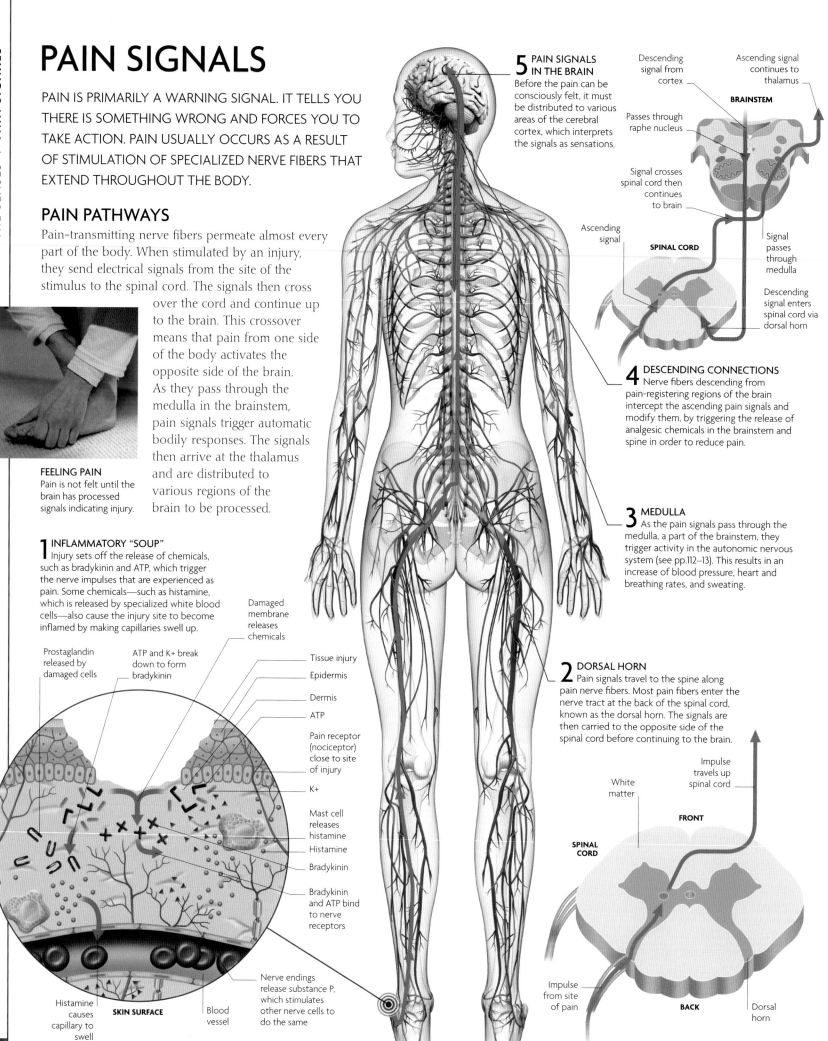

Prostaglandin released by damaged cells

ATP and K+ break down to form bradykinin

Damaged membrane releases chemicals

Tissue injury

Epidermis

Dermis

ATP

Pain receptor (nociceptor) close to site of injury

K+

Mast cell releases histamine

Histamine

Bradykinin

Bradykinin and ATP bind to nerve receptors

Histamine causes capillary to swell

SKIN SURFACE

Blood vessel

Nerve endings release substance P, which stimulates other nerve cells to do the same

5 PAIN SIGNALS IN THE BRAIN
Before the pain can be consciously felt, it must be distributed to various areas of the cerebral cortex, which interprets the signals as sensations.

Descending signal from cortex

Ascending signal continues to thalamus

BRAINSTEM

Passes through raphe nucleus

Signal crosses spinal cord then continues to brain

Ascending signal

SPINAL CORD

Signal passes through medulla

Descending signal enters spinal cord via dorsal horn

4 DESCENDING CONNECTIONS
Nerve fibers descending from pain-registering regions of the brain intercept the ascending pain signals and modify them, by triggering the release of analgesic chemicals in the brainstem and spine in order to reduce pain.

3 MEDULLA
As the pain signals pass through the medulla, a part of the brainstem, they trigger activity in the autonomic nervous system (see pp.112–13). This results in an increase of blood pressure, heart and breathing rates, and sweating.

2 DORSAL HORN
Pain signals travel to the spine along pain nerve fibers. Most pain fibers enter the nerve tract at the back of the spinal cord, known as the dorsal horn. The signals are then carried to the opposite side of the spinal cord before continuing to the brain.

Impulse travels up spinal cord

White matter

FRONT

SPINAL CORD

Impulse from site of pain

BACK

Dorsal horn

THE CHEMISTRY OF PAIN RELIEF

The body has a natural opioid (pain relief) system that acts in much the same way as opiate drugs, such as heroin and morphine. Natural opioids, which include endorphins and encephalins, are produced by the thalamus and pituitary gland during stress and pain. These substances are also produced in situations associated with feeling a natural "high," such as strenuous exercise and sexual activity. Nerve endings in the brain and throughout the body have special receptors on them that bind to opiate substances. The opiates then dampen the pain signals carried in those nerve endings, thus reducing pain.

OPIOID RECEPTORS
This PET scan shows the concentration of opioid receptors in a normal brain. Red areas show where they are highest, through yellow and green, to blue, which indicates the lowest concentration.

PAIN FIBERS

There are two main types of nerve fiber that detect pain: A-delta and C. A-delta fibers are thin and carry sharp, localized pain signals to the brain. The site of the injury will be within a millimeter of these nerve fibers, so the site is easily identified. These nerve fibers are covered in a fatty myelin sheath that aids the transmission of signals. C-fibers are not insulated by a myelin sheath. The source of pain transmitted by a C-fiber is difficult to pinpoint because its nerve endings are spread out over a relatively large area.

Myelin sheath

A-DELTA FIBER   **C-FIBER**

C-FIBERS AND A-DELTA FIBERS
A-delta fibers are found mostly in subcutaneous tissue. C-fibers accompany all the blood vessels, lymphatic, sensory, and motor nerves, and the peripheral autonomic nerves.

TYPES OF PAIN

Pain usually arises when pain receptors are stimulated by heat, cold, vibration, overstretching, or by chemicals released from damaged cells. Specialized nerve fibers (see panel, above) transmit this information to the brain. However, certain types of pain are processed and experienced in different ways, for example the facial nerves connect directly to the cranial nerves (see below), whereas visceral pain, from internal organs such as the heart (see right), can be difficult to locate. Damage to the nervous system itself, such as a trapped nerve, is known as neuropathic pain (see bottom).

FACIAL PAIN

Stimulation of trigeminal nerves usually causes facial pain. It often affects only one side of the face and can be felt on the skin or in the mouth and teeth. It comes and goes unpredictably and its nature is variously described as stabbing, lacerating, like an electric shock, and shooting. It can range in severity from mild to excruciating. There are frequently "trigger points" on the skin, which, if touched, will bring on a violent pain spasm. People may experience pain daily for weeks and months, then it may disappear for months or even years.

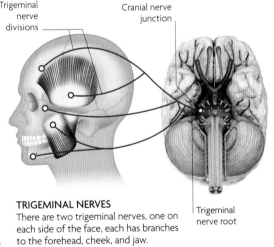

Trigeminal nerve divisions

Cranial nerve junction

Trigeminal nerve root

TRIGEMINAL NERVES
There are two trigeminal nerves, one on each side of the face, each has branches to the forehead, cheek, and jaw.

REFERRED PAIN

Referred pain occurs when nerve fibers from areas of high sensory input (such as the skin) and nerve fibers from areas of low sensory input (such as internal organs) enter the spinal cord at the same location. Since the brain expects to be receiving the data from high-sensory areas, it misinterprets the location of the pain.

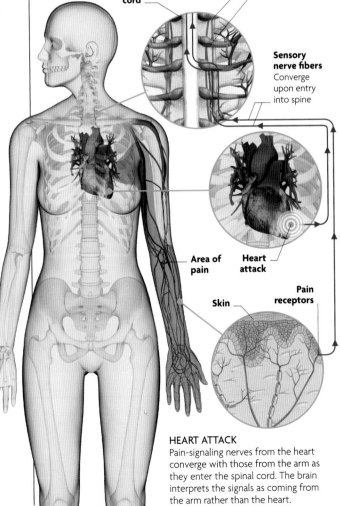

Spinal cord

Ganglion

Sensory nerve fibers
Converge upon entry into spine

Area of pain

Heart attack

Skin

Pain receptors

HEART ATTACK
Pain-signaling nerves from the heart converge with those from the arm as they enter the spinal cord. The brain interprets the signals as coming from the arm rather than the heart.

NEUROPATHIC PAIN

Pain that is caused by damage or malfunction in the nervous system itself rather than injury is known as neuropathic pain. A pain-transmitting nerve may be severed, or be stimulated so often that it gets into the "habit" of sending pain signals to the brain. Pain-registering neurons in the cortex can become sensitized so that they produce the experience of pain even when there is no external cause.

SEVERED NERVE BUNDLE
This colored electron micrograph shows a severed bundle of nerves. These may continue to send pain signals to the brain even when the cause of the damage itself is long gone.

EXPERIENCING PAIN

THE FEELING OF PAIN IS NOT ACTUALLY CAUSED BY AN INJURY IN ITSELF. IN ORDER TO EXPERIENCE PAIN, IT MUST BE MADE CONSCIOUS. THIS REQUIRES ACTIVITY IN BRAIN AREAS INVOLVED IN EMOTION, ATTENTION, AND ASSESSING SIGNIFICANCE. SUCH ACTIVITY CAN CREATE THE PAIN EXPERIENCE IN THE ABSENCE OF A CAUSE.

PATHWAY OF PAIN

Pain signals are transmitted to several areas of the cortex, where they activate neurons that monitor the state of the body. Two such areas are the somatosensory cortex, which lets the brain know which part of the body the pain stems from, and the insular cortex–the deep fold that divides the temporal and frontal lobes. The other cortical site associated with pain experience is the anterior (front) of the cingulate cortex (ACC), which lies in the groove between the hemispheres. The ACC seems to be particularly concerned with the emotional significance of pain and with determining how much attention an injury should command.

PAIN ROUTES
Pain signals from the body ascend to the brain via the spinal cord, then rise through the brainstem to the thalamus. Thereafter, they are distributed to various cortical areas for processing.

PAIN CENTERS
The somatosensory cortex (green) and the insular cortex (red) are responsible for pinpointing the exact site of the pain stimulus.

A WHOLE-BRAIN AFFAIR

Pain is so important to our survival that it may involve practically every part of the brain. Three main "pain areas" (see above) register and assess pain signals, and pinpoint the site of their source, but other areas also come into play. The supplementary motor area and motor cortex may plan and execute movement aimed at escaping the pain stimulus. Parts of the parietal cortex may direct attention to the threat, and several parts of the frontal cortex may be involved in working out the significance of the pain and what to do about it.

PAIN STUDY
The fMRI scans above show various "slices" through the brain of a healthy person who is being subjected to a painful stimulus on the arm. The regions highlighted in yellow show areas of neural activity in response to the stimulus, revealing how widespread the effects of pain are on the brain.

PAIN CIRCUITS
Pain signals travel along many different neural circuits to hit their targets. Some follow the paths of nerves that ascend from areas of the body, while others stem from brain nuclei, such as those in the hypothalamus, which are concerned with combating the effects of the pain stimulus.

KEY

→ **DIRECT SPINAL INPUT** to areas that monitor the state of the body, direct attention, and prioritize response.

→ **DIRECT SPINAL INPUT** to areas involved in automatic response to pain, such as arousal and movement.

→ **CIRCUIT THROUGH** cortical and limbic areas involved in evaluation and monitoring of pain.

→ **CIRCUIT THROUGH** cortical and limbic areas that affect pain, including intensity, emotion, and pain memory.

BRAIN OVER PAIN

Part of the role of higher brain areas is to modify pain. Nerve signals that travel from the brain into the body interrupt pain signals traveling up from the site of the injury before they reach the brain. This reduces the number of pain signals reaching the brain and, therefore, the amount of pain felt. Also, our thoughts, expectations, and emotions can all have a profound effect on the degree to which a person is "pained" by pain. People can affect pain consciously by directing attention away from it, or imagining that they are pain-free. An intensely imagined experience generates almost identical brain activity to the equivalent "real" experience, so an imagined state of physical ease may be achieved even as pain fibers in the body are being stimulated.

PLACEBO AND NOCEBO
Pain may be exacerbated or reduced as a result of the way in which we think about it. Believing that pain is being alleviated, by surgical intervention or a drug, for example, can help ease the pain. This is known as the placebo effect. Expecting pain to be intractable or bad does the opposite, known as the nocebo effect.

FREEZING OUT PAIN

The cingulate cortex is an area of the brain that is partly concerned with determining how much attention to give to a pain stimulus. People can develop the ability to tone down activity in this region by learning to shift attention away from the pain stimulus, creating an analgesic effect. Using virtual reality as a focus point has been found to help distract attention away from pain.

DISTRACTING ATTENTION
Burns victims have been found to experience pain relief when immersed in a cooling virtual environment, which is thought to work by distracting attention away from pain.

VIRTUAL ENVIRONMENT
Virtual reality is so distracting, it leaves less attentional resources available for the brain to process pain signals.

NO VIRTUAL REALITY   **USING VIRTUAL REALITY**

PAIN-RELATED BRAIN ACTIVITY
The areas colored yellow in these images show activity related to pain. The distraction provided by virtual reality significantly reduces activity in these areas (right).

Anxiety signals from the amygdala—pain-related or otherwise—spark brain activity in a way that is associated with the experience of pain.

Pain stimulus arrives in the brain via the spinal cord, causing levels of anxiety to become increased.

PAIN

Nocebo effect
Anxiety plus pain input from the body produces a pain-related experience that is more intense than if either factor occurred alone. Anxiety is therefore an example of the nocebo effect—an intensification of pain due to the effects of negative thoughts, beliefs, or expectations.

Placebo effect
The belief that an intervention such as a drug or a medical procedure will alleviate pain is itself able to reduce a pain experience. This is because experience is subjective so, if you think you do not feel pain, you don't. The process by which belief becomes fact is known as the placebo effect.

Descending signals from the prefrontal cortex of the brain can interrupt incoming pain signals. This can be unconscious or consciously controlled.

The anterior cingulate cortex can play a role in directing attention away from pain. Deliberately diverting attention from pain reduces activity here.

PAIN AND THE BRAIN

Although the brain is responsible for the experience of pain, it does not feel pain itself because it contains no pain receptors. This fact becomes very useful during brain surgery, because it allows surgeons to operate while the patient is conscious. The patient can report their experiences when different areas of the brain are stimulated and, therefore, help the surgeons recognize areas of the brain that have crucial functions. In this way, surgeons can carefully work their way toward, say, a brain tumor without damaging important and healthy brain tissue.

BRAIN SURGERY
Patients who remain conscious during brain operations can tell surgeons when the scalpel is close to a crucial area by responding to questions.

LIFE WITHOUT PAIN

A very few people–probably about one in 125 million–are born without the ability to feel pain. The condition is caused by a genetic disorder, congenital analgesia, that results in a lack of pain-sensitive nerve endings in the body. Some people with this condition are able to feel touch or pressure, which relies on different types of nerves. Although the idea of not feeling any pain may, at first, sound rather desirable, the effect is disastrous. Pain normally warns people that they are in danger and forces them to take action to protect themselves. Without it, physical perils are likely to be unnoticed or ignored, leading to lethal injuries and often to premature death.

THE BRAIN IS IN CONSTANT COMMUNICATION WITH THE
REST OF THE BODY, CONTROLLING EVEN ITS MOST BASIC
PROCESSES. IN DOING SO, IT INITIATES MANY MOVEMENTS
THAT WE ARE NOT AWARE OF, SUCH AS SPEEDING UP OR
SLOWING DOWN OUR RATE OF BREATHING. SOME OTHER
MOVEMENTS ARE MADE AS REFLEX ACTIONS, WITHOUT
ANY SIGNALS REACHING THE BRAIN AT ALL. SUCH
UNCONSCIOUS ACTION LEAVES THE CONSCIOUS BRAIN
FREE TO DIRECT ITS ATTENTION TO OTHER THINGS,
INCLUDING MOVEMENTS THAT REQUIRE GREAT
CONCENTRATION AS WELL AS CAREFUL PLANNING.

MOVEMENT AND CONTROL

REGULATION

THE BODY'S BASIC FUNCTIONS ARE CAREFULLY CONTROLLED IN ORDER TO MAINTAIN A STABLE INTERNAL ENVIRONMENT. THE HYPOTHALAMUS AND BRAINSTEM WORK WITH CHEMICAL MESSENGERS CALLED HORMONES TO KEEP THE BODY TICKING—MOSTLY WITHOUT US BEING AWARE OF IT.

THE RETICULAR FORMATION

The reticular formation is located in the brainstem and is made up of a series of long nerve pathways that modulate sensory inputs and carry information to and from the cerebral cortex. It also plays an important role in regulating the autonomic nervous system (ANS), which is responsible for maintaining a balanced internal environment. The reticular formation contains neuronal centers that manage various functions, such as controlling the heart rate and rate of respiration. It is also involved in regulating other basic functions such as digestion, salivation, perspiration, urination, and sexual arousal.

The reticular formation and its connections constitute the reticular activating system (RAS), an arousal mechanism that keeps the brain alert and awake.

THE RETICULAR ACTIVATING SYSTEM
The RAS receives incoming sensory information and transfers it to the cortex to keep it alert and primed for environmental changes.

Activating signals
Various areas of cerebral cortex receive signals from RAS via thalamus

Thalamus

Cerebral cortex

Medulla

Excitatory area of reticular formation (transmits and amplifies signals)

Inhibitory area of reticular formation (suppresses unwanted signals)

Reticular formation

Impulses from spinal cord

GENERAL ANESTHETICS

A cornerstone of modern medicine, general anesthetics allow surgeons to carry out operations that were previously unfeasible. Yet the way in which an anesthetic causes loss of consciousness in a controlled and reversible way is still not fully understood. Ether, chloroform, and halothane act on neurons in the reticular activating system, suppressing alertness and awareness, and also on neurons in the hippocampus, temporarily wiping out memories. These substances also affect the nuclei in the thalamus, by interrupting the flow of sensory information from the body to the brain. Together, the actions of anesthetics on the brain produce an experience of deep oblivion.

REGULATION OF HEART RATE

The heart rate is regulated by the hormonal action of the ANS, which, in turn, is regulated by the reticular formation. The sympathetic branch of the ANS speeds up the heart rate and the parasympathetic branch slows it down. The medulla in the brainstem contains a hub of neurons that constitute the cardioregulatory center, which, in response to information from the ANS, sends signals to the sinoatrial node and the atrioventricular node in the heart. These signals set the heartbeat according to the body's need for oxygen.

Hypothalamus

Medulla

Cardioregulatory center

VAGUS NERVE

CARDIAC NERVES

Sinoatrial node
Sets regular heartbeat of 60–70 beats per minute

SPEEDING UP THE HEART RATE
The hypothalamus performs an executive function, sending signals via the sympathetic nerves to speed up the heart rate if needed.

Atrioventricular node
Relays electrical impulses from upper to lower chambers of heart

KEY
Parasympathetic nerves
Sympathetic nerves

To coronary arteries

To heart muscle

REGULATION OF BREATHING

The rate of breathing in and out is regulated by collections of neurons in the reticular formation, called the dorsal and ventral respiratory groups. These respond to levels of oxygen and carbon dioxide in the blood and regulate the breathing rate accordingly to maintain constant levels. The basal rate of breathing can also be adjusted (in response to increased activity or metabolism) through electrical impulses sent by the pontine respiratory center.

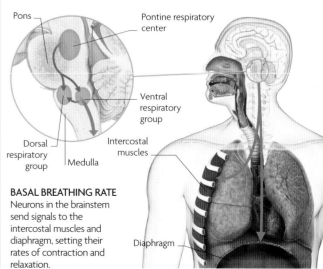

Pons

Dorsal respiratory group

Ventral respiratory group

Intercostal muscles

Medulla

Pontine respiratory center

Diaphragm

BASAL BREATHING RATE
Neurons in the brainstem send signals to the intercostal muscles and diaphragm, setting their rates of contraction and relaxation.

FUNCTIONS OF THE HYPOTHALAMUS

The hypothalamus contains many minute clusters of neurons, called nuclei, which perform specific functions, including controlling body temperature, eating and drinking behavior, water balance, hormonal levels, and sleep–wake cycles. Among other things, the hypothalamus is regarded as the major coordinating center of the limbic system, and it has extensive connections with the pituitary gland and autonomic nervous system. Through these connections, it produces vital responses to body conditions and initiates feelings such as hunger, anger, and fear. The functions of the hypothalamus are essential to life, so even subtle damage can have dramatic effects on behavior and survival.

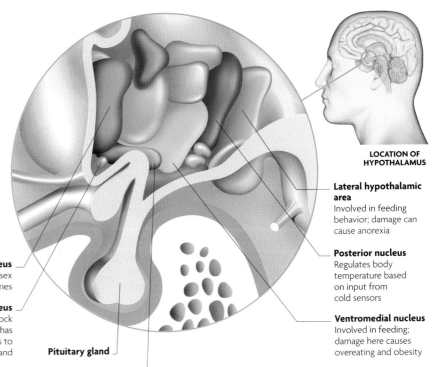

LOCATION OF HYPOTHALAMUS

Lateral hypothalamic area
Involved in feeding behavior; damage can cause anorexia

Posterior nucleus
Regulates body temperature based on input from cold sensors

Ventromedial nucleus
Involved in feeding; damage here causes overeating and obesity

Medial preoptic nucleus
Regulates production of sex hormones

Suprachiasmatic nucleus
Helps regulate body clock and circadian rhythms; has numerous connections to pituitary gland

Pituitary gland

Anterior nucleus
Neurons in this region are concerned with temperature control and process data from body's heat sensors

Hypothalamus

HYPOTHALAMUS
This illustration shows the location of the hypothalamus. It lies beneath the thalamus, near the brainstem, and is about the size of a sugar cube.

HYPOTHALAMIC NUCLEI
Groups of neurons (nuclei) within the hypothalamus have specialized roles in controlling specific responses and regulating the body's systems. Their complete range of functions is not fully known, but some functions have been identified and isolated to specific regions.

THE BODY'S THERMOSTAT

The skin has a number of thermoreceptors that convey information to the hypothalamus about the surrounding temperature. There are six types of receptor, each responding to a specific temperature range; some are sensitive to ranges of heat, others to ranges of cold, but none is sensitive to both. Information from these receptors travels via the spinal cord to the hypothalamus, where specialized nuclei receive the information and initiate various responses to bring the core temperature back to around 99°F (37°C). Some of the thermoregulatory responses are voluntary, arising as a result of conscious activity in the cerebral cortex, while others are involuntarily triggered by the autonomic nervous system.

THE BODY'S RESPONSE TO COLD
When the hypothalamus detects a drop in skin temperature, it responds by triggering heat production and conservation measures.

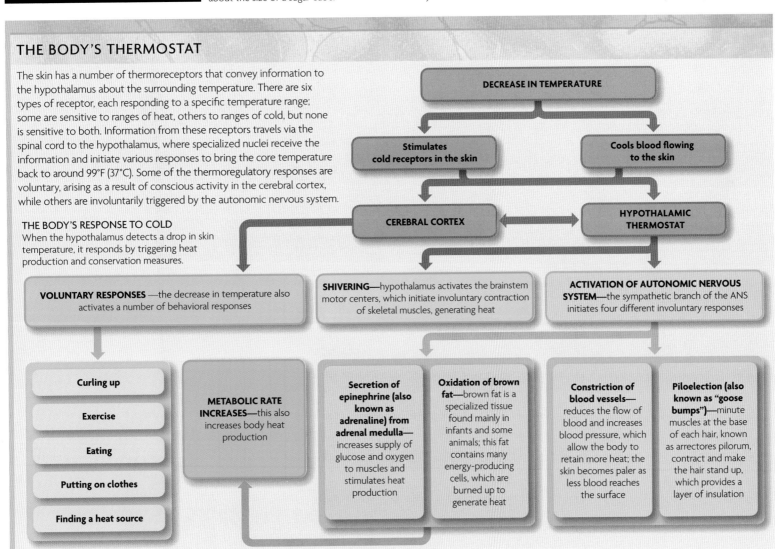

DECREASE IN TEMPERATURE

Stimulates cold receptors in the skin

Cools blood flowing to the skin

CEREBRAL CORTEX

HYPOTHALAMIC THERMOSTAT

VOLUNTARY RESPONSES—the decrease in temperature also activates a number of behavioral responses

SHIVERING—hypothalamus activates the brainstem motor centers, which initiate involuntary contraction of skeletal muscles, generating heat

ACTIVATION OF AUTONOMIC NERVOUS SYSTEM—the sympathetic branch of the ANS initiates four different involuntary responses

Curling up

Exercise

Eating

Putting on clothes

Finding a heat source

METABOLIC RATE INCREASES—this also increases body heat production

Secretion of epinephrine (also known as adrenaline) from adrenal medulla—increases supply of glucose and oxygen to muscles and stimulates heat production

Oxidation of brown fat—brown fat is a specialized tissue found mainly in infants and some animals; this fat contains many energy-producing cells, which are burned up to generate heat

Constriction of blood vessels—reduces the flow of blood and increases blood pressure, which allow the body to retain more heat; the skin becomes paler as less blood reaches the surface

Piloelection (also known as "goose bumps")—minute muscles at the base of each hair, known as arrectores pilorum, contract and make the hair stand up, which provides a layer of insulation

THE NEUROENDOCRINE SYSTEM

THE BRAIN MAINTAINS THE BODY'S STABLE INTERNAL STATE, KNOWN AS HOMEOSTASIS, THROUGH THE ACTION OF HORMONES. NEURAL-CONTROL CENTERS IN THE BRAIN INFLUENCE THE BODY'S GLANDS TO PRODUCE AND RELEASE THE HORMONES THAT ARE NEEDED TO MAINTAIN THIS VITAL BALANCE.

HORMONE SYNTHESIS AND CONTROL

Glands are organs that respond to imbalances in the body in order to regulate internal activities, such as the absorption of nutrients, and influence activities such as the intake of food or water. They react by increasing or decreasing their production of hormones, which then travel to a target organ, where they lock onto specialized receptors on the surface of cells. This binding triggers a physiological change that restores homeostasis. The hypothalamus is the crucial link between the nervous system and endocrine system, releasing hormones that, in turn, trigger the pituitary gland to either stop or start secreting its hormones.

HORMONES RELEASED BY THE PITUITARY GLAND

Melanocyte-stimulating hormone (MSH)	Stimulates the production and release of melanin, the determinant of skin and hair color
Adrenocorticotropic hormone (ACTH)	Triggers the adrenals to produce steroid hormones that control stress response
Thyroid-stimulating hormone (TSH)	Increases the activity of thyroid gland, which controls metabolism
Growth hormone (GH)	Acts on entire body, but especially important for growth and development in children
Luteinizing and follicle-stimulating hormone	Triggers the sex glands in males and females to make their own hormones
Oxytocin	Causes contractions during labor; also involved in the release of milk from the mammary glands
Prolactin	Stimulates the production of milk from the mammary glands
Antidiuretic hormone (ADH)	Controls amount of water removed from the blood by microfilters in the kidneys

FEEDBACK MECHANISMS

Imbalances in the body are detected and corrected using feedback mechanisms, or loops. Levels of a hormone within the bloodstream are gauged and the information is sent to the control unit in charge of that hormone, which in most cases is the hypothalamus–pituitary unit. If the level of a hormone is high, the control unit responds by reducing the production of that hormone to achieve balance. If the level is low, the control unit initiates an increase in production. Feedback mechanisms are also used to trigger rare homeostatic functions, such as contractions during labor.

Hypothalamus
Detects rising blood glucose levels; produces fewer hormones for pituitary gland

Pituitary gland
Reacts to drop in hormone levels by releasing fewer hormones for thyroid

Thyroid gland
Produces fewer hormones that stimulate glucose production

NEGATIVE FEEDBACK
In response to a rise in blood glucose, the hypothalamus triggers a chain reaction of reduced hormone production that results in a fall in glucose levels, which restores balance.

Pineal gland
Pea-sized gland that makes melatonin, a hormone crucially involved with the sleep–wake cycle

Hypothalamus
The vital link between the nervous system and endocrine system; produc two of its own hormones

Pituitary gland
Known as the "master gland" because it controls many other endocrine glands; manufactures eight hormones and receives two hormones directly from hypothalamus

Thyroid gland
Controls metabolic and heart rates; can store hormones, unlike the other glands

Thymus gland
Produces hormones involved in development of white blood cells

Heart
Produces hormone atriopeptin, which reduces blood volume and pressure

Stomach
Makes hormones that stimulate production or release of enzymes that aid digestion

Adrenal gland
Produces hormones that regulate metabolism of glucose, sodium, and potassium; also makes epinephrine

Kidney
Secretes erythropoietin, which stimulates production of red blood cells in bone marrow

Pancreas
Produces insulin and glucagon, which raise and lower blood glucose levels

Intestines
Manufactures hormones that stimulate production or release of enzymes that aid digestion

Ovary
Produces female sex hormones estrogen and progesterone

HORMONE PRODUCERS
Each part of the neuroendocrine system has a unique role to play, synthesizing specific hormones for specific purposes. The action of these hormones helps maintain an optimal internal environment.

HUNGER

The body maintains its weight at a set point by using hormones to trigger the sensations of either hunger or satiety. To stimulate the appetite, the stomach produces the hormone ghrelin, while fat tissues decrease their production of leptin and insulin. These changes signal to specific neurons (referred to as neuron type B on the chart below) to start producing more neuropeptide (NPY) and agouti-related peptide (AgRP), which stimulate eating. The production of these peptides also causes other neurons (referred to below as neuron type A) to inhibit the production of the hormone melanocortin, which usually works to suppress the appetite. These signals are transmitted to the lateral

hypothalamic nucleus (via other neurons), which generates the sensation of hunger. To suppress the appetite, the body's fat tissues increase production of leptin and insulin. These hormones signal to neuron type B to inhibit production of NPY and AgRP. At the same time, the increased leptin and insulin trigger neuron type A to produce melanocortin. These signals reach the ventromedial nucleus in the hypothalamus, which creates the feeling of satiety.

Lateral hypothalamic nucleus creates sensation of hunger

Neurons pass on stimulus

Neuron type A inhibits production of melanocortin

Neuron type B stimulates production of neuropeptide (NPY) and agouti-related peptide (AgRP)

Increased production of **ghrelin**

Decreased production of **leptin** and **insulin**

Stomach

Fat tissues

KEY
➡ INHIBITS
➡ STIMULATES

THE SENSATION OF HUNGER
Feeling hungry is caused by a chain reaction that begins in fat tissues, which reduce the production of leptin and insulin, and in the stomach, which increases production of the hormone ghrelin.

SUGAR ADDICTION

As a "reward" for performing functions essential for the survival of both the individual and the species, such as eating or reproducing, the brain releases opiates, which create sensations of pleasure. Sugar-rich diets generate heightened reward signals, so that the more sugar you have, the more you want. This can override self-control mechanisms and lead to addiction.

Nucleus accumbens

Basal ganglia

Dopamine flow

Ventral tegmental area (VTA)

REWARD SYSTEM
The VTA in the midbrain processes information about how well various needs are being met and transfers this data to the nucleus accumbens in the basal ganglia, via the neurotransmitter dopamine. The more dopamine, the greater the pleasure, and the more likely the action will be repeated in the future.

THIRST

When the body's water levels fall, salt concentration increases and blood volume decreases. Pressure receptors in the cardiovascular system and salt-concentration-sensitive cells in the hypothalamus detect these changes. In response, the pituitary gland releases antidiuretic hormone (ADH), which acts on the kidneys to retain water and produce less urine. The kidneys secrete the enzyme renin into the blood which, through a series of reactions, forms the hormone angiotensin II. This is detected by the subfornical organ, which is connected to the hypothalamus, which in turn activates more ADH-producing cells and creates the sensation of thirst, leading to drinking.

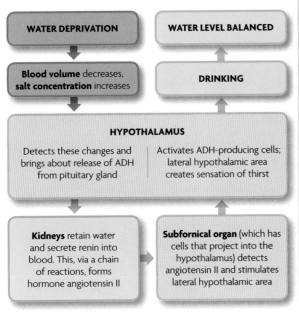

WATER DEPRIVATION
The decrease in blood volume and increase in salt concentration that are caused by dehydration have a detrimental effect on the body's biochemistry. The neuroendocrine system responds swiftly with a series of chain reactions that stimulate the sensation of thirst in an effort to restore balance in the body.

WATER DEPRIVATION

Blood volume decreases, **salt concentration** increases

HYPOTHALAMUS

Detects these changes and brings about release of ADH from pituitary gland

Activates ADH-producing cells; lateral hypothalamic area creates sensation of thirst

Kidneys retain water and secrete renin into blood. This, via a chain of reactions, forms hormone angiotensin II

Subfornical organ (which has cells that project into the hypothalamus) detects angiotensin II and stimulates lateral hypothalamic area

WATER LEVEL BALANCED

DRINKING

SLEEP–WAKE CYCLES

The suprachiasmatic nucleus (SCN) in the hypothalamus plays a key role in sleep–wake cycles. Light levels are sensed by the retina, and this information is relayed to the SCN, which then sends a signal to the pineal gland. This triggers the release of melatonin, the hormone that tells the body when to sleep. At this point, the brain becomes less alert and fatigue starts to take over. When melatonin levels fall in response to increased light, the waking part of the cycle begins.

PINEAL GLAND
The circle on this lateral MRI scan of the brain pinpoints the pineal gland, a pea-sized gland located beneath the thalamus. It is responsible for the secretion of melatonin.

MELATONIN
Falling levels of light trigger the production of melatonin, which forms a link between the external environment and the brain's sleep-wake cycles.

KEY

🟦 NIGHT
⬜ DAY
▬ MELATONIN LEVELS

% OF AVERAGE MELATONIN LEVEL

300

200

100

0

0   24   48   72   96   120   144

TIME IN HOURS

PLANNING A MOVEMENT

MOVEMENTS MAY BE PLANNED EITHER CONSCIOUSLY OR UNCONSCIOUSLY, AND BOTH TYPES MAY PRODUCE COMPLEX ACTIONS THAT LOOK VERY MUCH ALIKE. ALL PLANNED MOVEMENTS INVOLVE THE BRAIN, ALTHOUGH CONSCIOUS MOVEMENTS ARE HATCHED IN A DIFFERENT AREA FROM UNCONSCIOUS MOVEMENTS. THE MORE SKILLED WE ARE AT MAKING A PARTICULAR MOVEMENT, THE LESS LIKELY IT IS TO REQUIRE CONSCIOUS PLANNING.

CONSCIOUS AND UNCONSCIOUS MOVEMENT

Many of our actions are conscious—thinking about picking up an object, for example, and then actually picking it up. However, there are many actions that take place without our awareness, such as blinking. Some unconscious actions may be triggered directly by environmental stimuli—the sight of food may trigger an automatic reaching movement, for example. Whether a complex movement is conscious or unconscious depends largely on the individual's level of skill. As an action becomes increasingly familiar, it can become "automatic." However, these movements can also be performed consciously if the individual turns attention to them.

COMPLICATED ACTIONS
Even advanced movements, such as juggling and unicycling simultaneously, can be performed unconsciously.

SKILL AND FAMILIARITY
The chart to the left shows that a skilled driver on a familiar route will carry out all of the individual actions involved with turning the car unconsciously, while a learner will be conscious of all the actions. A skilled driver on an unfamiliar route will only be conscious of looking for the turn.

SKILLED DRIVER familiar route	SKILLED DRIVER unfamiliar route	LEARNING DRIVER
LOOKING FOR THE TURN	LOOKING FOR THE TURN	LOOKING FOR THE TURN
CHECK MIRROR	CHECK MIRROR	CHECK MIRROR
CHANGE GEAR	CHANGE GEAR	CHANGE GEAR
TURN WHEEL	TURN WHEEL	TURN WHEEL

KEY

CONSCIOUS	UNCONSCIOUS

COMPLEX PLANNING
Some actions require lengthy conscious deliberation. If a person is highly skilled at doing something—a professional golfer putting a ball, for example—the execution of the action will be relegated to unconscious areas of the brain. This "frees up" higher cognitive regions to concentrate on planning where to strike the ball and how hard to strike it.

REFLEX ACTIONS

Reflex actions are motor actions that are programmed into the spinal cord. The brain is not involved, and the actions cannot be controlled consciously. Most reflex actions protect the body by producing rapid reactions to escape from potentially damaging stimuli. In each case, the stimulus causes sensory nerve endings to fire; these signals pass through the nerve fibers to the spine, and trigger firing in the adjacent motor neurons, which then feed back to the relevant area and cause it to move.

Spinal cord

Nerve rootlets

Sensory nerve fiber
Each sensory nerve impulse is sent directly to the spinal cord

Stimulus

Motor nerve fiber

Patellar tendon

Direction of kick

Thigh muscle (rectus fermoris)

Fiber ends of sensory neurons
Relay impulses from sensory nerve endings in muscle and tendon directly to motor neuron via synapses

Cell body of motor neuron
Receives impulses from sensory fibers; starts its own impulses, which pass along fiber and back to muscle

PATELLAR SPINAL REFLEX
The "knee jerk" is a well-known example of a reflex action. It is used by doctors to test spinal-nerve function. Tapping the tendon just under the patella (kneecap) stretches the thigh muscle above, causing the lower leg to kick automatically.

BRAIN AREAS AND MOVEMENTS

Both conscious and unconscious actions involve the primary motor cortex, which sends the "go" signals that contract the muscles (via the spinal cord and motor nerves). However, while unconscious movements are planned by areas in the parietal lobe, conscious actions involve "higher" frontal brain areas, including the premotor and supplementary motor cortices. They may also involve prefrontal areas, such as the dorsolateral prefrontal cortex, where actions are consciously assessed. It may feel as though conscious actions result from a decision. In fact, unconscious areas of the brain plan and start to execute movements before we consciously decide to do them. The "decision" may, therefore, merely be the conscious recognition of what the unconscious mind is planning to do.

READINESS POTENTIAL

Unconscious activity in the SMA and PMA starts two seconds before an action. The "decision" to act occurs only a fraction of a second before the action.

ACTIVITY

0

-3   -2   -1   0   1

SECONDS

KEY —— SUPPLEMENTARY MOTOR AREA (SMA)
—— PREMOTOR AREA (PMA)

Posterior parietal cortex
Supplementary motor area (SMA)
Part of the dorsolateral prefrontal cortex
Premotor area (PMA)
Primary motor cortex
Somatosensory cortex

CORTICAL INVOLVEMENT
Unconscious and conscious actions involve slightly different areas; the former uses parietal regions, while the latter uses the supplementary motor area and prefrontal cortex.

THE BASAL GANGLIA

Action plans that are made in the parietal and frontal brain areas are fed down to the basal ganglia and then routed, via the thalamus, back up to the SMA and PMA before execution. The basal ganglia are thought to act as a filter, blocking plans that are inappropriate, for example, inhibiting automatic, environment-triggered responses such as grasping food.

RESPONSE CONTROL

As action plans are routed around the basal ganglia, the information is made more or less potent—and thus likely to be executed—by the action of various neurotransmitters.

KEY
—— BASAL GANGLIA LOOP
—— MODULATING CIRCUITS

Globus pallidus
Relays information to the thalamus

Putamen
Receives signals from frontal cortex

LOCATION OF BASAL GANGLIA

SMA

Thalamus
Passes signals back to SMA

Substantia nigra
Modulates actions, making them stronger or weaker

Subthalamic nucleus
Also responsible for modulating actions

Frontal cortex

THE CEREBELLUM

For the body to make any complex movement, the sequence and duration of each of its elements must be coordinated very precisely. This is controlled by the cerebellum, via a circuit that connects it to the motor cortex. It also modulates the signals that the motor cortex subsequently sends to the motor neurons. The cerebellum ensures that when one set of muscles initiates a movement, the opposing set acts as a brake, so that the body part in question arrives accurately at its target.

PRECISE TIMING

The cerebellar circuits include a system that measures time. It feeds its calculations to the primary motor cortex, which sends the signals to the muscles.

KEY
—— SIGNALS FROM CEREBELLUM
—— SIGNALS TO CEREBELLUM

Primary motor cortex

Red nucleus
Receives feedback from cerebellum

Pontine nucleus
Receives signals about impending movement and sends them to cerebellum

Dentate nucleus
Sends signals back to motor cortex

Cerebellar cortex
Motor programs are stored here

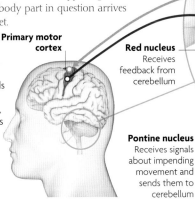

EXECUTING A MOVEMENT

ONCE A MOVEMENT HAS BEEN PLANNED, THE BRAIN AREAS RESPONSIBLE SEND SIGNALS TO THE MUSCLES TO EXECUTE THE ACTION. SOME OF THESE SIGNALS ARE SENT FIRST TO THE MOTOR CORTEX, AND THEN ONWARD THROUGH THE SPINAL CORD. OTHERS TRAVEL BY MORE DIRECT ROUTES. MOVEMENT OCCURS WHEN THE SIGNALS REACH THE MUSCLE FIBERS, CAUSING THEM TO CONTRACT.

SPINAL TRACTS

Action plans generated in the supplementary, premotor, and parietal cortices are forwarded to the motor cortex for execution. The motor cortex is made up of about one million neurons, which send long axons down the spinal cord. These are bundled together, along with axons that come directly from the somatosensory cortex, to form the lateral corticospinal tract. Just before entering the spinal cord, the nerves from each hemisphere of the brain separate and cross over, so the fibers from the left hemisphere of the cortex go down the right side of the spinal cord, and vice versa. The rubrospinal tract originates from the red nucleus in the midbrain, and helps to produce fine movements. The vestibulospinal and reticulospinal tracts start lower down in the brainstem and help control balance and orientation.

Primary motor cortex
The starting point for the lateral corticospinal tract

Thalamus

Inferior colliculus

Red nucleus

Reticular formation

Vestibular nucleus

Pyramidal decussation
Lateral corticospinal tract branches cross over here

Spinal cord
Most nerve fibers from the brain synapse onto motor neurons in the spinal cord

KEY

- ┄┄┄ VESTIBULOSPINAL TRACT
- ─── RUBROSPINAL TRACT
- ─── LATERAL CORTICOSPINAL TRACT
- ─── RETICULOSPINAL TRACT

LIMB CONTROL
The lateral corticospinal tract is the only spinal tract to originate in the cerebral cortex and is mostly responsible for controlling limb movements.

BALANCING ACT
The reticulospinal and vestibulospinal tracts help control balance and orientation, and neutralize the effects of gravity.

SPINE TO MUSCLE

The axons of the motor neurons, which receive signals from the spinal tracts, emerge from between the vertebrae and travel to the muscles. The nerve endings infiltrate the muscle fibers at neuromuscular junctions, and when they fire they release the neurotransmitter acetylcholine. This diffuses across the narrow "synaptic cleft" connecting the muscle to the nerve and binds to acetylcholine receptors in the muscle cell membrane, which, by a series of reactions, makes the specific muscle contract. Muscles required to carry out fine movements have correspondingly higher numbers of neurons than those required to perform gross movements.

muscle fiber

motor neuron

NEUROMUSCULAR JUNCTION
When stimulated by a motor nerve, electrical changes in the muscle cause the release of calcium ions inside the muscle. This causes the filaments of the muscle to slide against each other and contract.

PRECISE SEQUENCE
After receiving the order to move from the primary motor cortex, a rapid, precisely timed sequence of motor-neuron firings causes specific muscles to contract.

MOTOR DISORDERS

Motor disorders can be divided into two principal groups: hyperkinesia (overactivity) and hypokinesia (too little movement). The former includes a wide range of motor disorders, from involuntary, slow shaking of various body parts to tics, which are uncontrollable, rapid, disjointed movements and/or sounds. Sudden, shocklike muscle contractions are symptoms of myoclonus, while quick, random, usually jerky limb movements are caused by chorea and ballism. Hyperkinesia disorders include: general slowness of movement (bradykinesia); "freezing" or inability to begin a movement or involuntary arrest of a movement; rigidity—an increase in muscle tension when a limb encounters force; and postural instability, which is the loss of ability to maintain an upright posture.

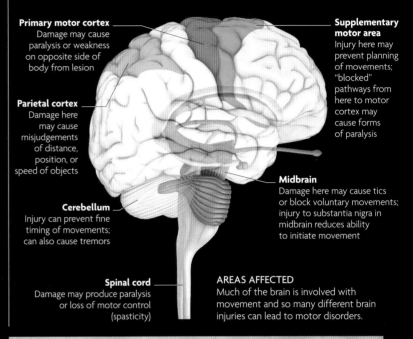

Primary motor cortex
Damage may cause paralysis or weakness on opposite side of body from lesion

Supplementary motor area
Injury here may prevent planning of movements; "blocked" pathways from here to motor cortex may cause forms of paralysis

Parietal cortex
Damage here may cause misjudgements of distance, position, or speed of objects

Midbrain
Damage here may cause tics or block voluntary movements; injury to substantia nigra in midbrain reduces ability to initiate movement

Cerebellum
Injury can prevent fine timing of movements; can also cause tremors

Spinal cord
Damage may produce paralysis or loss of motor control (spasticity)

AREAS AFFECTED
Much of the brain is involved with movement and so many different brain injuries can lead to motor disorders.

MOTOR RECOVERY

Movement disorders may result from damage to many different areas of the brain, and it is very common for one of these to follow a stroke. Damage to the motor cortex, for example, may cause whole or partial paralysis of the opposite side of the body, and strokes in subcortical areas may lead to loss of control of voluntary movements. The affected neural pathways can, however, rebuild to a certain extent, reducing the long-term effect of the damage. Studies show that damaged midbrain-cortical motor pathways form new connections in as little as three months after remedial therapy.

STROKE REHABILITATION
The neural pathways damaged by a stroke do rebuild themselves to a limited degree. Physical therapy encourages the rewiring of motor circuits, and recovery is often directly related to the intensity of the therapy.

STROKE
This CT scan shows the extent of internal bleeding in the brain caused by a stroke.

UNCONSCIOUS ACTION

THE BRAIN REGISTERS EVENTS VIA THE SENSE ORGANS ALMOST IMMEDIATELY, BUT IT TAKES UP TO HALF A SECOND TO BECOME CONSCIOUS OF THEM. IN ORDER TO GENERATE EFFECTIVE RESPONSES IN A FAST-CHANGING ENVIRONMENT, THE BRAIN MUST PLAN AND EXECUTE MOMENT-BY-MOMENT ACTIONS UNCONSCIOUSLY.

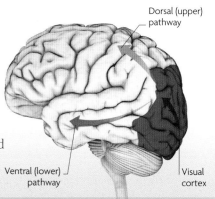

Dorsal (upper) pathway

Ventral (lower) pathway

Visual cortex

REACTION PATHWAYS

It takes up to 400 milliseconds (ms) for the brain to process incoming information to the stage where it may become conscious. It takes a similar length of time to prepare the body for action. So if we waited to be conscious of a sight or sound before starting to respond to it, our behavior would lag almost a second behind the events to which we are responding. By the time we leapt out of the path of a speeding car, it is likely to have run us over. The brain speeds up our physical responses by fast-tracking sensory information to the motor-

DORSAL AND VENTRAL ROUTES

Visual stimuli are processed along parallel pathways. The unconscious dorsal route generates physical responses while the ventral route creates conscious perception.

RETURNING A SERVE

Professional tennis players can plan and initiate the complex moves required to return a fast service before they are consciously aware that the ball is on its way. Unlike novice players, they do not have to think consciously about each muscle movement because practice has turned the relevant action sequences into automated motor programs that are stored and run unconsciously. Familiarity with their opponents' body language also allows them to make well-informed unconscious predictions about where the ball will land.

EVENTS IN RECEIVER'S BRAIN

🕐 0ms Attention

The player's brain prepares for action by focusing attention on his opponent. This prevents the brain from responding to irrelevant stimuli and amplifies information coming from the part of the visual field containing the target of attention. If the player is familiar with the opponent's playing style, his brain will register the movements made by the opponent as he serves and compare them with previous observations to help predict where the ball will land. Attention to such cues may speed up reactions by 20–30 milliseconds.

LOCKING ON

The thalamus directs attention to the target, while the frontal lobes inhibit distracting thoughts.

Frontal lobes

Thalamus

🕐 70ms Body memory

The ball is not yet consciously visible to the player, but unconsciously his brain is already planning the actions he must make to return it. At this stage he is mainly using information about his opponent's movements to decide how his own body should move. A skilled player processes fewer visual cues than an inexperienced one because the brain identifies irrelevant signals at a very early stage and ignores them. The visual information from his opponent's movements activates the player's parietal cortex, which in turn calls up relevant procedural memories. These are learned actions –such as how to return a serve–that have become encoded as automatic motor programs. They are stored in an unconscious brain module called the putamen, which replays them as the situation demands.

MOVEMENT MEMORY

Part of the basal ganglia, the putamen acts as a store of memories about deeply ingrained habits of movement. Signals from the putamen are passed to the parietal cortex.

Signals are sent from putamen to parietal cortex along a complex loop of nerves

Parietal cortex

Putamen

SERVER

planning areas along an unconscious pathway. A visual stimulus such as a moving object prompts neural activity that works out where it is in relation to the body. Various parts of the occipital and parietal cortex, between them, calculate the object's shape, size, relative motion, and trajectory. This information is then brought together and used to form an action plan, which might involve hitting (swatting a fly, for example), avoidance (ducking or jumping out of the way of a missile), or grabbing (a falling fruit or a stumbling child). The chosen response is largely learned; for example, a skilled athlete is likely to catch or hit a speeding ball while an unpracticed player might just duck it.

TENNIS PLAYERS UNDER OBSERVATION

Tennis players watching a video of another player serving a ball imagine themselves making the action. These fMRI images show that watching a moving ball (left) activates areas of the brain that track visual objects, but watching someone serve a ball (right) activates visual areas plus large parts of the parietal cortex. The additional activation shows the viewer's brain is "acting out" the moves seen in the video. This information helps the viewer predict where the ball will go.

WATCHING A MOVING BALL — FRONT / BACK / RIGHT / LEFT

WATCHING A SERVE — FRONT / BACK / RIGHT / LEFT

🕐 250ms Action plan
The receiving player's brain brings together the information that has been registered so far to construct a response to the fast-approaching ball. The plan is informed by information gathered from the opponent's body movements, the (still unconscious) knowledge of the ball's speed and trajectory, and the procedural memories triggered by these stimuli. The plan is held in the premotor area, which lies just in front of the motor cortex. This is like a rehearsal stage, allowing action to be played out as a pattern of neuronal activity without affecting the muscles.

Motor cortex — Visual cortex

REHEARSAL
Unconscious knowledge is brought together to create an action plan. This is formed and rehearsed in the premotor area, adjacent to the motor cortex.

🕐 355ms Sending signals
The action plan held in the premotor cortex is transmitted to the neighboring motor cortex. The neurons in this strip of brain connect via the spine to skeletal muscles, and when they fire they cause the muscles to contract. In this case, the firing of neurons about halfway down the right side of the motor strip move the player's left arm and hand to position the racket to connect with the ball. Other neurons control the rest of the body. The sequence in which these neurons fire—and therefore the sequence of limb movement—is controlled by the cerebellum.

Motor cortex

Cerebellum

Signal from motor cortex travels to player's hand

INSTRUCTION TO MOVE
Neural signals from the motor cortex are sent along the spine, causing muscles to contract and leading to overt movement.

🕐 500ms Conscious act
If the player's conscious perception of the ball's trajectory differs markedly from his earlier, unconscious prediction he may veto the earlier action plan and start to construct an alternative, or try to adjust the current plan to take into account the new information. It takes another 200–300ms, however, to incorporate the new, conscious information into a revised action plan and by then the ball has traveled too far for any player to be able to return it.

The situation is similar to the one that occurs when a person steps forward onto what the brain predicted was flat ground, but which is actually a downward step. The resultant physical catastrophe, in both cases, triggers a further cascade of signals that may generate a wide range of emotions, including anger, embarrassment, and a feeling of failure.

🕐 285ms Conscious thought starts
The player's brain becomes consciously aware-belatedly-of the ball moving away from the opponent's racket. But his brain has already (unconsciously) predicted its real-time position, and –providing the two information streams do not clash–the player is likely to think he sees the ball where it really is.

Ball comes into conscious view

RECEIVER

MIRROR NEURONS

CERTAIN NEURONS ARE ACTIVATED WHEN YOU MOVE, AND ALSO WHEN YOU SEE SOMEONE ELSE MOVING. THIS MEANS WE UNCONSCIOUSLY MIMIC THE ACTIONS OF OTHERS, AND THUS SHARE, TO SOME EXTENT, THEIR EXPERIENCE. MIRROR NEURONS ALSO ALLOW US TO KNOW WHAT ANOTHER PERSON IS FEELING, WITHOUT HAVING TO THINK ABOUT IT. THESE FINDINGS ARE AMONG THE MOST SIGNIFICANT NEUORSCIENTIFIC DISCOVERIES IN RECENT YEARS.

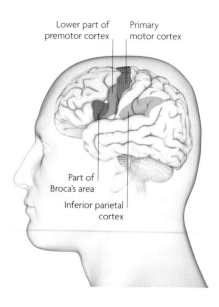

Lower part of premotor cortex

Primary motor cortex

Part of Broca's area

Inferior parietal cortex

WHAT ARE THEY?

Mirror neurons were first discovered in the motor-planning area in the brains of macaques (a species of monkey) and subsequent brain-imaging studies suggest that they exist in humans too. The human mirror system seems to be broader in scope than that of monkeys, in that mirror neurons exist not only in movement areas, but also in areas concerned with emotions, sensations, and even intentions. They provide people with immediate knowledge of what is going on in another's mind; this ability to know what another person is feeling or doing is thought to be the basis of mimicry.

HOW THEY WERE DISCOVERED

Mirror neurons were discovered in a monkey whose brain was wired up to show which nerve cells lit up as it reached out to grasp food. When laboratory staff made the same movement while the monkeys sat and watched, the same neurons lit up.

WHERE THEY ARE

In humans, mirror neurons seem to extend into the areas of the frontal lobe that are concerned with intentions, such as part of the premotor cortex. They are also found in the parietal lobe, which is involved with sensations. However, the full extent of these neurons is still being researched.

MIRRORING TOUCH

Mirror neurons also seem to operate in the somatosensory cortex–the area of the brain that registers touch. In one study, subjects' brains were scanned, first while their leg was brushed, and then while they watched a video of someone else's leg being touched. Activity in their brains revealed that some parts of the somatosensory areas are activated only by direct touch and others are activated by the sight of another being touched. A third group of neurons, however, are activated both by direct touch and by seeing others being touched. These mirror neurons–shown in white on the scans below–were limited to the left hemisphere in this study, though in other experiments they have been detected in both hemispheres.

MIRRORING SPEECH

Mirror neurons may help people communicate by "syncing" their brains when they talk together. Partners in a conversation unconsciously imitate one another, adopting a similar rate of speaking and the same sort of grammatical structures. This helps one person predict what the other is going to say next, making communication quicker and smoother. Speech is combined with body movements and facial expressions to convey full meaning, and these tiny movements amplify the perception of another's voice. Watching a speaker's face is equivalent in effect to turning up the volume by 15 decibels.

Somatosensory areas in left hemisphere activated by both touch and vision-of-touch

Activity only arises in the right hemisphere from direct touch, but mirror neurons have been detected here in similar experiments

ACTIVATED AREAS

These MRI scans are coronal sections taken from the same brain. They show the areas stimulated by touch, watching another being touched, and the overlap between the two.

KEY

▓	AREAS ACTIVATED BY TOUCH
■	AREAS ACTIVATED BY VISION-OF-TOUCH
☐	AREAS ACTIVATED BY BOTH

BODY LANGUAGE

As well as mirroring speech patterns and speed, people unconsciously adapt their body language to match whoever they are speaking to. Partners in a conversation focus on each other's faces, picking up minute movements that help express meaning.

KNOWING HOW IT FEELS
To mirror another's actions, the brain must "know" how it feels to do it. For example, to mirror expert dance moves, you would have to have some idea of how to go about doing them, even if you could not reproduce them perfectly.

MIRRORING MOVEMENT

Recent studies have found that a certain, as yet unknown, proportion of mirror neurons are active both when moving and when watching movement. Neurons in the premotor cortex concerned with planning to move the legs are activated when you watch a person running, for example. In other words, when you see someone doing something, in your brain you do it too. However, in order to mirror another's action, the sight of the action must "resonate" with a motor program that the brain has already learned.

WATCHING CHEWING
Simply watching another person chewing shows activity in both the premotor cortex and the part of the primary motor cortex concerned with mouth and jaw movements.

ACTING ON AN OBJECT
When the movement involves acting on an object—biting an apple, for example, rather than just simply chewing—areas of the parietal cortex also light up.

MIRRORING EMOTIONS

When one person sees another expressing an emotion, the areas of the brain that are associated with feeling that emotion are activated, making emotions transmittable. In one study, volunteers inhaled a disgusting smell, and later, watched a video of someone else smelling something and expressing disgust. Both produced neuronal activity in the area of the brain associated with feeling disgust. Emotion mirroring is thought to be the basis of empathy.

Autistic people, who tend to lack empathy, have been found to show less mirror-neuron activity.

HORROR MOVIE
Seeing someone else looking frightened makes you feel scared yourself. Mirror neurons, therefore, help whip up emotion in audiences.

MIRRORING INTENTIONS

Two movements may be identical, but may signal very different things in different contexts. Human mirror neurons seem to take this into account. When one person sees another picking up a cup in order to drink from it, a different set of neurons are activated from those that light up at the sight of a person making the identical movement but in a context that suggests they are clearing the cup away. Hence, the observer's brain does not just generate a faint idea of what the other person is doing with their body, but also an echo of their intention in doing it. This allows us to get a glimpse of another individual's plans and thought processes without consciously having to work it out.

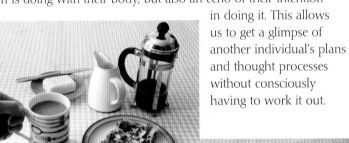

DRINKING AND CLEANING UP
The top image shows a table set for breakfast, while the image at the bottom shows the table after the meal has been finished. The action of grasping the cup can be exactly the same in both, but our brains take into account the difference in contexts and therefore we automatically "know" that each one signals a different intention.

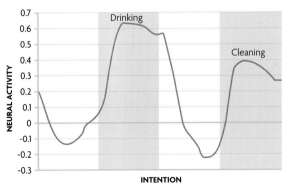

LEVEL OF ACTIVITY
The increased activity associated with watching the intention to drink is thought to be because it is more commonly practiced than the intention to clear up.

EMOTIONS CAN BE THOUGHT OF AS BODY CHANGES
THAT PROMPT US TO ACT. THEY HAVE EVOLVED TO GET
US TO DO WHAT WE HAVE TO IN ORDER TO SURVIVE
AND PASS OUR GENES ON TO THE NEXT GENERATION.
TO REINFORCE THEIR EFFECTIVENESS, EMOTIONALLY
TRIGGERED ACTIONS ARE ASSOCIATED WITH PLEASANT
OR UNPLEASANT CONSCIOUS FEELINGS. EMOTIONS TEND

EMOTIONS AND FEELINGS

THE EMOTIONAL BRAIN

EMOTIONS MAY SEEM TO BE CONSCIOUS FEELINGS, BUT THEY ARE, IN FACT, "INNER MOTIONS"—PHYSIOLOGICAL RESPONSES TO STIMULI, DESIGNED TO PUSH US AWAY FROM DANGER AND TOWARD REWARD. EMOTIONS ARE GENERATED CONSTANTLY, BUT MUCH OF THE TIME WE ARE UNAWARE OF THEM.

ANATOMY OF EMOTION

Emotions are generated in the limbic system: a cluster of structures that lies beneath the cortex. The system evolved very early in mammalian history. In humans, it is closely connected with the more recently evolved cortical areas. The two-way traffic between the limbic system and the cortex allows emotions to be consciously felt and conscious thoughts to affect emotions. Each emotion is produced by a different network of brain modules, including the hypothalamus and pituitary gland; these control the hormones that produce physical reactions such as increased heart rate and muscle contraction.

Cingulate cortex
This part of the cortex is closest to the limbic system. Performing difficult tasks, or experiencing intense love, anger, or lust, causes activity in the anterior cingulate cortex (ACC) to increase; this area has been found to be active when mothers hear infants cry. The ACC contains unusual neurons called spindle cells (right), which may be particularly concerned with detecting how others feel and reacting to their emotions.

Stria terminalis
This is part of the network of pathways that link the amygdala to other parts of the brain. The stria terminalis plays a part in anxiety and stress responses. Cell density differs in men and women, and may play a part in gender identification—for example, transsexuals have been found to have a cell structure that matches the typical pattern of the sex to which they are changing.

Frontal cortex
Information from the limbic system is fed to the frontal cortex to produce conscious feelings, while conscious knowledge about the environment is fed from the cortex back to the limbic system in a continuous loop. The effect of emotion on thought is stronger than vice versa, probably because there are more nerve tracts carrying signals up from the limbic system than passing signals back down.

Olfactory complex
The olfactory bulbs carry messages about smell straight to the limbic areas—unlike the pathways serving the other senses, which pass signals via the thalamus to the cortex for processing. This is why scents create such an intense, instant emotional response. The olfactory complex is thought to be the brain's original "emotional" center, and probably evolved before sight and hearing.

Nasal bones

Corpus callosum
The corpus callosum (CC) plays an important role in transmitting emotions between the left and right hemispheres. Women, on average, have a greater density of fibers in the CC than men; this may account for some differences between the sexes in emotional response.

Thalamus
The thalamus acts as a distribution center for incoming information and is therefore involved in more or less every activity. However, some of the thalamic nuclei (dark green) have a particularly strong influence on emotions because they shunt emotionally salient stimuli to the appropriate limbic areas, such as the amygdala and the olfactory cortex, for further processing.

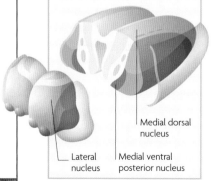

Lateral nucleus | Medial ventral posterior nucleus | Medial dorsal nucleus

Hippocampus
The hippocampus is mainly concerned with encoding and retrieving memories. Personal or "episodic" memories include an emotional component, so the hippocampus, by calling these up, creates a replay of emotions from the past. These may blend with current emotions, or they may override them—as when a sudden memory of something sad "blights" a happy moment.

Amygdala
The amygdala is a tiny part of the brain that is most centrally and exclusively concerned with emotion. This area assesses both external and internal information for threat level and emotional significance (see opposite page).

Hypothalamus and mammillary body
The hypothalamus is a tiny part of the brain but it has complex and widespread effects. It acts as a hormonal signaler and transmitter, affecting bodily reactions to the environment and causing the sensations we feel as emotion. It also mediates the fear reaction made by the amygdala. The mammillary bodies, which connect to the hippocampus via the fornix, lie at the interface between memory and emotion.

Hypothalamus | Mammillary body

AMYGDALA

The amygdala "tastes" all stimuli and signals other areas to produce appropriate emotional reactions. It contains distinct regions called nuclei, which generate different kinds of responses to fear. The central nucleus generates the fear response of freezing, while the basal nucleus generates the fear response of flight. The nuclei are affected by sex hormones, and are therefore different in men and women. Activation of the amygdala can be modulated by the hypothalamus (see right).

CORE OF EMOTION
Emotions engage widespread areas of the brain but the "core" network is centered on the red parts shown here —the amygdala and the dorsomedial and orbitofrontal cortices.

core limbic areas

MEDIATING AMYGDALA RESPONSE
The amygdala is activated by frightening stimuli (left). However, the hormone oxytocin, secreted by the hippocampus, damps down amygdala activity (right) and with it the feeling of fright.

FEAR RESPONSE

WITH OXYTOCIN

POSITIVE EMOTION

Limbic system structures next to the amygdala are involved in feelings of pleasure, mainly by reducing activity in the amygdala and in cortical areas concerned with anxiety. Anticipation and pleasure-seeking are influenced by the "reward" circuit. This acts on the hypothalamus and amygdala: it secretes dopamine, which provides anticipation and drive, and GABA, which inhibits neurons from firing.

PLEASURE AND THE BRAIN
Pleasurable stimuli, such as watching your soccer team score a goal, activate brain areas close to the limbic system.

FEELING FEAR

The amygdala acts as a store for good and bad memories, especially emotional traumas. It is also "hard-wired" to fear certain stimuli, such as low-flying birds, spiders, and snakes. For a phobia to develop, however, there also needs to be an environmental trigger, such as a nasty encounter with a "hard-wired" stimulus, or the sight of someone else being frightened by it. It is often very hard to get rid of a phobia because the amygdala is not under conscious control. It can, however, "learn" to reduce its reaction to the stimulus.

PANIC RESPONSES
The autonomic nervous system, responsible for automatic body functions, produces the physical responses felt in a phobic reaction.

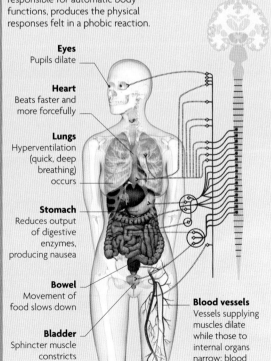

Eyes
Pupils dilate

Heart
Beats faster and more forcefully

Lungs
Hyperventilation (quick, deep breathing) occurs

Stomach
Reduces output of digestive enzymes, producing nausea

Bowel
Movement of food slows down

Bladder
Sphincter muscle constricts

Blood vessels
Vessels supplying muscles dilate while those to internal organs narrow; blood pressure rises

UNCONSCIOUS EMOTION

We have evolved a conscious emotional system, but we retain the primitive, automatic responses at the heart of emotion. A frightening sight or sound, for example, registers in the amygdala before we are even conscious of it. While the sensory information is sent to the cortex to be made conscious, the amygdala sends messages to the hypothalamus, which triggers changes that ready the body for flight, fight, or appeasement. This "quick and dirty" route allows us to take instant action to save ourselves. When we "start" at a loud noise, then relax on realizing that it is harmless, we are experiencing both stages–unconscious reaction and conscious response.

FACES OF FEAR
This series of images shows the onset of fear. The amygdala registers the emotional facial expressions of others, and produces a reaction before we even know we have seen them.

CONSCIOUS AND UNCONSCIOUS ROUTES
The amygdala picks up on emotional stimuli before we are also aware of them. This allows the body to react very quickly to threat or reward. Emotional stimuli are processed along a second route that does not involve the amygdala. This takes the information through cortical areas that produce conscious awareness and a more thoughtful response.

Sensory cortex
Sensory information is transmitted along this route to the sensory cortex for recognition. More information is extracted along this path, but it takes longer.

Hippocampus
Information that is consciously perceived is encoded in the hippocampus to form memories. The hippocampus also feeds back stored information confirming or modifying the initial response.

Thalamus
Sensory information is directed to the amygdala for quick assessment and action, and also to cortical areas for processing to conscious awareness.

Amygdala
The amygdala instantly assesses incoming information for emotional content, and sends signals to other areas for immediate body action. It operates unconsciously, and is thus liable to produce errors.

Hypothalamus
Signals from the amygdala are used to trigger hormonal changes that make the body ready to take action in response to emotional stimuli; these responses include muscle contraction and an increase in heart rate.

KEY

SLOW AND ACCURATE ROUTE

QUICK AND DIRTY ROUTE

CONSCIOUS EMOTION

EMOTIONS ARE GENERATED IN THE LIMBIC SYSTEM, WHICH DOES NOT SUPPORT CONSCIOUSNESS ITSELF. INTENSE EMOTIONS CREATE "KNOCK-ON" ACTIVITY IN THE CORTEX, ESPECIALLY IN THE FRONTAL LOBES, WHICH WE EXPERIENCE AS A CONSCIOUS "FEELING" OR MOOD. SOMETIMES, AN EMOTION IS CLEARLY LINKED TO AN EXPERIENCE. AT OTHER TIMES, THE CAUSE IS NOT OBVIOUS, BUT BEING AWARE OF THE EMOTION MAKES IT EASIER TO UNDERSTAND WHAT IS HAPPENING TO US.

FEELING EMOTION

Emotions are primarily unconscious physical reactions to threat or opportunity. The sight of a snake, for example, automatically prepares the body for flight. In humans, emotions are consciously experienced as powerful "feelings" that give our lives meaning and value. The unconscious physiological component of emotion is generated in deep brain areas as signals that are then sent to the body to prepare it for action. Some signals travel upward to activate cortical areas, and this activation produces the feeling of emotion. The type of emotion experienced depends on which parts of the cortical areas are activated.

EMOTIONS INITIATED
Emotions arise in the amygdala, brainstem, and hypothalamus (blue). Conscious feelings (red) involve the orbitofrontal and cingulate cortex.

CONSCIOUS EXPRESSION
The amygdala and hypothalamus (blue) are active in expressing emotion, while the thalamus (green) maintains consciousness.

RIGHT HEMISPHERE

The right hemisphere generates more negative emotions than the left, and recognition and consciousness of sadness and fear depend on signals from the right hemisphere being received and processed by the left hemisphere. If the signals do not get through, a person may remain unconscious of their emotions, even though their behavior may be affected by them.

INCREASED ACTIVITY
This PET scan shows brain activity in a volunteer who is watching a person display various emotional facial expressions and gestures. These stimulate far more activity in the right frontal cortex (targeted) than in the same area in the left hemisphere.

EMOTIONS BECOME CONSCIOUS
Large areas of the frontal and parietal lobes (green) are involved in making emotions conscious and mediating their intensity.

DISGUST
This cutaway shows the insula (red—also in top scan), part of which is active during the generation of emotion, particularly disgust.

EMOTION CIRCUITS

Information from the environment, and from the rest of the body, is constantly "tasted" for emotional content. The main emotion "sensor" is the amygdala, which is particularly sensitive to threat and loss. The amygdala takes in information both directly from the sense organs and via the sensory cortices, and connects to the cortex and also to the hypothalamus, creating a circuit. When the amygdala is activated, it sends signals around this circuit. These trigger body changes as they pass through the hypothalamus, and create conscious recognition of the emotion as they pass through the frontal lobe. Positive emotions are passed along a slightly separate circuit, which takes in an area of the brainstem that produces the mood-lifting neurotransmitter dopamine.

PROCESSING EMOTION
Information about the identification and orientation of emotion travels from the thalamus, ventral striatum, and amygdala to the rostral (lower) anterior cingulate cortex. Regulatory signals travel from areas of the frontal and prefrontal cortices to meet them.

Dorsal lateral prefrontal cortex
Dorsal anterior cingulate cortex
Ventral striatum
Thalamus
Ventral lateral prefrontal cortex
Rostral anterior cingulate cortex
Amygdala
Hippocampus
Medial prefrontal cortex

FEELING HATRED

Each emotion sparks a slightly different pattern of activity in certain brain areas. Hatred, for example, activates the amygdala (which responds to all negative emotion), the insula (which is associated with disgust and rejection), and also areas of the brain concerned with action and calculation.

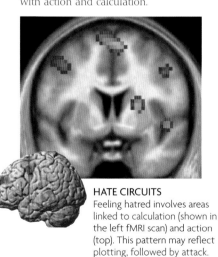

HATE CIRCUITS
Feeling hatred involves areas linked to calculation (shown in the left fMRI scan) and action (top). This pattern may reflect plotting, followed by attack.

TIMING EMOTION

Things that we find emotionally moving grab our attention rapidly (see illustrations, right) compared with things that we do not. The sight of something that poses a threat, for example, is brought to conscious awareness faster than a nonemotional stimulus. This may be because the amygdala unconsciously picks up the threat and primes the conscious brain to "expect" an important perception. Good things also attract attention fast. Research shows that people react as quickly to an image of a smiling baby as they do to one of an angry face—both elicit quicker reactions than nonemotional stimuli.

⏱ Less than 100ms
Initial awareness

Responses to emotional visual stimuli can travel in less than one-tenth of a second from the superior colliculus in the brainstem to the frontal cortex, where the emotion is consciously experienced.

Superior colliculus

Orbitofrontal cortex

Amygdala

WEARING YOUR EMOTIONS

Scientists have developed clothing that can project the emotion of the wearer. Biometric sensors that pick up minute changes or detect EEG signals are being incorporated into garments next to the skin. The clothes then change color according to the information received. This futuristic dress developed by Philips shines bright white when the wearer is happy but turns blue when she is sad. It has a corset layer containing sensors that send information to an outer skirt layer causing it to change color.

HAPPY

SAD

⏱ 100–200ms
Further information

A little later, information comes in from the sensory cortices and association areas—such as the face-recognition area in the fusiform gyrus—providing more detailed input to emotion-inducing parts of the brain, such as the amygdala.

Superior temporal colliculus

Orbitofrontal cortex

Amygdala

Fusiform gyrus

Primary visual cortex

⏱ 350ms
Full awareness

After about 350 milliseconds, the emotional meaning of a stimulus has been evaluated by the brain. Signals from the amygdala trigger a conscious response in the body, which in turn feeds back to areas such as the insula.

Insula

Superior temporal colliculus

Orbitofrontal cortex

Amygdala

Response signal from body

Fusiform gyrus

Primary visual cortex

EMOTIONS AND FEELINGS

An emotion is usually transient and arises in response to the thoughts, activities, and social situations of the day. Emotions act as cues that prompt adaptive behavior (see table, right). Moods, in contrast, may last for hours, days, or even months, in the case of some illnesses. Thus, the emotional state of distress, when extended over time, is called sadness; if it persists, unrelenting, for a period of weeks, it is referred to as depression (see p.239). Moods can be initiated very quickly by things that we are not even aware of. One study, for instance, found that flashing pictures of a disgusting nature for a split second–too fast to be seen consciously–made those who were subjected to them more sensitive to other stimuli of a similar nature afterwards. The feelings elicited by these unconscious stimuli were described by the volunteers as "moods" rather than emotions.

TELLING THE DIFFERENCE
Emotions are sudden, intense reactions to events, such as unexpected bad news, whereas moods are more diffuse and tend to last longer.

ADAPTIVE BEHAVIORS

EMOTION OR FEELING	POSSIBLE STIMULUS	ADAPTIVE BEHAVIOR
Anger	Challenging behavior from another person	"Fight" reaction prompts dominant and threatening stance or action
Fear	Threat from stronger or dominant person	Flight, to avoid the threat, or appeasement, to show a lack of challenge to the dominant person
Sadness	Loss of loved one	Backward-looking state of mind and passivity, to avoid additional challenge
Disgust	Unwholesome object (e.g. rotting food or unclean surroundings)	Aversion behavior—remove oneself from the unhealthy environment
Surprise	Novel or unexpected event	Focus attention on the object of surprise, ensuring maximum information input to guide further actions

DESIRE AND REWARD

DESIRE IS HARD TO DEFINE PRECISELY, BUT IT CAN BEST BE DESCRIBED AS WANTING OR YEARNING FOR
SOMETHING THAT YOU FEEL WILL BRING PLEASURE OR SATISFACTION ONCE YOU OBTAIN IT. THERE ARE
SPECIFIC BRAIN CIRCUITS LINKED TO DESIRE AND REWARD (PLEASURE). DESIRE FOR FOOD AND SEX HAS
A SURVIVAL VALUE, BUT DESIRE CAN ALSO BE DESTRUCTIVE IF IT FUELS AN ADDICTION.

DESIRE

Desire is a complex drive that strongly reflects personal preferences.
It is made up of two different components–liking and wanting. Put
simply, liking is linked to getting pleasure, while wanting is linked to
an actual need for something. With some activities, such as eating,
sleeping, and sexual activity, liking and wanting overlap, and the
resulting desire has survival value. However, an individual with an
addiction may want and "need" a drug, but not particularly like or
enjoy it, so the resulting pleasure is tainted with destruction. Liking
and wanting seem to use somewhat different brain circuits, although
dopamine is the most important neurotransmitter in both cases.

1. Stimulus This can originate outside the body, for example the sight of food, or from within, for example falling glucose levels.

STIMULUS AND REWARD
An external or internal stimulus is registered by the limbic system, which creates a feeling of desire; the cortex acts on this, and the resultant activity sends messages back to the limbic system, which creates a reward and sense of satisfaction.

2. Urge The incoming stimulus is registerred by the limbic system, which creates an urge.

3. Desire The urge is registered as a conscious desire in the cortex, which then instructs the body to act.

LIMBIC SYSTEM

CORTEX

5. Reward The activity triggers signals back to the limbic system, which releases opioid-like neurotransmitters.

6. Satisfaction The neurotransmitters raise circulating dopamine levels and create a feeling of satisfaction.

4. Action On instructions from the cortex, the body acts to achieve its desire.

ANTICIPATION

Learning and memory clearly play an important role in shaping
desires and preferences. This leads to the possibility of anticipation,
which is the expectation of a reward. Anticipation has been studied
by researchers using a game of chance. In the anticipation phase,
where participants were told they might win money, fMRI scans
showed that cerebral blood flow in the amygdala and orbitofrontal
cortex increased, indicating activity
in the nucleus accumbens and the
hypothalamus–all rich in dopamine
receptors. The bigger the potential
reward, the greater the brain activity.

LEFT INTRAPARIETAL CORTEX

REWARD ANTICIPATION
This fMRI scan shows activity in the left intraparietal cortex. Activity in the anterior cingulate cortex and intraparietal cortex show that greater attention is paid to a task when a person is anticipating a reward.

PLEASURE-SEEKING AND ADDICTION

Addictive substances can activate the dopamine reward system,
providing pleasure, even though the substances are not essential to
survival. Chronic exposure to drugs leads to the suppression of reward
circuits, increasing the amounts needed to get the same effect. The
opiate system is involved in pain and anxiety relief. Heroin and
morphine lock onto the opiate
receptors, creating a sense of
euphoria. The cholinergic
circuits–where nicotine acts–are
involved in memory and learning.
Cocaine acts at the noradrenergic
receptors, which are involved in
stress responses and anxiety.

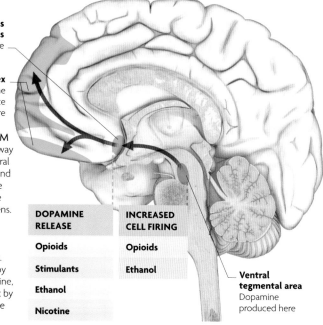

CULTURAL EXPOSURE
Smoking is regarded as a highly social
activity in many cultures. Prolonged
exposure to addictive substances may lead
to increasing dependence, drug-seeking
behavior, and withdrawal problems.

Nucleus accumbens
Releases dopamine

Prefrontal cortex
Involved in the
conscious experience
of pleasure

REWARD SYSTEM
The reward pathway
starts in the ventral
tegmental area, and
dopamine release
is triggered in the
nucleus accumbens.
From there the
reward pathway
extends to the
prefrontal cortex.
Some drugs act by
triggering dopamine,
while others work by
also increasing the
rate of cell firing.

DOPAMINE RELEASE	INCREASED CELL FIRING
Opioids	Opioids
Stimulants	Ethanol
Ethanol	
Nicotine	

Ventral tegmental area
Dopamine produced here

HUMANS ARE EXCEPTIONALLY SOCIAL CREATURES. WE NEED
EACH OTHER FOR MUTUAL SUPPORT AND PROTECTION,
AND TO THIS END WE HAVE EVOLVED BRAINS THAT ARE
EXQUISITELY SENSITIVE TO OTHERS OF OUR KIND. THE
SOCIAL BRAIN IS A SET OF FUNCTIONS THAT BETWEEN
THEM ENSURE THAT WE CAN OPERATE IN A TIGHTLY KNIT
COMMUNITY. IT INCLUDES THE ABILITY TO COMMUNICATE
WITH AND TO UNDERSTAND OTHER PEOPLE, AND TO KEEP
TRACK OF OUR SOCIAL POSITION IN RELATION TO THEM.
IN ORDER TO ACHIEVE THIS, WE ALSO NEED TO BE ABLE
TO GENERATE A SENSE OF BEING A DISTINCT SELF

THE SOCIAL BRAIN

SEX, LOVE, AND SURVIVAL

SEX HAS A SURVIVAL VALUE IN THAT IT DRIVES REPRODUCTION. SEXUAL ACTIVITY STIMULATES THE BRAIN'S REWARD SYSTEM—IF IT DID NOT, PEOPLE MIGHT NOT BOTHER WITH IT AND HUMANITY WOULD DIE OUT. RECENT RESEARCH HAS SHED LIGHT ON THE BRAIN CIRCUITS INVOLVED IN SEX AND LOVE. ROMANTIC LOVE, WHICH BRINGS COUPLES TOGETHER, AND MATERNAL LOVE, WHICH BINDS MOTHER AND CHILD, ALSO HAVE SURVIVAL VALUE.

DIFFERENT TYPES OF LOVE

Love is a complex phenomenon, encompassing sex, friendship, intimacy, and commitment. Not only does it have a survival value for the individual as well as the species, it also adds greatly to quality of life. As far as sex is concerned, humans engage in it whenever they wish, unlike most other species who undertake sex only when the female is ready to conceive. Therefore, sex has become disconnected from reproduction in humans. Romantic love, which is what many people mean by "love," has a survival advantage because it promotes pair bonding–an ideal setting for the care and protection of young children. Friendship and social networks are also important for promoting health and well-being. We know a little about the neurotransmitters involved in "falling in love," but not much about corresponding brain circuits. Phenylethylamine and dopamine are involved in the initial euphoria, which probably act in the pathways between the limbic system (concerned largely with emotions) and cortical areas (concerned with reason).

LIKING
INTIMACY

ROMANTIC LOVE
PASSION AND INTIMACY

COMPANIONATE
INTIMACY AND COMMITMENT

CONSUMMATE LOVE
INTIMACY + PASSION + COMMITMENT

INFATUATION
PASSION

FATUOUS LOVE
PASSION AND COMMITMENT

EMPTY LOVE
COMMITMENT

LOVE-TRIANGLE THEORY
Love has three components—passion, intimacy, and commitment—which can be blended in various ways to produce the spectrum of human love experiences. Passion was a strong factor between archetypal lovers Romeo and Juliet (right).

FEMALE — MALE

MACAQUE — EUROPEAN — HADZA

HIGH SYMMETRY   LOW SYMMETRY   HIGH SYMMETRY   LOW SYMMETRY

GENDER AND SYMMETRY
These composite faces, from photos of individuals from three groups, represent high- and low-symmetry faces for each group. High-symmetry faces are often selected as most gender-typical.

SEXUAL ATTRACTION

An individual's face is an important element in how attractive they appear to others and whether they are instinctively considered a good mating prospect. The degree of symmetry, which is linked to how masculine or feminine they appear, has been shown to be an important aspect of facial attractiveness. A recent study shows that these properties are involved in sexual pairings in groups of Europeans, African hunter-gatherers, and one group of nonhuman primates (see below and left). Because the relationship is common to two human groups and one primate group, it may be universal. It seems, therefore, that symmetry and how masculine or feminine a face appears are linked to an underlying biological mechanism that could advertise a person's level of attractiveness and genetic fitness as a mate.

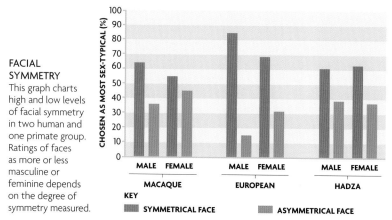

FACIAL SYMMETRY
This graph charts high and low levels of facial symmetry in two human and one primate group. Ratings of faces as more or less masculine or feminine depends on the degree of symmetry measured.

CHOSEN AS MOST SEX-TYPICAL (%)

MALE   FEMALE   MALE   FEMALE   MALE   FEMALE
MACAQUE   EUROPEAN   HADZA

KEY

SYMMETRICAL FACE   ASYMMETRICAL FACE

TWO-WAY BOND
The desire to keep baby happy appears to be wired into a mother's brain (see below). Babies signal when they want to be cuddled by making a grasping action. The cuddle makes the baby happier, bringing a sense of reward to the parents —thereby reinforcing cuddling behavior.

OXYTOCIN—THE FEEL-GOOD FACTOR

Oxytocin is a hormone produced by the hypothalamus and released by stimulation of the sex and reproductive organs, during orgasm and in the final stages of childbirth. It produces a pleasurable feeling that promotes bonding. This could be because, like the closely related hormone vassopressin, oxytocin helps the processing of social cues involved in the recognition of individuals, and may play a role in laying down shared memories. It is possible that oxytocin has a somewhat "addictive" effect, like dopamine. This may explain why people feel anguish at being parted from loved ones–they miss the oxytocin "rush" involved in being with them.

OXYTOCIN
This light micrograph shows oxytocin crystals. In women, this hormone is secreted naturally by the pituitary gland during childbirth, breastfeeding, and sex.

PITUITARY GLAND

FEELING CLOSE
Kissing and cuddling trigger the release of oxytocin into the bloodstream. This may help heighten feelings of closeness and strengthen the bond between partners.

ATTACHMENT

Humans form attachments –bonds of intimacy and affection–with people, animals, and objects. The importance of attachment was underlined by the observation of babies in orphanages during World Wars I and II. They were provided with food and shelter, but not the care and attention of a parent. Many experienced long-term problems: they did not gain weight, became emotionally and physically stunted, or simply died. They were not held, smiled at, kissed, or talked to, so no attachments could form. A mother's instinct to bond with her baby appears to be built into the brain. Imaging studies have shown that when a woman sees a picture of her own baby smiling, it triggers strong activity in the dopamine reward system (see p.130) of her brain. Pictures of other babies smiling produced a weaker response here, but crying or neutral expressions in the mothers' own babies did not activate the system at all.

HEALTHY DEVELOPMENT
Attachment encourages babies to trust their parents as a source of support and comfort, helping them become confident. It is vital for healthy development.

EXPRESSION

HUMANS ARE HIGHLY INTERDEPENDENT—WHAT ONE DOES INVARIABLY AFFECTS WHAT HAPPENS TO OTHERS. IT IS THEREFORE VERY USEFUL FOR US TO BE ABLE TO READ EACH OTHERS' EMOTIONS IN ORDER TO PREDICT WHAT SOMEONE MIGHT DO NEXT. WE ALSO NEED TO SIGNAL OUR OWN EMOTIONS IN ORDER TO NUDGE OTHERS TO DO WHAT WE WANT.

EXPRESSING EMOTION

Expressions are more than just signals, they are an extension of the emotion itself. When we feel something, the neural activation pattern associated with the emotion includes the firing of neurons which, if not inhibited, cause face and body muscles to contract in characteristic ways. There are six basic, or universal emotions (see bottom). Recent studies have looked at the range of expressions used by people who have been blind since birth and found that they are similar or identical to those displayed by sighted people. This suggests that learning plays quite a small part in expression.

BABIES AND PETS

One way that expressions work to our advantage is that we can use them to manipulate others. The need to persuade other people to behave in ways that benefit us is greatest among those who are powerless. This is probably why babies are born with a range of facial and aural expressions, such as gurgling and crying. These help the babies get what they want or need in the way of attention and food. Typical pet animals, such as dogs and cats, also have expressions that we read and respond to. The most popular pets tend to be those that best mimic human expressions.

TRUE EXPRESSION?
The left hemisphere controls movement on the right side of the face, while the more emotional right brain controls the left side.

RIGHT AND RIGHT
The two right sides of former US president Richard Nixon's face hint at his unconscious feelings. Here the eyes appear less engaging.

LEFT AND LEFT
The two left halves together give a clearer picture of the intended or "social" facial expression that looks more eager to please.

SIX EMOTIONS
Surprise, anger, disgust, fear, happiness, and sadness are all universal emotions. Each produces a distinct facial expression, which is almost identical across every culture.

ANATOMY OF A SMILE

There are two fairly distinct types of human smile: the conscious "social" smile, and the genuine "Duchenne" smile, which is named after the French neurologist Guillame Duchenne, who first described it. The first involves consciously activating the muscles that stretch the mouth sideways. The second involves an additional set of muscles, which are mainly controlled by unconscious brain processes. These muscles make the lower lids of the eyes swell and the edges crinkle into "crows' feet." Expressions not only show what a person is feeling, they can also actually bring about the feeling that they are associated with. In laboratory tests, consciously producing a smile was found to produce a weak, but detectable, sense of happiness in those who displayed it. So, even producing a "fake" social smile can promote a faint but real sensation of happiness in the person expressing it.

READING EMOTIONS

When we read somebody's expression, we automatically make it ourselves. We can hide this echo by consciously inhibiting the muscular change. Because expressions cause, as well as transmit, our feelings this mimicry creates an echo of the emotion we see and tells us how the other person is feeling. This is shown by experiments in which people are stopped from echoing expressions by temporarily paralyzing an area of the motor cortex with transcranial magnetic stimulation. When volunteers were unable to mimic expressions, they were less accurate at reading them in others.

TMS coil

Induced current

Motor area

SMILING

A heartfelt smile is hard to produce on demand because it requires and is controlled by emotion. The real smile, with both mouth and eye areas (top) activated, is usually a true reflection of a happy mood.

Motor cortex

Orbicularis occuli, controls eyelid movement

In "genuine" smile, signals from unconscious areas of brain, such as amygdala, are transmitted to motor cortex

Amygdala

Signal causes small muscles surrounding eye socket to contract, creating characteristic "wrinkles"

Premotor cortex

In "social" smile, signals are sent from conscious areas of brain to premotor and motor cortices

Motor cortex

Frontal cortex

Signal bypasses eyes

Zygomaticus minor muscle

Signal causes large muscles around mouth to contract, pulling lips sideways

Zygomaticus major muscle

HAPPINESS

Raised mouth corners

SADNESS

Raised inner brows

Lowered mouth

CONFLICTING EMOTIONS

Expressions have a direct effect on those who see them (see pp.122–23), so they are useful to get others to serve our needs. However, in social situations we sometimes have to make a conscious effort to stop making the expression that matches either what we spontaneously feel or what we see in others. Because expressing an emotion creates that emotion, when we do this we have to override one emotion with another, creating emotional conflict. Humans are probably unique in using facial expressions dishonestly, and we have become experts at doing so, but we are also very good at scrutinizing the expressions of others to discern the genuine from the fake.

Supplementary motor cortex
Constructs alternative expression

Insula
Suggests emotional effort

Superior temporal gyrus
Monitors effect of forced expression

Orbito-frontal cortex
May inhibit natural mimicry

AREAS OF CONFLICT
Trying to override natural mimicry of an emotion by expressing a conflicting one engages various brain areas.

THE SELF AND OTHERS

THE HUMAN ANIMAL IS AN INTENSELY SOCIAL SPECIES, AND OUR SURVIVAL DEPENDS LARGELY ON SUCCESSFUL INTERACTIONS WITH OUR NEIGHBORS. AS WITH OTHER SOCIAL ANIMALS, WE HAVE EVOLVED DISTINCT BRAIN CIRCUITS DEDICATED TO BONDING, COOPERATION, AND PREDICTING THE ACTIONS OF OTHERS. WE CAN ALSO RECOGNIZE THAT OTHER PEOPLE HAVE THEIR OWN THOUGHTS AND FEELINGS.

MADE TO BE SOCIABLE

One of the most distinctive features of the human brain is the large area of neocortex, its relatively recently developed outer layer. The frontal cortex (the part of the neocortex that surrounds the frontal lobe) is responsible for abstract reasoning, conscious thought and emotion, planning, and organization, and is highly developed in humans. One reason for the substantial growth of the neocortex may be that humans adapted this way in response to the demands of living in large, close-knit groups. Social living creates challenges such as moderating one's own behavior in order to accommodate others, competing subtly for reproductive rights, and predicting how others will behave, all of which need neocortical activity. Spending time in social activity also seems to grow the areas of the brain responsible for understanding and dealing with others. People who have large numbers of friends on social networking sites have correspondingly large social brain regions.

GROUP SIZE MATTERS
In primates, the size of the neocortex relative to other brain areas increases in almost direct proportion to the average size of the social group.

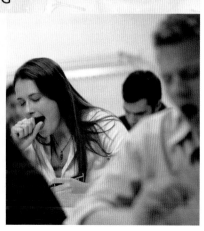

SOCIAL ANIMAL
Animals that live in large groups are socially smarter than those that don't. A study found that ring-tailed lemurs, which live in big groups, learned to steal food from people only when they were not looking. Other animals with comparable intelligence failed to do this.

CONTAGIOUS YAWNING

Social behaviors can be deliberate or unconscious. For example, it is thought that "catching" a yawn is an unconscious way of synchronizing group behavior. One theory about yawning is that, when one person does it, it signals that it is time for the entire group to sleep. By mimicking the yawn, other members implicitly agree. Another theory is that yawning keeps the brain alert. Its contagious nature ensures that each member of the group sharpens up.

SOCIAL AWARENESS

Social awareness covers a wide range of cognition that generates a sense of a "self" as well as of that self in a social context. For example, we adapt our behavior to cooperate with others, we predict what other people are likely to do and their reasons for doing it, we understand that others may hold different ideas and beliefs from our own, we are able to imagine how other people see us, and we can scrutinize our own minds. The range and diversity of skills required means that several areas of the brain are involved.

Anterior cingulate cortex
Selects actions, correcting intentions according to social context; registers social rejection

Medial prefrontal cortex
Controls own emotions in social situations

THE SELF-AWARE AND SOCIAL BRAIN
The "self" is sensed in different ways: we are aware of ourselves as physical beings, as agents of our actions, as objects in the world, and as components of a social system. Each type of self-awareness is generated by activity in different areas, and the information is combined to decide on socially appropriate actions.

THE INSULA
The insula may be responsible for humans experiencing the feeling of a "self" and having a sense of the boundary of that self, allowing for the distinction between "me" and "you." According to a school of thought known as "embodied cognition," which proposes that rational thought cannot be separated from emotions and their impact on the body, the insula detects body states that are induced by emotions as part of a process that brings our emotional experiences into our consciousness.

OBSERVING PAIN
Tests using fMRI scans show insula activity (green) in participants watching a person in pain, suggesting that the insula triggers empathic feelings.

THE PAIN OF REJECTION

In one study, fMRI scans were conducted on people playing a virtual ball game from which they were progressively excluded. Upon awareness of rejection, the anterior cingulate cortex (ACC) was activated, an area that also registers body pain, suggesting that the emotional impact of the two is similar. Part of the prefrontal cortex that helps control emotions was also activated, which seemed to reduce feelings of rejection.

ANTERIOR CINGULATE CORTEX
Social rejection causes the same type of activity in the anterior cingulate cortex (ACC) as physical pain.

PREFRONTAL CORTEX
The ventral prefrontal cortex then interacts with the ACC, which seems to reduce the pain of social rejection.

CONGRUENCE

Our brains are highly sensitive to the movements of other animals, especially other humans. The mirror neuron system (see pp.122–23) automatically makes us mirror the actions of others. The effect is so strong that when one person notices another not mirroring their own actions, it often makes them falter in their own actions. This "interference effect" applies only to biological motion–when participants observe a robot, no such interference occurs, even if the actions are humanlike.

MIRRORING
A person is discomfited if someone fails to mirror their actions, but whether or not a robot does so has no effect.

THEORY OF MIND

Theory of mind (ToM) refers to the instinctive "knowledge" that other people may hold different beliefs than one's own, and that it is those beliefs, not the facts of a situation, that inform and determine their behavior. One way to test for ToM is the Sally-Ann test (see diagram, below). Recent studies have shown that infants as young as 10 months may "pass" the Sally-Ann test.

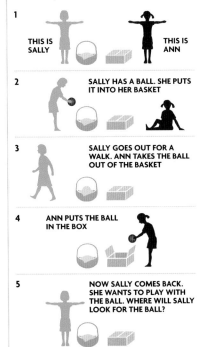

1. THIS IS SALLY / THIS IS ANN
2. SALLY HAS A BALL. SHE PUTS IT INTO HER BASKET
3. SALLY GOES OUT FOR A WALK. ANN TAKES THE BALL OUT OF THE BASKET
4. ANN PUTS THE BALL IN THE BOX
5. NOW SALLY COMES BACK. SHE WANTS TO PLAY WITH THE BALL. WHERE WILL SALLY LOOK FOR THE BALL?

SALLY-ANN TEST
If children indicate that, on her return, Sally will look in the place she expects the ball to be (in the basket), they appear to have ToM.

Motor cortex
Controls physical actions (making physical actions confirms sense of self)

Temperoparietal junction
Holds a "map" of body and constantly monitors physical self in relation to rest of world

Posterior temporal sulcus
A sense of one's own presence is triggered by activity here

Insula
Activity here correlates with self-reflection

Amygdala
Registers emotion in self and others

Fusiform face area
Face-recognition area within fusiform gyrus recognizes familiar faces, and analyzes faces for emotional signals

NONEXPRESSIVE
Neutral expressions produce less amygdala activity. The circuit from amygdala to face-recognition area is toned down and the brain takes in less information.

Amygdala
Face-recognition area

EXPRESSIVE
The amygdala reacts to facial expressions by "mirroring" the emotion. A smile, for example, triggers signals that begin the process of smiling back.

Amygdala
Face-recognition area

RESPONDING TO EMOTION

Facial expression is a signal–of intention and state of mind–and also a means of achieving empathy between people. Expressions are initially processed unconsciously by the amygdala, which monitors incoming data for emotional content. It responds by generating the emotion that has been observed. A fearful expression, for example, produces amygdala activation that triggers fear in the observer. Soon after the amygdala activation, the expression registers in the face-recognition area situated in the fusiform gyrus. Studies suggest that if a face expresses emotion, the amygdala signals this area to scrutinize it for meaning.

AUTISM AND THE MIND

Autism is marked by the absence of ToM. Rather than just "knowing" why Sally acts according to a false belief, people with Asperger's syndrome (a form of autism) consciously "work out" what is happening using part of the brain (yellow) that is thought to be more recently evolved than the area that generates ToM (red).

Normal

Asperger's

THE MORAL BRAIN

NORMAL PEOPLE BROUGHT UP IN A NORMAL ENVIRONMENT DEVELOP AN INSTINCTIVE SENSE OF RIGHT AND WRONG THAT SEEMS TO BE, AT LEAST IN PART, "HARD-WIRED" INTO THE BRAIN. THIS NATURAL "MORALITY" IS NOT NECESSARILY RATIONAL OR FAIR, AND PROBABLY EVOLVED BECAUSE BEHAVIOR PROMOTING SOCIAL COHESION ALSO, INDIRECTLY, AIDS SELF-SURVIVAL.

EMPATHY AND SYMPATHY

"Feeling" for another person–experiencing a faint version of their sorrow or flinching when you see them hurt–seems to be largely instinctive. It depends partly on theory of mind (see pp.138–39), which ensures that we "know" what is likely to be going on in other people's minds. Empathy goes a step further, in that it also involves "echoing" the emotions of another person. When a person is told a

story about someone experiencing emotional trauma, the activated areas in the listener's brain come into play when he or she is in such a situation.

SYMPATHETIC STANCE
Being able to put yourself into someone else's situation, to experience an echo of what they feel, and sympathize with them appears to be an instinctive human trait.

WITNESSING ACCIDENTAL PAIN
This fMRI scan shows that seeing someone hurt by accident produces similar brain activity as if the viewer was accidentally hurt.

WITNESSING INTENTIONAL INJURY
When witnessing someone hurt intentionally, brain areas concerned with judgments and moral reasoning (above) are also activated.

MORALITY

Our sense of right and wrong permeates all our social perceptions and interactions. Moral decision-making is partly learned, but it also depends on emotions, which give "value" to actions and experiences. When making moral judgments, two overlapping but distinct brain circuits come into play. One is a "rational" circuit, which weighs up the pros and cons of an action objectively. The other circuit is emotional. It generates a fast and instinctive sense of what is right and wrong. The two circuits do not always arrive at the same conclusion, because emotions are biased toward self-survival and/or protecting those who are loved or related to oneself. Emotional bias in moral judgments seems to rely on activity in the ventromedial and orbitofrontal prefrontal cortex. Studies of people with damage to this area have found that their moral judgments are more rational than those of others, suggesting that human "morality" is hard-wired into the brain, and evolved more to protect ourselves than to "do good."

MORAL JUDGMENT CIRCUITS
Emotions play a crucial role in moral decision-making (see p.169 and p.172). In order to arrive at moral decisions, areas of the brain associated with emotional experience work alongside those that register facts and consider possible actions and outcomes.

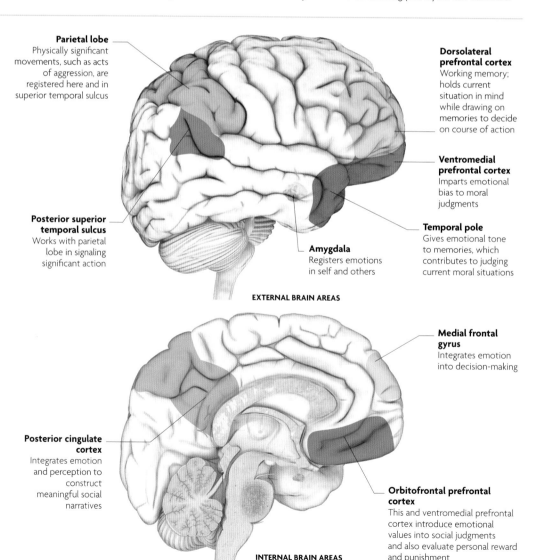

Parietal lobe
Physically significant movements, such as acts of aggression, are registered here and in superior temporal sulcus

Dorsolateral prefrontal cortex
Working memory; holds current situation in mind while drawing on memories to decide on course of action

Ventromedial prefrontal cortex
Imparts emotional bias to moral judgments

Posterior superior temporal sulcus
Works with parietal lobe in signaling significant action

Amygdala
Registers emotions in self and others

Temporal pole
Gives emotional tone to memories, which contributes to judging current moral situations

EXTERNAL BRAIN AREAS

Medial frontal gyrus
Integrates emotion into decision-making

Posterior cingulate cortex
Integrates emotion and perception to construct meaningful social narratives

Orbitofrontal prefrontal cortex
This and ventromedial prefrontal cortex introduce emotional values into social judgments and also evaluate personal reward and punishment

INTERNAL BRAIN AREAS

ALTRUSIM

The notion of altruism assumes that people can do things for others with no motivation of a direct reward for themselves. However, brain scans show that doing "good" things is personally rewarding. One fMRI study was conducted while participants made or withheld donations to real charities. The participants could keep any donations they refused to make. The result showed that both keeping the money and giving it away activated the brain's "reward" pathways. Giving away money also enhanced activity in areas concerned with belonging and group bonding.

RECEIVING   **GIVING**

REWARD AREAS
Giving and receiving activate areas linked to pleasure and satisfaction. Areas linked to bonding and social cohesion are active when giving.

Emotional conflict

Emotion

INTERNAL BRAIN AREAS

Cognition

Understanding intention

EXTERNAL BRAIN AREAS

BRAIN DAMAGE AFFECTS MORALS
Damage to any one of several brain areas can affect moral judgment. They include: areas involved in feeling emotion and assessing emotional intent and conflict; the frontal areas involved in thinking about current situations and assessing action; and the area at the junction of the parietal and temporal lobes, which allows for understanding others' intentions.

PHINEAS GAGE

The idea that our moral sense may have a biological basis in the brain arose largely as a result of a freak accident in 1848. A well-respected rail worker called Phineas Gage blew a hole in the front of his brain with a tamping rod that he was using to compress explosive powder. He survived with remarkably little damage to most of his faculties. His behavior, however, changed dramatically. From being a conscientious, polite, and thoughtful man he became reckless, rude, and socially irresponsible. Acquaintances remarked that he was "no longer Gage." The change was linked by his doctor to his brain damage, and modern reconstructions of the injury show that it affected the areas now known to be central to moral sensitivity.

RECONSTRUCTION
Computer-generated images reveal the exact location of the damage to Phineas Gage's brain. Apart from going blind in one eye, he suffered few physical effects, but his behavior changed dramatically.

Tamping rod

Frontal lobe

Entry point

MORALITY VERSUS RATIONALITY

The two cognitive circuits that generate moral judgments do not always arrive at the same conclusion. The one that engages emotions almost certainly evolved first, in an environment in which survival depended on protecting tribal units rather than adhering to a social code that includes, for example, the right to justice and equal rights. Hence the instinctive, or "natural," judgments we make may vary from those we arrive at after consideration. Our behavior often reflects this inner conflict. For example, we tend to help people who are close or similar to us more than those who are distant and strange.

CONFLICTING MORAL VALUES

NATURAL MORALITY	RATIONAL MORALITY
Favor those nearest and most similar to self.	Treat all people in same way.
Judge committed acts, such as murder, more harshly than acts of omission, for example, failing to stop a murder.	Judge by result of action/inaction rather than by whether the act is active or passive.
Less concerned about acts of violence that involve causing pain at a distance, for example, less inhibited about killing by launching missiles than killing by hand-to-hand combat.	Judges acts involving local and distant consequences as equal.

PSYCHOPATHS AND BULLIES

Psychopaths are defined as people who use manipulation, intimidation, and violence to control others and satisfy selfish needs. They display an inability to feel guilt, remorse, or anxiety about their antisocial behavior. This may result from damage or developmental problems involving the moral circuits of the brain. Imaging studies have found that psychopaths show low levels of activity in the amygdala when faced with stimuli that would be emotionally traumatic to others and normally generate amygdala activation.

CONTROL   **PSYCHOPATH**

DIMINISHED REACTION
These fMRI scans show that, when seeing pictures they had learned to associate with fear, psychopaths showed much less activity in the amygdala than normal people.

CONTROL   **PSYCHOPATH**

WE SIGNAL OUR INTENTIONS TO EACH OTHER IN VARIOUS
WAYS. A SURPRISINGLY LARGE AMOUNT OF INFORMATION
CAN BE TRANSMITTED BY GESTURES AND BODY LANGUAGE.
THIS IS AN ABILITY THAT HUMANS SHARE WITH MANY
OTHER ANIMALS, BUT WE CAN ALSO COMMUNICATE IN
WAYS THAT ARE UNIQUE TO OUR SPECIES. ONLY THE
HUMAN BRAIN HAS AREAS DEDICATED TO LANGUAGE. WE
USE THESE TO SPEAK AND TO READ AND WRITE. ALTHOUGH
READING AND WRITING HAVE TO BE LEARNED, WE SEEM
TO BE BORN WITH THE ABILITY TO SPEAK AND TO FOLLOW
COMPLEX RULES OF GRAMMAR.

LANGUAGE AND COMMUNICATION

GESTURES AND BODY LANGUAGE

WE SIGNAL OUR THOUGHTS, FEELINGS, AND INTENTIONS BY GESTURE AND BODY LANGUAGE AS WELL AS BY SPEECH. HALF OF OUR COMMUNICATION IS TYPICALLY NONVERBAL, AND WHEN THEY CONFLICT, GESTURES "SPEAK" LOUDER THAN WORDS.

EYE TALK

Human eyes convey information through facial expression and movement. Unlike in most species, the visible white of the human eye makes it easy to see in which direction a person is looking and thus where their attention is directed. People have a strong instinct to follow another's eye gaze, and this simple mechanism ensures that when someone is in sight of another person, they can manipulate each other's attention and share information without even having to communicate with words.

STRONG SIGNALERS
Pupils dilate when a person has an emotional reaction. Some drugs have a similar effect—belladonna was once used by women to send signals of sexual excitement.

MIRRORING PARENTS

By three months old, babies have the ability to follow another person's eye gaze, and they are quick to pick up any emotion contained in a look. Experiments show that if a parent looks toward something and displays fear, for example, by widening their eyes, the child is very likely to mirror this reaction and be scared too, even if the object is clearly harmless.

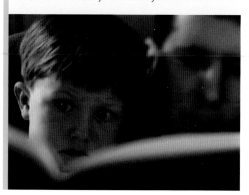

BODY LANGUAGE

Body language is mostly instinctive, consisting largely of unconscious "breakthrough" acts. Some of these are remnants of primitive reflexes, when other living things were often seen primarily as either predator or prey. These ancient reflexes program us to approach small, soft stimuli, which suggest prey, and to withdraw from strong, hard stimuli, which suggest a predator. Aggression is usually shown through tensed muscles and an upright or forward-leaning stance, indicating that a predator is ready to pounce. Fear is displayed by a softer body contour and backward stance, indicating that the prey is preparing to flee. When emotions are mixed,

EXPRESSION AND BODY LANGUAGE STUDY
When body language and facial expression do not match each other, we are biased toward the emotion signaled by the body, rather than the expression on the face.

a person may take up a midway stance from which they can shift quickly from one posture to another.

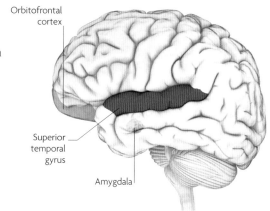

BRAIN PROCESSES
Giveaway eye, mouth, hand, and body movements, as well as deliberate gestures, are registered in the superior temporal sulcus, a brain area concerned with the self in relation to others. The amygdala notes the emotional content, and the orbitofrontal cortex analyzes it.

Orbitofrontal cortex
Superior temporal gyrus
Amygdala

ANGRY EXPRESSION; ANGRY BODY LANGUAGE
FEARFUL EXPRESSION; ANGRY BODY LANGUAGE
ANGRY EXPRESSION; FEARFUL BODY LANGUAGE
FEARFUL EXPRESSION; FEARFUL BODY LANGUAGE

REACTING TO BODY LANGUAGE

Body language showing fear or anger sparks activity in brain areas involved in movement, while that expressing happiness stirs activity in the visual cortex. In one study, subjects' brains were scanned while they were shown images of actors with blurred faces in fearful, happy, or neutral poses. Happy gestures, such as arms spread in welcome, spurred activity in the visual cortex. Fearful ones, like cowering, caused activity in emotional centers and in areas involved in movement. This might explain how fear spreads in a crowd and prepares the body to flee.

HAPPINESS
FEAR

GESTURES

Although body language is mostly unconsciously performed, we have a greater degree of conscious control over its more refined form–gestures. Many parts of the body can be involved with making gestures, but most tend to include hand and finger movements, which can display complex spatial relations, issue directions, and show the shape of imagined objects. They can help convey emotions and thoughts, insults, and invitations. Gestures are used throughout the world, although they by no means have universal meanings. Even

simple gestures, such as pointing at a person, which is commonly used in many parts of the world, can be highly offensive in parts of Asia.

THREE MAIN CATEGORIES

"Natural" gestures tend to be used for three main purposes: to tell a story, to convey a feeling or idea, or to emphasize a spoken statement. Invented gestures, such as the Masonic handshake, may be completely arbitrary or developed from natural body language.

INTRICATE GESTURES
Statues of Hindu deities often convey symbolic meanings through the specific positioning of their hands. With his outward-facing palm, the god Shiva is assuring protection.

THE GRAMMAR OF GESTURE

Unlike the rules of speech, which vary from language to language, gesturing seems to have a universal "grammar". Asked to communicate a simple statement using words of their native languages, English, Chinese, and Spanish speakers started with the subject, then the verb and finally the object, whereas Turkish speakers used the subject, object, then the verb. However, when just using gestures, speakers of all of these languages placed the subject, object, and verb in that order.

Arms wide and hands open, with the body exposed says: "I'm not hiding anything or deceiving you"

This hand movement may either be comforting or an attempt to suppress a scream

Aggressive, rigid hand movement suggests anger or rejection of another person

PROTESTING INNOCENCE

SHOCK

ANNOYANCE

Raising to full height with clenched fists suggests victory

Pulling fingertips together suggests accuracy, cohesion, and concentration; may be used to focus listener's attention on words

JUBILATION

MEASURING WITH HANDS

Hands may convey a more precise measurement than the speaker might be able to get across verbally

REINFORCING A POINT

THE ORIGINS OF LANGUAGE

HUMANS HAVE AN INNATE CAPACITY FOR LANGUAGE—A FACULTY THAT SEEMS TO RELY ON ONE OR MORE GENES THAT ARE UNIQUE TO OUR SPECIES. IT IS NOT KNOWN, THOUGH, WHETHER LANGUAGE AROSE AS A DIRECT RESULT OF GENETIC MUTATION, OR AS A RESULT OF THE INTERACTION BETWEEN SUBTLE BIOLOGICAL CHANGES AND ENVIRONMENTAL PRESSURES.

HEMISPHERE SPECIALIZATION

Compared to the brains of other species, human brains are less symmetrical in terms of functions. Language is the most obvious example of this lopsidedness, and the vast majority of people have the main language areas on the left side of the brain, although a few seem to have language functions distributed on both sides, and some have it only on the right. Generally, language is associated with the "dominant" side of the brain—that is, the one that controls the most competent hand. Language is thought by some to be the mechanism that elevates the brain to full consciousness, and before language evolved it is possible that our ancestors were not consciously aware of themselves. Because language is so important, disruptions have awful consequences, so brain surgeons have to be very careful to avoid damaging the language areas. This is one of the reasons for the Wada test.

LEFT HEMISPHERE　　**RIGHT HEMISPHERE**

LANGUAGE FUNCTIONS

The three principal language areas are usually found in the left hemisphere, while four other important language areas are located in the right hemisphere.

HEMISPHERE	FUNCTION
Left	Articulating language
Left	Comprehending language
Left	Word recognition
Right	Recognizing tone
Right	Rhythm, stress, and intonation
Right	Recognizing the speaker
Right	Recognizing gestures

AREAS INVOLVED
The main language skills of recognizing, understanding, and generating speech are situated in the left hemisphere in most people. The right hemisphere, however, processes aspects of language that are needed to obtain "full" comprehension.

THE WADA TEST
The Wada test, named after Canadian neurologist Juhn Wada, involves anesthetizing one hemisphere of the brain while leaving the other fully active. This is possible because each hemisphere of the brain has its own blood supply. If the patient is able to speak when one brain hemisphere is asleep, the principal language areas must be on the conscious side. This information is vital for surgeons to plan operations. The Wada test will eventually be replaced by advanced scanning techniques.

Left internal carotid artery　　Right internal carotid artery

CAROTID ARTERIES
This colored magnetic resonance angiogram (MRA) shows the arteries that supply the head and neck. The Wada test involves injecting one of the internal carotid arteries to put one brain hemisphere to sleep.

SILBO LANGUAGE

Most languages use words—that is, noises made by exercising muscles in the throat and mouth that chop up (articulate) and vary the sound of the passage of air from the lungs. Silbo, however, is a language made up entirely of whistles, used by the inhabitants of La Gomera in the Canary Islands. Brain-imaging studies show that Silbo-users process the whistles in the main language areas of their brains, whereas those who do not know the language process the whistles simply as a collection of sounds, which are registered in other areas of the brain.

WHISTLE WHILE YOU WORK
Silbo developed among islanders who needed to communicate in a landscape where deep ravines made shouting impractical—their whistles carry farther than words and with less distortion.

WHAT IS LANGUAGE?

Language is not just a matter of stringing symbols together to convey meaning. Language is governed by a complex set of rules, known as grammar. The details of these rules differ from language to language, but they share a similar type of complexity. Simple, wordlike sounds do not engage language areas in the same way that words that form part of a language do—the brain just treats them as noises. Some theorists believe that the overarching rules of language–the structure that is common to them all–is embedded in the human brain and is instinctive rather than learned. Although primates have learned how to link visual symbols on keyboards to objects and some can understand sign language, it has not been possible to teach another species spoken language.

LEFT HEMISPHERE

SENTENCES AND CONSONANT STRINGS
Several areas in the brain's left hemisphere become active when people hear a familiar language spoken to them, compared to a small area of the right hemisphere that is active when they hear strings of consonants that do not make any sense.

RIGHT HEMISPHERE

COLOR STUDY

Brain scans show that discriminating easy-to-name colors (top row) activates similar regions as hard-to-name colors (bottom row). However, the additional activity in language areas in the top scans suggests that language retrieval plays a part in visual perception.

LANGUAGE AND PERCEPTION

Language is much more than just a way of signaling things to one another—evidence shows that it shapes the way we perceive the world. If your language makes a distinction between blue and green, for example, you will be less likely to confuse a blue color chip with a green one when recalling them, because you will have been able to attach a mental label to each of them. If a language does not distinguish between colors in the same way, it will be more difficult to recall which is which. Similarly, the Amazonian Piraha tribe do not have words for numbers above two, and are unable to reliably tell the difference between four and five objects placed in a row.

THE EVOLUTION OF LANGUAGE

Spoken language leaves no traces in the historic record, so we shall probably never know how or even exactly when it originated. The ability to generate speech and understand language is something only humans possess, although some primates' brains have regions that may function as primitive language areas. An important factor in the evolution of language took place in the throat and larynx, around the time that our ancestors started walking upright. These changes affected the variety and intricacy of the sounds they could produce. This improved ability to communicate probably increased the chances of survival for those who used it most effectively and therefore the chances of it being passed on to subsequent generations.

THE ANATOMY OF SPEECH

The altered larynx in upright hominids allowed them to make more inventive noises. It also meant they could no longer swallow and breathe at the same time, leading to an increased risk of choking. The descended hyoid bone is also thought to facilitate the production of a wide range of sounds.

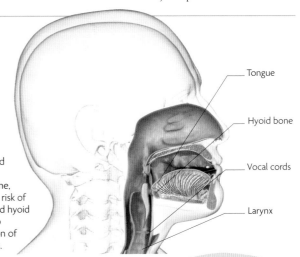

Tongue

Hyoid bone

Vocal cords

Larynx

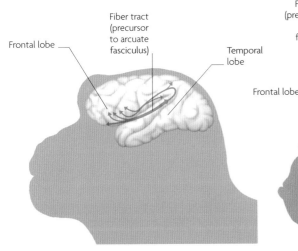

Frontal lobe

Fiber tract (precursor to arcuate fasciculus)

Temporal lobe

Fiber tract (precursor to arcuate fasciculus)

Frontal lobe

Temporal lobe

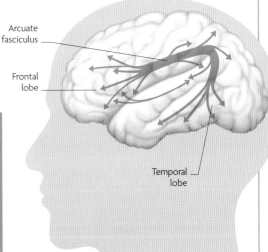

Arcuate fasciculus

Frontal lobe

Temporal lobe

MACAQUE FIBER TRACT

Macaques have simple language areas. A crucial part of this region is a thick bundle of fibers, which links the areas associated with understanding language in the temporal lobe with the areas that generate it, in the frontal lobe.

CHIMPANZEE FIBER TRACT

The connections between the frontal lobe and the temporal lobe are more advanced than in macaques, allowing for improved cognitive abilities, but they do not have such prominent temporal-lobe projections of the fiber tract.

HUMAN FIBER TRACT

In the human brain, the tract is known as the arcuate fasciculus, connecting two areas crucial for speech and comprehension. It is one of the specializations thought to have led to the evolution of language.

KOKO THE GORILLA

Koko is a female lowland gorilla who has been taught to understand more than 1,000 signs based on American sign language and about 2,000 words of spoken English. She initiates the majority of conversations with her human companions and typically constructs meaningful statements with average lengths of 3–6 words. She has an IQ of between 70 and 95.

SKILLED SIGNER

In addition to knowing more than 1,000 signs, Koko makes up her own signs to convey metaphor, humor, and affection.

SIGNING "EAT"

RECEIVING REWARD

TEACHING KOKO HOW TO SIGN

THE LANGUAGE AREAS

THE HUMAN BRAIN DIFFERS FROM THAT OF OTHER SPECIES BY
HAVING A REGION THAT IS DEDICATED TO LANGUAGE ALONE.
IN THE VAST MAJORITY OF PEOPLE, THIS IS SITUATED IN THE
LEFT HEMISPHERE, BUT IN ABOUT 20 PERCENT OF LEFT-
HANDED PEOPLE, IT IS IN THE RIGHT HEMISPHERE.

MAIN LANGUAGE AREAS

Language processing occurs mainly in Broca's
and Wernicke's areas. Broadly speaking, words
are comprehended by Wernicke's area and
articulated by Broca's. A thick band of tissue
called the arcuate fasciculus connects these
two areas. Wernicke's area is surrounded by
an area known as Geschwind's territory.
When a person hears words spoken,
Wernicke's area matches the sounds to their
meaning, and special neurons in Geschwind's
territory are thought to assist by combining
the many different properties of words
(sound, sight, and meaning) to provide full
comprehension. When a person speaks, the
process happens in reverse: Wernicke's area
finds the correct words to match the thought
that is to be expressed. The chosen words
then pass to Broca's area via the arcuate
fasciculus (or, possibly, via a more circuitous
route through Geschwind's territory). Broca's
area then turns the words into sounds by
moving the tongue, mouth, and jaw into the
required position and by activating the larynx.

Arcuate fasciculus
Nerve fibers linking
Wernicke's and Broca's
areas; thicker than in
other primates.

Geschwind's territory
Located in lower part
of parietal lobe, where
information from sound,
sight, and body sensation
come together; is one
of last parts of brain
to mature.

Broca's area
Lies in frontal lobe; back
region moves mouth to
form words, while front
part is thought to be
concerned with aspects
of word meaning.

Wernicke's area
Lies in upper temporal lobe,
adjacent to occipital and parietal cortices;
heard and seen words are understood here,
and also selected for articulation.

LOCATING LANGUAGE AREAS
Together, the main language areas generate comprehension
and articulation, but full language appreciation requires input
from areas concerned with tone, emotion, and rhythm.

Part of
visual cortex

Part of Broca's
area

Wernicke's
area

Geschwind's
territory

SEEING WORDS PASSIVELY

LISTENING TO WORDS

AREAS ACTIVATED IN DIFFERENT TASKS
These fMRI scans show
distinct patterns of
activity in the three
main language areas,
depending on whether
the person undertaking
the task is listening to
speech or pronouncing
words. Simply looking
at words passively
does not involve
much activity
in the language areas.

Area activated
includes part of
Broca's area

PRONOUNCING WORDS

LANGUAGE TASKS

Different types of language tasks
activate a number of different areas of
the brain. However, the key language
areas only become active when
language is turned into meaning. So
merely looking at words as marks on
a page involves areas of the brain
such as the visual cortex, which is
responsible for processing incoming
visual information, whereas listening
to spoken words triggers activity in
Wernicke's area and Geschwind's's
territory, signifying that the sounds
are being turned into meaningful
information. Broca's area is
significantly involved in listening,
too, because understanding words
involves, to some extent, articulating
them "in your head" (also referred to
as "sounding out"). Broca's area is
strongly activated when the task
involves pronouncing words, while
generating words involves both
Wernicke's and Broca's areas, as
well as Geschwind's territory.

SHIFTING GROUND

Wernicke's and Broca's areas are now well defined,
but immediately around them lie large regions of the
cortex that become active during a variety of different
language studies. Their precise functions remain unclear,
and their shapes and locations differ from person to
person. Even with a single individual, the peripheral
areas engaged in language may shift over the course of
that person's life.

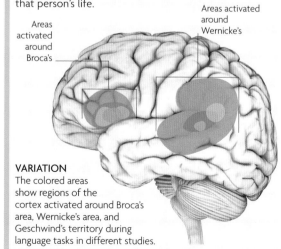

Areas
activated
around
Broca's

Areas activated
around
Wernicke's

VARIATION
The colored areas
show regions of the
cortex activated around Broca's
area, Wernicke's area, and
Geschwind's territory during
language tasks in different studies.

THE MULTILINGUAL BRAIN

Being fluent in two languages, particularly from early childhood, enhances various cognitive skills and might also protect against the onset of dementia and other age-related cognitive decline. One reason for this may be that speaking a second language builds more connections between neurons. Studies show that bilingual adults have denser gray matter, especially in the inferior frontal cortex of the brain's left hemisphere, where most language and communication skills are controlled. The increased density was most pronounced in people who learned a second language before the age of five.

Dorsolateral prefrontal cortex
Broca's area
Caudate nucleus
Dorsolateral prefrontal cortex
Inferior frontal cortex
Caudate nucleus
Inferior frontal cortex

LEFT HEMISPHERE   **RIGHT HEMISPHERE**

BILINGUALS   **MONOLINGUALS**

CONTRASTING ACTIVATION
These scans show the brains of bilingual and monolingual individuals when hearing the same language.

KEY
- Areas used when speaking one language
- Areas activated in bilinguals when switching languages

NEURAL SIGNATURE OF BILINGUALISM
The purple area is used by both mono- and bilingual individuals when speaking one language; areas in green are activated when bilingual speakers switch languages. The caudate nucleus is also activated during the switch.

LANGUAGE PROBLEMS

There are a wide range of speech and language problems that can arise from a correspondingly varied number of injuries and impairments. Some problems only affect comprehension, whereas others specifically hinder expression; learning disabilities, such as dyslexia (see p.153) and specific language impairment (see p.248), can affect both. Traumatic brain injuries and strokes can lead to aphasia, which is the loss of the ability to produce and/or comprehend language. By contrast, dysphasia is the partial loss of the ability to communicate, although these terms are often incorrectly used interchangeably.

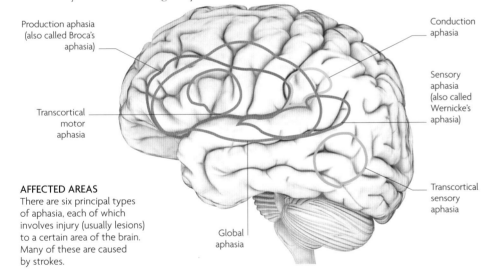

Production aphasia (also called Broca's aphasia)
Transcortical motor aphasia
Conduction aphasia
Sensory aphasia (also called Wernicke's aphasia)
Transcortical sensory aphasia
Global aphasia

AFFECTED AREAS
There are six principal types of aphasia, each of which involves injury (usually lesions) to a certain area of the brain. Many of these are caused by strokes.

STUTTERING

About 1 percent of people (75 percent of them men) stutter. In most cases, stuttering (also known as stammering) begins between the ages of two and six. Imaging studies have shown that the brains of stutterers behave differently from those of non-stutterers when processing speech, in that many more areas of the brain are activated during speech production. It may be that these interfere with one another and cause the stuttering, or it may be the result of stuttering.

NON-STUTTERER   **STUTTERER BEFORE TREATMENT**

TREATMENT FOR STUTTERING
Speech therapy is often successful, as these PET scans show. As treatment progresses, brain activity during speech dies down to near normal.

EARLY STAGE OF TREATMENT   **LATER STAGE OF TREATMENT**

TYPES OF APHASIA

Aphasia is usually associated with a brain injury (such as a stroke), which affects the brain's language areas. Depending on the type of damage, the area affected (see right), and the extent of damage, those suffering from aphasia may be able to speak, yet have little or no comprehension of what they or others are saying. Or they may be able to understand language, yet be unable to speak. Sometimes, sufferers can sing but not speak, or write but not read.

Production aphasia (damage to Broca's area) Inability to articulate words or string them together; if words can be uttered, they tend to be verbs or nouns, with abnormal tone and rhythm.

Conduction aphasia (damage to link between Wernicke's and Broca's areas) Speech errors include substituting sounds, but good comprehension and fluent speech production.

Global aphasia (widespread damage) General deficits in comprehension, repetition, naming, and speech production; automatic phrases (e.g. reeling off numbers) may be spared.

Transcortical sensory aphasia (damage to temporal-occipital-parietal junction) Inability to comprehend, name, read, or write, but with normal ability to recite previously learned passages.

Transcortical motor aphasia (damage around Broca's) Good comprehension but nonfluent speech, often limited to two words at a time. Sufferers retain the ability to repeat words and phrases.

Sensory aphasia (damage to Wernicke's area) Inability to understand language, often combined with general comprehension problems and lack of awareness of own deficiency.

A CONVERSATION

CONVERSATION COMES NATURALLY TO MOST OF US, BUT IN TERMS OF BRAIN FUNCTION IT IS ONE OF THE MOST COMPLICATED CEREBRAL ACTIVITIES WE ENGAGE IN. BOTH SPEAKING AND LISTENING INVOLVE WIDESPREAD AREAS OF THE BRAIN, REFLECTING MANY DIFFERENT TYPES AND LEVELS OF COGNITION.

LISTENING

The sound of spoken words take a short time–about 150 milliseconds–to pass from the speaker's mouth to the listener's ear, for the ear to turn this stimulus into electrical signals, and for this to be processed as sound by the auditory cortex. Words are decoded in Wernicke's area in the left hemisphere, but other areas are also at work to provide full comprehension, including parts of the right hemisphere concerned with tone, body language, and rhythm. If any of these areas are damaged, a person may be left with an incomplete understanding of what is being communicated.

MORE THAN WORDS
Face-to-face conversations involve more than just decoding words—tone and body language are also part of "understanding."

◎1 50–150 MS
AFTER WORDS ARE SPOKEN
SOUND REGISTERED
Sound from the speaker registers in the auditory cortex and is distributed to areas concerned with decoding the words and other areas of the brain involved with emotion, tone, and rhythm.

◎3 250–350 MS
STRUCTURE OF WORD STREAM ANALYZED AND MEANING OF WORDS EXTRACTED
Speech is decoded in Wernicke's area (orange, below right) in the left hemisphere. Then, the anterior temporal lobe (brown, below left) and inferior frontal cortex (purple, below left) in both hemispheres start to extract the meaning of the words.

Wernicke's area

LEFT HEMISPHERE

◎4 400–550 MS
MEANING CONSCIOUSLY COMPREHENDED
Turning the sound of speech into a stream of meaning requires more than just decoding the words—they also have to be associated with memories to give full comprehension. This takes place in part of the frontal lobe.

◎2 150–200 MS
EMOTIONAL TONE REGISTERED
The amygdala is quick to pick up on the emotional tone of the speech and subsequently produces an appropriate emotional reaction.

THE LISTENER
The illustration above highlights the areas of the brain involved in listening. Zero represents the time at which the words are spoken. The rest of the times are measured in milliseconds (ms) after that. It takes just over half a second for the brain to comprehend the meaning of the words.

SPEAKING

The speech process starts about a quarter of a second before words are actually uttered. This is when the brain starts to select the words that are to convey whatever the person wants to say. The words then have to be turned into sounds, and are finally articulated. Most of this complicated activity occurs in specific language areas, which in most people are on the left side of the brain. However, in a minority of people they are situated in the right, or spread between both hemispheres. Right-hemisphere language dominance is more prevalent among left-handers (see p.199).

SHIFTING FUNCTIONS

Speech and comprehension problems often result from strokes, which damage the language areas. If the damage happens early in life, the speech functions may shift to the opposite hemisphere. In older people, this is less likely to be successful, but undamaged areas can still take on some functions of the damaged areas.

SPEECH AND LANGUAGE THERAPY
It is possible for people who suffer from aphasia as a result of a stroke to recover some language functions through intense speech and language therapy.

CRUCIAL PATHWAY
"Prepared" words are transmitted to Broca's area via a bundle of nerve fibers called the arcuate fasciculus. It is much thicker and better developed in humans than in other species, and is thought to be key to the development of language.

◎ 2 –200 MS
WORDS TO PHONOLOGY
Shortly after they have been retrieved from memory, the words are matched to the sounds in Wernicke's area, which is adjacent to the auditory cortex, where sounds are distinguished.

◎ 3 –150 MS
PHONOLOGY TO SYLLABLES
Broca's area is the part of the brain most closely associated with speech. It matches the sounds of words to the specific mouth, tongue, and throat movements required to actually voice them.

◎ 4 –100 MS
ARTICULATION
The mouth, tongue, and throat movements needed to articulate the selected words are directed by the part of the motor cortex that controls these parts of the body.

◎ 1 –250 MS
BEFORE SPEAKING
CONCEPTS TO WORDS
Words are attached to memories and ideas and act as "handles" by which the brain can grasp the correct ones to express an idea. The matching of words to concepts happens in the temporal lobe.

◎ 5 UNDER 100 MS
FINE CONTROL OF ARTICULATION
The cerebellum is concerned with orchestrating the timing of speech production. The right cerebellar hemisphere connects to the left cerebral hemisphere, and this shows greatest activation during speech, whereas the left cerebellar hemisphere is more active during singing.

THE SPEAKER
The illustration above highlights the six crucial brain areas that are activated immediately before speaking. Zero is the point on the timescale when words are actually uttered; the timings of the stages before this are therefore indicated by negative values.

READING AND WRITING

OUR ABILITY TO SPEAK AND TO UNDERSTAND THE SPOKEN WORD HAS EVOLVED SO THAT OUR BRAINS ARE WIRED FOR SPEECH. READING AND WRITING, HOWEVER, DO NOT NATURALLY COME TO US IN THE SAME WAY. IN ORDER TO LEARN TO READ AND WRITE, EACH INDIVIDUAL HAS TO TRAIN THE BRAIN TO DEVELOP THE NECESSARY SKILLS.

LEARNING TO READ AND WRITE

To learn how to read and write, a child has to translate the shapes of letters on the page into the sounds they make if they are spoken aloud. The word "cat," for instance, must be broken down into its phonological components–"kuh," "aah," and "tuh". Only when the word on the page is translated into the sound that is heard when the word is spoken, can the child match it to its meaning. Learning to write uses even more of the brain. In addition to the language areas concerned with comprehension, and the visual areas concerned with decoding text, writing involves integrating the activity in these areas with those concerned with manual dexterity, including the cerebellum, which is involved with intricate hand movements.

VISUAL DISTINCTIONS
Distinguishing between written letters uses a part of the brain that evolved to make detailed visual distinctions between natural objects. This may be why many letters resemble shapes seen in nature.

3 THE AUDITORY CORTEX
Written words are broken into their phonological elements and "sounded out" so they can be "heard"; the auditory cortex allows the reader to recognize each word by the way it sounds.

4 BROCA'S AREA
Once a word has been recognized, it is also "sounded out" in Broca's area, linking the written word to the spoken word.

5 THE TEMPORAL LOBE
This area helps match the words to their meanings by retrieving memories. Full appreciation of written text—especially fiction—may involve recalling personal memories from the hippocampus.

BRAIN AREAS USED IN READING
Reading uses various areas across the brain, from the visual cortex at the back, to areas of the frontal lobes so that the sound, spelling, and meaning of a word are linked together.

Hippocampus

2 THE VISUAL WORD-RECOGNITION AREA
This area, which evolved to make fine visual distinctions between different objects, is "hijacked" by the reader's brain when it is trained to recognize written text.

1 THE VISUAL CORTEX
The text is initially processed in the visual cortex, which sends the information along the "recognition"-processing route toward the language areas of the brain.

SKILLED READERS
While we are learning to read, our brains have to work very hard to translate the symbols on the page into sounds. This activates an area in the upper rear of the temporal lobe, in which sounds and vision are brought together. The process becomes automatic with practice, and the brain becomes more concerned with the meaning of the words. Hence, the areas concerned with meaning are more active in a skilled reader's brain (usually an adult's) during reading.

6–9 YEARS

9–18 YEARS

20–23 YEARS

READING DEVELOPMENT
These fMRI scans show that children learning to read rely on a brain area that matches written symbols to sounds (top). As skill develops, areas involving meaning (middle and bottom) become more active.

HOW LITERACY AFFECTS THE BRAIN

Literacy may improve the ability to make fine distinctions between spoken sounds. Tests have shown that when literate people hear a spoken sound they do not recognize as a word, a wider network of brain areas becomes active than in those who cannot read or write. This enables them to compare the unknown word with a greater number of possible matches, as they hear the word's phonological components more accurately.

READING IN YOUR MOTHER TONGUE

Languages are stored in separate areas in the brains of bilingual people, which means that different groups of neurons are used to generate each language. This prevents the two languages from interfering with one another. Damage to one area of the brain can result in the complete loss of one language, while the other remains intact. The brain treats a second language learned later in life differently from the mother tongue. A language that has been absorbed from infancy has wider and more intense associations than a second language, so the brain is more active when the person reads in the mother tongue than in any other language.

REVEALING THE MOTHER TONGUE
These colored electron micrographs of a bilingual person reading in the mother tongue (left) and a second language (right) show that the former sparks more brain activity, which suggests that it has a greater amount of associations and creates a more intense and meaningful experience.

READING IN MOTHER TONGUE   **READING IN SECOND LANGUAGE**

DYSLEXIA

Dyslexia is a language–development disorder with a genetic basis. It may affect 5 percent of the population, and is most obvious when a language such as English, has a complex mapping system between speech sounds and letters of the alphabet. One explanation for dyslexia, known as the phonological deficit hypothesis, is that dyslexics cannot analyze and remember the sounds contained in words. This slows down the learning of spoken language and makes it very difficult to map sounds to their corresponding letters of the alphabet when learning to read.

TREATING DYSLEXIA?

There is no cure for dyslexia, but dyslexics can improve reading skills through compensatory learning, using the help of specialist teachers to find ways to remember spellings. While reading is likely to remain slow and spelling error-prone, audio books, spell-checkers, and voice-recognition programs can help circumvent the problems of dyslexia.

VISUAL TECHNIQUES
Some cases of dyslexia are thought to be improved by using colored glasses or by wearing a patch over one eye.

HOW DYSLEXICS DIFFER
Dyslexics differ mostly in the brain area in which words are translated from visual symbols into sounds (shown in green on this fMRI scan). Research has found that dyslexics have more gray matter in this area than nondyslexics, but the significance of this finding is not fully understood.

REMEDIATION
Early studies suggest that a process of listening to slowed-down sounds can aid dyslexics. The circles in the left-hand scan show inactivity in crucial reading areas of a dyslexic's brain; the more detailed right-hand scan shows greater activity in reading areas after training.

frontal region   temporo-parietal region   frontal region   temporo-parietal region

DEVELOPMENTAL DYSLEXIC   **DEVELOPMENTAL DYSLEXIC AFTER TRAINING**

LANGUAGE DIFFERENCES

English speakers have a particularly hard time learning to read. English spelling rules are notoriously difficult to master, and skilled readers know that they cannot rely on letter-to-sound decoding rules, as there are too many exceptions–for example, "i" is pronounced differently in "ice" and "ink". For dyslexics, these exceptions are difficult to master, and learning to read and spell takes years longer than it does for non-dyslexics.

HYPERLEXIA

Hyperlexic children exhibit extremely advanced reading and writing skills, but may experience difficulty in understanding spoken words. They often have problems with social interaction and may have symptoms of autism. Some hyperlexics learn to spell fairly long words before the age of two, and to read sentences by three. Brain scans of one such child suggest that hyperlexia is neurologically opposite to dyslexia in that, when the child was reading, brain areas that are sluggish in dyslexic children were overactive.

ENGLISH-SPEAKING DYSLEXICS
Learning to read English can be challenging for dyslexics due to the number of words that do not follow standard spelling rules.

ITALIAN-SPEAKING DYSLEXICS
Italian dyslexics are more accurate at word recognition than their English counterparts, as Italian spelling rules are less complex.

PRECOCIOUS READERS
Hyperlexic children are fascinated by letters and numbers and learn how to read from an early age, but sometimes find it hard to understand spoken language.

MOST OF OUR MOMENT-TO-MOMENT EXPERIENCES PASS
RAPIDLY INTO OBLIVION, BUT A TINY FEW ARE ENCODED IN
THE BRAIN AS MEMORIES. WHEN WE REMEMBER AN EVENT,
THE NEURONS INVOLVED IN GENERATING THE ORIGINAL
EXPERIENCE ARE REACTIVATED. HOWEVER, RECOLLECTIONS
ARE NOT REPLAYS OF THE PAST, BUT RECONSTRUCTIONS
OF IT. THE PRIMARY PURPOSE OF MEMORY IS TO PROVIDE
INFORMATION TO GUIDE OUR ACTIONS IN THE PRESENT, AND
TO DO THIS EFFICIENTLY WE GENERALLY RETAIN ONLY THOSE
EXPERIENCES THAT ARE IN SOME WAY USEFUL. OUR RECALL

MEMORY

THE PRINCIPLES OF MEMORY

MEMORY IS A BROAD TERM USED TO REFER TO A NUMBER OF DIFFERENT BRAIN FUNCTIONS. THE COMMON FEATURE OF THESE FUNCTIONS IS THE RE-CREATION OF PAST EXPERIENCES BY THE SYNCHRONOUS FIRING OF NEURONS THAT WERE INVOLVED IN THE ORIGINAL EXPERIENCE.

WHAT IS MEMORY?

A memory may be the ability to recall a poem or recognize a face on demand; a vague vision of some long past event; the skill required to ride a bike; or the knowledge that your car keys are on the table. What all these phenomena have in common is that they involve learning, and total or partial reconstruction of a past experience.

Learning is a process in which neurons that fire together to produce a particular experience are altered so that they have a tendency to fire together again. The subsequent combined firing of the neurons reconstructs the original experience, producing a "recollection" of it. The act of recollecting makes the neurons involved even more likely to fire again in the future, so repeatedly reconstructing an event makes it increasingly easy to recall.

MEMORY PROCESS

The process of memory formation has several natural stages, from the initial selection and retention of information to recollection and, sometimes, eventual change or loss of the memory. Each stage has particular characteristics—and things that can go wrong.

STAGE	WHAT'S MEANT TO HAPPEN	WHAT CAN GO WRONG
Selection	The brain is designed to store information that will be useful at a later date and allow the rest to pass by unnoted.	Important events are neglected or irrelevant ones retrieved. You might fail to recall a person's name, but remember the mole on their nose.
Lay-down	Experience selected for memorizing is stored so that it is associated with relevant pre-existing memories and retained for an appropriate period.	Information may be "mis-filed," with faulty links between items. Or new items are not laid down, so it is hard to learn or to retain new memories.
Recollection	Current events should stimulate the recollection of appropriate memories—i.e. information that can guide future actions.	Current events fail to prompt useful memories, such as words, names, events—you know the information is there but you cannot grasp it.
Change	Each time a memory is recalled it is altered slightly to accommodate new information.	Alteration may create false memories.
Forgetting	Items start to be forgotten as soon as they have been registered, unless they are regularly refreshed. Unnecessary information is deleted.	Important or useful information is forgotten. Alternatively, unnecessary or even damaging memories are not.

SHORT- AND LONG-TERM MEMORY

Short-term memories generally stay with us only as long as we need them. A telephone number you use just once is an example. Short-term memories are held in the mind by a process of "working" memory (see opposite page). Long-term memories, in contrast, can be recalled years or even decades later. The address of your childhood home may be such a memory. In between these extremes, we have many medium-term memories, which may last for months or years and finally fade away.

Many different factors determine whether an experience or item of knowledge is destined to be a short- or a long-term memory. These include their emotional content, novelty, and the amount of effort that we make to practice recalling them.

Parietal lobe
Associated with spatial memories

Caudate nucleus
Associated with memories of instinctive skills

Mamillary body
Mamillary bodies are associated with episodic memories

Frontal lobe
Seat of working memory

Thalamus
Directs attention

Putamen
Associated with procedural skills

Amygdala
Emotional memories may be stored here

Cerebellum
Associated with conditioned memories—events linked by time

Hippocampus
Experiences are turned into memories here

Temporal lobe
Holds general knowledge

MEMORY AREAS
Memory involves a wide range of facets and functions, from deeply rooted instincts to conscious factual knowledge. These are associated with different areas throughout the brain.

FIRST AND LAST
If we are asked to learn a list of words, we are more likely to remember the first and last items than those in the middle. This is thought to be because we give the first greater attention, so it "sticks," while the last may be repeated more than the others because we can do this without another item crowding in behind.

TYPES OF MEMORY

We have five different types of memory, for particular purposes. Episodic memory comprises reconstructions of past experiences, including sensations and emotions; these usually unfold like a movie and are experienced from one's own point of view. Semantic memory is non-personal, factual knowledge that "stands alone." Working memory is the capacity to hold information in mind for just long enough to use it. Procedural "body" memories comprise learned actions, such as walking, swimming, or riding a bicycle. Implicit memories are those we don't know we have. They affect our actions in subtle ways; for example, you might take an inexplicable dislike to a new person because they remind you of someone nasty.

LEARNING IS GOOD FOR YOU

Learning involves making new connections between clusters of neurons in different parts of the brain. This builds up the brain, making it fitter. For example, practicing spatial skills such as finding your way around a city has been shown to increase the size of the rear hippocampus. The more connections you create, the better you can use what you learn and the longer it takes you to forget it.

ENLARGED AREAS
This image shows areas to do with implicit learning (red) and explicit skills (yellow) that have grown denser with practice.

Frontal lobe
Activity here ensures that episodic memories are not mistaken for real life

Cortical areas
Episodic memories activate the areas originally involved in the experience that is being recalled

Hippocampus
Events are turned into memories here

EPISODIC MEMORY
The parts of the brain involved in episodic memories depend on the content of the original experience. Highly visual experiences, for example, will activate visual areas of the brain, while remembering a person's voice will activate the auditory cortex.

Frontal lobe
Semantic memories are activated by frontal lobe areas that draw on stored knowledge to guide current behavior

Temporal lobe
The temporal lobes encode factual information, and activity here is a marker of facts being recalled

SEMANTIC MEMORY
Semantic memories are facts that may once have had a personal context but now stand as simple knowledge. The fact that a man once walked on the Moon, for example, may once have been part of your personal experience, but now it is just "knowledge."

Central executive
Holds entire plan, including language component

Language scratch pad
Uses Broca's area as "inner voice" that repeats information

Visual scratch pad
Maintains an image of what needs to be done, by activating areas near visual cortex

Central executive
Holds entire plan, including visual element

Phonological loop
"Inner ear" where the sounds of words are kept in mind

Visual cortex

LEFT SIDE　　**RIGHT SIDE**

WORKING MEMORY
One part of the frontal lobes, the central executive, holds a plan of action while calling up items from the rest of the brain. There are also two neural loops, for visual data and for language; these act as scratch pads, temporarily holding data until it is erased by the next job.

Caudate nucleus
Instinctive actions such as grooming are stored here

Putamen
Learned skills such as riding a bike are stored here

Cerebellum
Body skills depend on the cerebellum to direct timing and coordination

PROCEDURAL MEMORY
"Body" memories allow us to carry out ordinary motor actions automatically, once we have learned them. Such skills are stored in brain areas that lie beneath the cortex. They can be recalled to mind, but usually remain unconscious.

THE MEMORY WEB

MEMORIES ARE STORED IN FRAGMENTS THROUGHOUT THE BRAIN. ONE WAY TO ENVISAGE THE PATTERN OF MEMORIES IN THE BRAIN IS AS A COMPLEX WEB, IN WHICH THE THREADS SYMBOLIZE THE VARIOUS ELEMENTS OF A MEMORY THAT JOIN AT THE NODES, OR INTERSECTION POINTS, TO FORM A WHOLE, ROUNDED MEMORY OF AN OBJECT, PERSON, OR EVENT.

BRAIN–WIDE WEB

"Declarative" memories–episodes and facts you can bring to mind consciously– are laid down and accessed by the hippocampus but are stored throughout the brain. Each element of a memory–the sight, sound, word, or emotion that it consists of–is encoded in the same part of the brain that originally created that fragment. When you recall the experience, you recreate it in essence by reactivating the neural patterns generated during the original experience that was encoded to memory. Take, for example, the memory of a dog you once owned. Your recall of his color is created by the "color" area of the visual cortex; the recollection of walking with him is reconstructed (in part at least) by the motor area of your brain; his name is stored in the language area, and so on.

RECALLING MEMORY

The fMRI scan to the left shows activity in the sensory cortex when sensory aspects of a memory are recalled. The scan to the right shows the hippocampus, which plays a central role in memory management. Here, the person being scanned is actively suppressing a memory—note the lack of activity in the sensory cortex.

FACETS OF A MEMORY

Once a memory is sparked off, the hippocampus triggers various aspects of it in unison. If you remember a pet dog, different brain areas recall a variety of memories of the dog and peripheral items such as dog bowls, as well as memories of things connected to the idea of "dog."

FORMING MEMORIES

The initial perception of an experience is generated by a subset of neurons firing together. Synchronous firing makes the neurons involved more inclined to fire together again in the future, a tendency known as "potentiation," which recreates the original experience. If the same neurons fire together often, they eventually become permanently sensitized to each other, so that if one fires, the others do as well. This is known as "long-term potentiation."

Neuron
Existing synapse
Input
Nucleus

1 INPUT
An external stimulus triggers two neurons to fire simultaneously. In future, if one fires, the other is likely to fire, too.

Input
New link forged
Increasing activity
New synapse

New link established
Regular input
Facilitated synapse

2 CIRCUIT FORMATION
A third neuron fires. One of the initial pair is stimulated to fire with it, triggering the second, so the three become linked.

3 INCREASING ACTIVITY
The three neurons are now sensitized to one another, so that if one fires, the other two are likely to fire as well.

DISTRIBUTED MEMORIES

Our memories are distributed throughout the brain, so even if one part of an experience is lost, many others will remain. One benefit of such a distributed storage system is that it makes long-term memories more or less indestructible. If they were held in a single brain area, damage to that place–for example, from a stroke or head injury–would eradicate the memory completely. As it is, brain trauma and degeneration may nibble away at memories but rarely destroy them entirely. You may lose a person's name, for example, but not the memory of their face.

Neighboring neuron
Circuit joins network of neurons
Input
New neuron assimilated

EXPANDING WEB

The memory web spreads through the brain as existing neurons make connections with new neurons by firing together.

ACCESSING MEMORIES

Events that are destined to be recalled are more strongly encoded to begin with than events that are later forgotten. In one study, 16 people viewed 120 photographs and answered which pictures were taken indoors or outdoors. Each image was then shown once again. After 15 minutes, the subjects were shown the photos again, along with some new ones, and asked if they remembered them. Scans taken during the test show strong activation of the hippocampus in response to recalled photos at the first viewing, but less activity in this area when the photos were repeated. This pattern is a "marker" for familiarity (see below).

— NOVEL REMEMBERED   — NOVEL FORGOTTEN
— REPEATED REMEMBERED   — REPEATED FORGOTTEN

HIPPOCAMPAL ACTIVITY AND MEMORY FORMATION
Things that get remembered are marked by high activity in the hippocampus when they are first experienced but less activity when they are seen a second time. This distinguishes the recalled scenes from those that are new or forgotten.

PARAHIPPOCAMPAL ACTIVITY
When you recall an episode from your life, the hippocampus and the area around it (shown in yellow on this fMRI scan) are activated. During memory recall, the hippocampus is busy pulling together the various facets of the memory from widely distributed areas of the brain.

INABILITY TO STORE

In 1953 surgery was performed on a patient known as HM to relieve the symptoms of severe epileptic seizures. The operation involved removing a large part of the hippocampus. This controlled the seizures, but it also produced a severe memory deficit. From the time HM woke up from the operation he was unable to lay down conscious memories. Day-to-day events remained in his mind for only a few seconds or minutes. When he met someone, even a person he had seen many times a day, year after year, he did not recognize them. HM believed himself to be a young man right into his eighties, because the years since his operation did not, effectively, exist for him. His case shows how essential the hippocampus is for memory storage.

THE MISSING PIECE
The hippocampus is embedded deep in the temporal lobes. Experiences "flow through it" constantly, and some of them are encoded in memory through a process of long-term potentiation. Thereafter, the hippocampus is involved in retrieving most types of memory.

Hippocampus

Large areas of hippocampus removed from HM's brain in both hemispheres

3¼in (8cm)

SIDE VIEW

VIEW FROM BELOW

LAYING DOWN A MEMORY

MOST EXPERIENCES LEAVE NO PERMANENT TRACE. A FEW, THOUGH, ARE SO STRIKING THAT THEY ALTER THE STRUCTURE OF THE BRAIN BY FORGING NEW CONNECTIONS BETWEEN NEURONS. THESE CHANGES MAKE IT POSSIBLE FOR THE NEURAL ACTIVITY THAT GENERATED THE INITIAL EXPERIENCE TO BE RECONSTRUCTED, OR "RECOLLECTED," AT A LATER DATE.

THE ANATOMY OF MEMORY

Only experiences giving rise to unusually prolonged and/or intense neural activity become encoded as memories. It takes up to two years to consolidate the changes that create a long-term memory (see sequence below) but, once encoded, that memory may remain available for life. Long-term memories include events from a person's life (episodic memories) and impersonal facts (semantic memories). Together, these are termed "declarative memories," since they can be recalled consciously ("declared"). Procedural (body) memories and implicit (unconscious) memories may also be stored long-term.

Visual association cortex

Hippocampus
The hippocampus encodes new memories, and helps recall some others

Somatosensory cortex

Gustatory association cortex

Auditory association cortex

Amygdala

Olfactory cortex

MEMORY MAKERS
Experiences that become memories are usually prolonged or emotionally charged, and register strongly in the sensory cortices and hippocampus.

FORMING A LONG-TERM MEMORY

🕐 0.2 seconds Attention

The brain can absorb only a finite amount of sensory input at any point. It can sample a little input about several events at once, or focus attention on one event and extract lots of information from that alone. Attention causes the neurons that register the event to fire more frequently. Such activity makes the experience more intense; it also increases the likelihood that the event will be encoded as a memory. This is because the more a neuron fires, the stronger connections it makes with other brain cells.

MEMORABLE EVENT
Zooming in on an event helps capture it as a memory, like a camera taking a snapshot.

Thalamus
Maintains activity in brain regarding target of attention

Frontal lobe
Keeps attention locked to target by inhibiting distractions

INTENSE FOCUS
Attention helps us memorize events by intensifying our experience of them.

🕐 0.25 seconds Emotion

Intensely emotional experiences, such as the birth of a child, are more likely to be laid down in memory because emotion increases attention. The emotional information from a stimulus is processed initially along an unconscious pathway that leads to the amygdala; this can produce an emotional response even before the person knows what they are reacting to, as in the "fight or flight" response.

Some traumatic events may be permanently stored in the amygdala.

EMOTIONAL EVENTS
Personal interactions and other emotional events "grab" attention, so are more likely to be stored.

EMOTION PATHWAY
The amygdala helps keep an emotional experience "live" by replaying it in a loop, which begins the encoding of a memory.

Motor cortex

Auditory cortex

Frontal area

Amygdala
Triggers instant emotional reaction

Visual cortex

🕐 0.2–0.5 seconds Sensation

Most memories derive from events that included sights, sounds, and other sensory experiences. The more intense the sensations, the more likely it is that the experience is remembered. The sensational parts of such "episodic" memories may later be forgotten, leaving only a residue of factual knowledge. For example, a person's first experience of seeing the Washington Monument may be reduced to the simple "fact" of what the tower looks like. When it is recalled, it triggers a ghost of a visual image, encoded in the sight area of the brain.

Sensory cortices
Perceptions start to be formed in sensory cortices

Sensory signal
Information flows to hippocampus

Hippocampus

TASTE
Sensory perceptions, such as taste, sight, or smell, form the raw material of memories.

FORMING PERCEPTIONS
Sensations are combined in association areas, to form conscious perceptions.

HIPPOCAMPUS REPLACEMENT

Neuroscientists from the University of Southern California, in Los Angeles, have developed an artificial hippocampus that may one day help people with dementia halt memory loss. The researchers first devised a model of how the hippocampus performs by observing the input–output patterns of the real thing. Then they built the model into a silicon chip designed to interface with the brain, taking the place of damaged tissue. One side of the chip records the electrical activity coming in from the rest of the brain, while the other sends appropriate electrical instructions back out to the brain.

MEMORY CHIP
The chip is designed to be spliced into the hippocampus and communicate with the brain through two arrays of electrodes, placed on either side of the damaged area.

THE LOCATION OF MEMORIES

After consolidation, long-term memories are stored throughout the brain as groups of neurons that are primed to fire together in the same pattern that created the original experience. "Whole" memories are divided into their components (sensations, emotions, thoughts, and so on); each component is stored in the brain area that initiated it. Groups of neurons in the visual cortex, for instance, will encode a sight, and neurons in the amygdala will store an emotion. The simultaneous firing of all these groups constructs the memory in its entirety.

LASTING IMPRESSION
Some memories seem to be cast in stone. In fact, no recollection is ever perfectly sharp or complete.

Hippocampus
Auditory area
Amygdala

MEMORY STORE
Memories are encoded in the neurons that created them: for example, sounds in the auditory cortex and emotions in the amygdala. The hippocampus pulls them together.

⏱ 0.5 seconds–10 minutes
Working memory

Short-term, or "working," memory is like text on a blackboard that is constantly refreshed. It begins with an experience, and continues as that experience is "held in mind" by repetition. A telephone number, for example, may be repeated for as long as it takes to dial. Working memory is thought to involve two neural circuits (see p.157), around which the information is kept alive for as long as it is needed. One circuit is for visual and spatial information, and the other for sound. The routes of the circuits encompass the sensory cortices, where the experience is registered, and the frontal lobes, where it is consciously noted. The flow of information into and around these circuits is controlled by neurons in the prefrontal cortex.

Visual circuit
Loops between sensory and prefrontal cortices keep information "live"

Frontal lobe
Parts of the frontal lobe control flow and maintenance of working memory

Auditory circuit

MENTAL NOTES
Auditory and visual data circulates on two separate memory loops.

⏱ 10 minutes–2 years
Hippocampal processing

Particularly striking experiences "break out" from working memory and travel to the hippocampus, where they undergo further processing. They cause neural activity that loops around coiled layers of tissue; the hippocampal neurons start to encode this information permanently by a process called long-term potentiation (see p.158). The strongest information "plays back" to the parts of the brain that first registered it. A sight, for example, returns to the visual cortex, where it is replayed as an echo of the original event.

Hippocampus
Information circulates here, then returns to brain areas where it originated

Entorhinal cortex
Collects information from many different areas of brain

One-way system
Information follows a one-way path as it is encoded

PREPARATION FOR STORAGE
This activity in the hippocampus begins to turn short-term memories into those that might remain for life.

⏱ 2 years onward
Consolidation

It takes up to two years for a memory to become firmly consolidated in the brain, and even after that it may be altered or lost. During this time, the neural firing patterns that encode an experience are played back and forth between the hippocampus and the cortex. This prolonged, repetitive "dialogue" causes the pattern to be shifted from the hippocampus to the cortex; this may happen in order to free up hippocampal processing space for new information. The dialogue takes place largely during sleep. The "quiet" or slow-wave phase of sleep is thought to be more important to this process than rapid eye movement sleep (see p.188).

KEY
— CORTICAL SIGNALS
— HIPPOCAMPAL SIGNALS

AMPLITUDE (Z): 15, 14, 12, 10, 8, 6, 4, 2, 0, -2
TIME (S): 0, 1, 2, 3, 4, 5, 6, 7

Auditory cortex
Hippocampus

ECHOING SIGNALS
A hippocampal neuron (orange) talks to cells in the auditory cortex (purple), echoing their activity pattern. Hippocampal and cortical cells form almost identical copies of the same experience.

RECALL AND RECOGNITION

MEMORIES OCCUR WHEN THE BRAIN "REPLAYS" A PATTERN OF NEURAL ACTIVITY THAT WAS ORIGINALLY GENERATED IN RESPONSE TO A PARTICULAR EVENT. SO SIMILAR IS THE PATTERN TO THE ORIGINAL THAT THE MEMORY ECHOES THE BRAIN'S PERCEPTION OF THE REAL EVENT. BUT THESE REPLAYS ARE NEVER IDENTICAL TO THE ORIGINAL—IF THEY WERE, WE WOULD NOT KNOW THE DIFFERENCE BETWEEN THE GENUINE EXPERIENCE AND THE MEMORY.

THE NATURE OF MEMORIES

When we recall an event, we reexperience it–but only up to a point. Even when "lost" in reminiscence, we maintain some awareness of the present moment, so the neural activity is not identical to the one that produced the remembered event. Rather, the experience is that of the original mixed with an awareness of the current situation. This experience of remembering "overwrites" the memory, so each time an event is brought to mind it is really a recollection of the last time we remembered it. Hence, memories gradually change over the years, until eventually they might bear very little resemblance to the original event.

SENSORY MEMORY
Tests using fMRI scans show that objects we associate with specific smells spark activity in the olfactory cortex (largest yellow area). In this way, cues trigger all senses, conjuring detailed memories.

STATE-DEPENDENT MEMORY

If you learn or experience something when in a certain state of mind or while concurrently experiencing a particular sensation, you will subsequently recall it more readily when you are again in that state. For example, if you read a book on a sunny beach during a vacation, you may seem to forget it completely when you get home. But years later, on another sunny beach, the plot may come flooding back. Similarly, certain behaviors may be learned when in a particular situation or state of mind, and subsequently displayed only when in the same situation or state of mind, and "forgotten" at other times, giving the impression that the person has more than one personality.

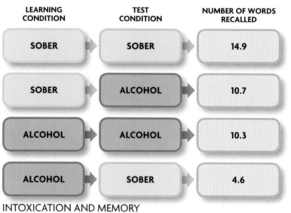

LEARNING CONDITION	TEST CONDITION	NUMBER OF WORDS RECALLED
SOBER	SOBER	14.9
SOBER	ALCOHOL	10.7
ALCOHOL	ALCOHOL	10.3
ALCOHOL	SOBER	4.6

INTOXICATION AND MEMORY
Subjects drank a nonalcoholic or alcoholic beverage prior to studying a list of words, later recalling them while sober or intoxicated. Those intoxicated in both phases recalled more words than those intoxicated in the study phase only.

MEMORY AIDS
Memories of past events are often "jogged" into consciousness when we re-encounter some of the sensations involved in the original experience. Photographs and similar memory aids work in this way. Even if the sensations they trigger are not identical to the original ones, they are likely to be similar enough to jog memories of the same period.

SPATIAL MEMORY

The structure of the human brain reveals just how important spatial orientation and memory are for our species. The whole parietal lobe of the brain–the area under the crown of the skull–is given over to "maps" of our bodies and of our position in space. Also, a sizeable part of the hippocampus is concerned with registering the landscape through which we travel and laying down memory maps. Damage to either of these areas can seriously affect a person's ability to find his or her way around. If the "navigation" area of the hippocampus is affected by stroke or injury, for instance, a person may lose the ability to remember new routes.

MAZE-MINDED
People who can find their way out of mazes use the hippocampus in both hemispheres. Those who remain lost use one side only.

"THE KNOWLEDGE"

Some people have better memories for places than others. In part, this is a matter of habit and training—those whose lives depend on their ability to find their way around vast tracts of land naturally attend more closely to landmarks. London taxi drivers, for example, are famously adept at finding their way around the city's labyrinthine streets. Their skill is developed during a two-year training, known as "the knowledge," during which time they "exercise" the part of the hippocampus responsible for spatial memory. The training seems to increase the size of the hippocampus, much as a muscle is enlarged by weight training.

NATURAL NAVIGATORS
A brain-scanning study found that the rear hippocampus, which encodes spatial memories, is larger in taxi drivers.

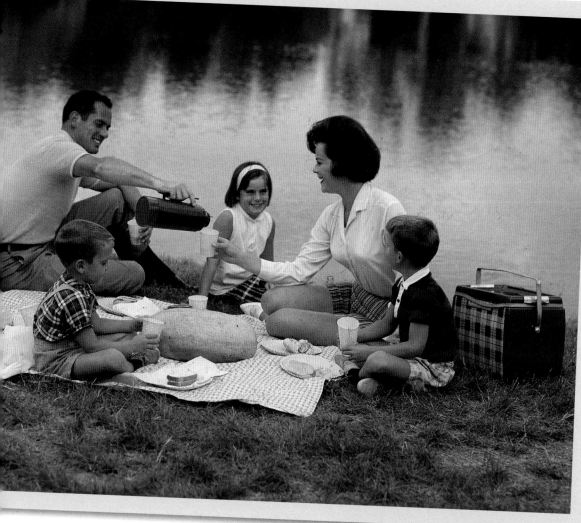

Déjà vu is characterized by a sudden, intense feeling of familiarity and the sense that you have experienced the same moment before. One explanation for this is that the new situation triggers a memory of a similar experience in the past, but the recollection is confused with the present as it is recalled, creating a sense of recognition without bringing to mind the previous event. Research suggests that déjà vu occurs when a new situation is mistakenly "marked" as familiar when processed in the limbic system. Jamais vu, by contrast, occurs when one is in a situation that should be familiar, but which seems strange. You might suddenly find your own home to be unfamiliar, for instance. Jamais vu is thought to be a glitch in recognition, whereby the emotional input that usually accompanies familiar experiences fails to occur.

RECOGNITION

Recognizing a person fully involves collating a huge number of memories. They include different types of facts about the person–I know him/he owns a dog/he walked right past me the last time I saw him/his name is Bill. At the same time, you have an emotional reaction to the person based on memories, which produces the feeling of familiarity. Most or all of this happens unconsciously– you see the person and immediately "know" who it is.

FACE-RECOGNITION AREA

SITE OF RECOGNITION
This area processes the sight of a face (see p.84) by extracting information about expression and familiarity.

EMOTIONAL RECOGNITION
When you spot someone you know, the information is first processed by the visual cortex, and is then shunted through the brain along different pathways (see pp.84–85) as shown on this diagram (right). One path travels through the limbic areas that generate a sense of familiarity–separate from conscious recognition–when a familiar person is seen. If this route is blocked, a person may recognize consciously that they know a person, but feel strangely detached from them. Without this input, even one's nearest relatives would feel like strangers.

RECOGNITION PATHWAYS
The cortical path (red) processes data about a person's movements and intentions. Another (purple) generates conscious knowledge of who a person is. The limbic path (yellow) generates a sense of familiarity.

Cortical path

Emotional and sensory signals combined

Limbic path

Frontal lobe

New signal compared with stored recollection

Hippocampus

Visual cortex

RECOGNITION ROUTE

RECOGNIZING A PERSON
Recognizing a person and assigning them their correct name is a complicated process. When it works properly, it seems easy, because it happens unconsciously and apparently instantly. But if the process fails at any stage, recognition is incomplete.

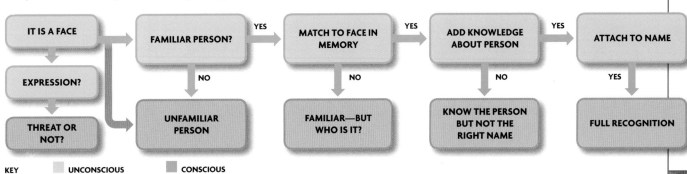

IT IS A FACE

EXPRESSION?

THREAT OR NOT?

FAMILIAR PERSON? — YES — MATCH TO FACE IN MEMORY — YES — ADD KNOWLEDGE ABOUT PERSON — YES — ATTACH TO NAME

NO — UNFAMILIAR PERSON

NO — FAMILIAR—BUT WHO IS IT?

NO — KNOW THE PERSON BUT NOT THE RIGHT NAME

YES — FULL RECOGNITION

KEY   UNCONSCIOUS   CONSCIOUS

UNUSUAL MEMORY

"BAD" MEMORY USUALLY MEANS FORGETTING. BUT THERE ARE MANY OTHER TYPES OF MEMORY PROBLEM: CLEAR BUT FALSE RECOLLECTION, BLURRED MEMORIES, AND INTRUSIVE FLASHBACK MEMORIES OF TRAUMATIC EVENTS. IT IS EVEN POSSIBLE TO REMEMBER THINGS TOO CLEARLY.

FORGETTING

The purpose of human memory is to use past events to guide future actions, and keeping a perfect and complete record of the past is not a useful way to achieve this. It is more important to be able to generalize from experience. When you first drive a car, for example, you learn the pedal positions of the first vehicle you use. Subsequently, when you get in any car, you assume that the pedal positions are the same. The specific memory of the layout of one particular car is lost while the general knowledge, the position of the pedals, is retained. Forgetting specifics is not a fault—it is essential.

FALSE MEMORY

Our brains sometimes lay down memories that are false from the start. This usually happens because an event is misinterpreted. For example, if you expect to see a particular thing, something similar may easily be mistaken for it. The memory will be of what was assumed to be there, rather than what really was. False memories can also be created during, what seems like recall. If a person is persuaded that a given thing happened, the event may be "patched together" from scraps of other memories and then experienced as a "real" recollection.

HIPPOCAMPAL ACTIVITY   **FRONTAL AND PARIETAL ACTIVITY**

CONFIDENT RECALL
True memory (left) sparks activity in the hippocampus, which "lays down" memory. Confident recall of false memory (right) activates frontal areas associated with familiarity rather than precise recollections.

TRAUMATIC MEMORY

Post Traumatic Stress Disorder (PTSD) is a condition in which people have vivid "flashback" memories of a traumatic experience (see page 233). Such memories can ambush a person out of the blue–the sound of a car back-firing, for example, may plunge a soldier back into the middle of a gunfight, complete with the emotions experienced at the time. Emotionally traumatic experiences are by their nature more likely to be remembered because emotion amplifies experience. Yet there is also a strong incentive to put such events "out of mind" and it seems the brain has a mechanism that can make this possible. Experts have found that the brain is able to block memories at will (see below).

ACTIVE SUPPRESSION   **ACTIVE RECALL**

ACTIVE MEMORY
Emotional memory recall activates the hippocampus and amygdala (emotion). If the memory is suppressed, there is less activity in these areas and in brain areas that recreate the sensations associated with the recalled event.

CHOOSING TO FORGET

You can, up to a point, choose to forget. In one study, two groups of volunteers studied a list of pairs of words. One group was invited to "block out" one half of the pairs. Later, both groups were shown the words again and asked if they recognized them. The blocking out group were worse at recognizing the words that they had tried to forget—even when offered money as an inducement to recall them. Brain images of the group suggested that the deliberate "forgetting" was achieved by frontal-lobe activity, which inhibited the process of laying down the memory.

DECIDING WHAT TO DO IN A COMPLEX WORLD TAKES
THOUGHT. BY THINKING WE CAN EXPLORE THE POTENTIAL
CONSEQUENCES OF OUR ACTIONS IN OUR IMAGINATION.
THIS, IN TURN, INVOLVES HOLDING ONE OR MORE IDEAS IN
MIND AND MANIPULATING THEM. THINKING IS AN ACTIVE,
CONSCIOUS, ATTENTION-DEMANDING PROCESS THAT
USUALLY DRAWS ON SEVERAL AREAS OF THE BRAIN.
THINKING UNDERPINS SOME PARTICULARLY HUMAN
ABILITIES AND TENDENCIES, INCLUDING CREATIVITY AND
THE CONSTRUCTION OF IMAGINATIVE EXPLANATIONS

THINKING

INTELLIGENCE

"INTELLIGENCE" REFERS TO THE ABILITY TO LEARN ABOUT, LEARN FROM, UNDERSTAND, AND INTERACT WITH ONE'S ENVIRONMENT. IT EMBRACES MANY DIFFERENT TYPES OF SKILLS, SUCH AS PHYSICAL DEXTERITY, VERBAL FLUENCY, CONCRETE AND ABSTRACT REASONING, SENSORY DISCRIMINATION, EMOTIONAL SENSITIVITY, NUMERACY, AND ALSO THE ABILITY TO FUNCTION WELL IN SOCIETY.

THE BRAIN'S SUPERHIGHWAY

The frontal lobes have long been considered the seat of intelligence since damage to them affects the ability to concentrate, make sound judgments, and so on. Yet frontal-lobe damage does not always affect a person's IQ ("intelligence quotient," measured by testing spatial, verbal, and mathematical dexterity), so other brain areas must also be involved. Recent research suggests that intelligence relies on a neural "superhighway" that links the frontal lobes, which plan and organize, with the parietal lobes, which integrate sensory information. The speed and efficiency with which the frontal lobes receive a stream of ready-to-use data via this route may affect IQ.

Pathway of data from parietal lobe to frontal lobe

Parietal-lobe areas in both hemispheres

Frontal-lobe areas in both hemispheres

Frontal-lobe areas in left hemisphere

Parietal-lobe areas in left hemisphere

WHY WE CAN'T DO TWO THINGS AT ONCE

If you try to do something while still working on a previous task, your brain stalls. This may be because the prefrontal cortex, which disengages attention from one task and switches it to another, cannot do so instantly, resulting in a short "processing gap." The brain is also unable to do two similar things simultaneously because the tasks compete for the same neurons. For example, listening to speech while reading words activates overlapping brain areas, so is difficult to achieve, but listening to speech while looking at a landscape is easy.

JUGGLING TASKS
The brain needs a minimum of 300 milliseconds to switch from one distinct task to the next. This "processing gap" makes a task combination such as talking on a phone while driving potentially lethal.

LOCATING INTELLIGENCE
There are regions in both sides of the brain (orange) as well as areas in the left hemisphere only (blue) that are strongly associated with intelligence and reasoning. The arcuate fasciculus (green), a thick bundle of nerve fibers, provides a neural link between the parietal and frontal lobes.

FACTORS IN INTELLIGENCE

Many different factors, relating to both "nature" and "nurture," affect IQ. One is physical development. A brain that has received optimum nutrition during gestation and infancy is primed to work well. Genes influence intelligence, but so do social factors—good nutrition, for example, is clearly less achievable in poverty. Children from poor and/or culturally deprived homes who are moved into a more privileged environment have shown an increase in IQ by up to 16 points (see panel, right). This is thought to be due to increased talking and reading, and interacting in a positive way with family members.

GENETIC LEGACY
The influence of genes is said to account for about half of the difference in IQ between two people. Identical twins are more likely than others to have the same, or very similar, IQ.

WHAT CONTRIBUTES TO INTELLIGENCE?

Tests for IQ measure general intelligence rather than quantity of knowledge or the level of a specific skill. A score of 100 is average, and the vast majority of people fall in the range of 80–120. High scores are correlated with a number of both social and physical factors.

FACTOR	EFFECT
Genes	There are thought to be about 50 different genes related directly to IQ, but so far very few have been identified. Identical twins raised apart typically have very similar IQs, even when raised in strikingly different environments.
Brain size	Those with bigger brains compared to other members of the same sex seem to have a slight intelligence advantage. Overall size, however, may be less important than the size, or neural density, of areas concerned with reasoning.
Signaling efficiency	The smoothness and speed of neural signaling may determine how much information is available for action and how well it can be integrated into plans. Depression, fatigue, and some types of illness reduce efficiency.
Environment	A stimulating social environment in infancy is essential for normal brain development and continues to be important throughout childhood. Verbal interaction seems to be especially useful for IQ.

MAKING DECISIONS

Intelligence is largely the ability to make sensible decisions, which involves calculating pros and cons. First, the brain assesses the "goal value"–the reward expected as a result of the decision. Next, it calculates the "decision value"–the net outcome, or the reward minus the cost. Finally, the brain makes a prediction of how likely it is that the decision will deliver the reward envisaged, which can be compared with the actual outcome, giving a "prediction error." The more complex the problem, the more the frontal areas of the brain are involved.

Decision values · Goal values · Prediction errors

ACTIVATION MAP
Activity in the medial orbito-frontal cortex correlates with goal values (red); activity in the central orbitofrontal cortex (yellow) correlates with decision values; and activity in the ventral striatum, part of the caudate nucleus and putamen, correlates with prediction errors (green).

Step 1 The premotor cortex (where actions are prepared) is activated first, to make basic decisions about unconscious physical movements.

PREMOTOR CORTEX

Step 2 If more than a simple physical action is needed, an area of cortex slightly farther forward is brought in, to plan and refine a course of action.

PREMOTOR CORTEX

Step 3 If the decision is made in a complicated context, prefrontal areas concerned with comparing past and present situations are activated.

LATERAL PREFRONTAL CORTEX

Step 4 Finally, the most frontal area of the brain kicks in, combining all the information gathered so far into a single, fully integrated plan.

FRONTAL LOBE

THE ROLE OF EMOTIONS

Decision-making and judgment are profoundly affected by emotions. This is because emotion "drives" action–without it, the brain is like a car with steering but no power. Moods may have a profound effect on the outcome of decision-making. Being in a pleasant, anxious, or neutral mood, or experiencing extreme emotion, can have a significant short-term influence on areas of the brain that are critical for reasoning, intelligence, and other types of higher cognition.

MOODS
The ventrolateral prefrontal cortex is shown in fMRI scans to work harder if a person is in the "wrong" mood for a task, perhaps by stifling emotions.

Active areas

STATES OF MIND
Research shows that mild anxiety improves performance in some mental tasks, but makes it worse in others. For example, word tasks are performed better in an anxious mood, while face-recognition tasks come easier to those in a pleasant state of mind.

TASK SUCCESS RATE

WORDS · FACES

KEY ■ PLEASANT ■ NEUTRAL ■ ANXIOUS

THE NUMERICAL BRAIN

Number sense seems "hard-wired" into the human brain. Babies as young as six months can spot the difference between one and two. One study recorded electrical activity from babies' brains while they watched a pair of soft toys. The toys were then momentarily screened and one was removed, then the screen was lifted to reveal just one toy. The babies' brains registered the "error" by activating the same circuit known to mark error detection in adults, suggesting that even very young babies are able to recognize such discrepencies.

TESTING BABIES
When two toys in this test "become" one, the brains of babies register an error, showing they can discriminate between one and two.

TWO STUFFED TOYS DISPLAYED

TOYS SCREENED MOMENTARILY

ONLY ONE TOY IS REVEALED WHEN SCREEN IS REMOVED

Mid-frontal area · Intraparietal sulcus · Superior temporal sulcus

NUMBER ACTIVITY
Several brain areas deal with numbers: estimates come from the intraparietal sulcus; the superior temporal sulcus deals with numerical values in abstract form; and the mid-frontal area notes when numbers seem wrong.

FMRI SCANS OF ADULT BRAINS

FMRI SCANS OF CHILDREN'S BRAINS

NUMBER DEVIATION
When confronted with a numerical "error," such as the number of items on view unexpectedly changing, children's brains register the change in an area that estimates quantities of what is seen. Adults engage both this area and one concerned with abstract numbers. This suggests that the ability to "guesstimate" develops earlier than the ability to think of numbers in the abstract, and also that, as numeracy develops, our brains deal with numbers in different ways.

CREATIVITY AND HUMOR

CREATIVITY IS THE ABILITY TO RECONFIGURE WHAT YOU KNOW, OFTEN IN THE LIGHT OF NEW INFORMATION, AND COME UP WITH AN ORIGINAL CONCEPT OR IDEA. IN ORDER TO BE CREATIVE, A PERSON MUST BE CRITICAL, SELECTIVE, AND GENERALLY INTELLIGENT.

THE CREATIVE PROCESS

Our brains are bombarded with stimuli, much of which is filtered out before it reaches consciousness. Focusing on immediate tasks is vital in day-to-day life, but to be creative it is necessary to open our minds to new inputs and memories that may not seem useful. This process allows us to connect things that otherwise stay apart. The brain state most conducive to kindling new ideas is relaxed attentiveness, or the resting state (see p.184), characterized by alpha waves (see p.181). Being creative involves connecting information and reconfiguring it to make something new. The resting state allows information to flow around the brain. The "eureka moment" that occurs when several thoughts combine into a new idea is marked by a change in brain activity involving a shift to the temporal lobe and anterior cingulate cortex. A period of critical assessment may follow, marked by a switch from the resting state to a task-oriented pattern centered on frontal lobe activity.

Anterior cingulate cortex (ACC)

Right superior temporal gyrus

WHOLE BRAIN CONNECTIVITY
When the brain defocuses, information flows more freely around its highways of connecting fibers, as shown in this DTI scan.

"EUREKA MOMENT" AREAS
Activity in the superior temporal sulcus in "eureka moments" signifies recognition of a new association of ideas. Critical analysis of new ideas sparks ACC activity.

CREATIVE INDIVIDUALS

Everyone is creative, but those who can put their brains into "idle" on demand are more likely to open up their minds to new possibilities and generate original ideas. This process only works, however, if the brain is already "primed" with knowledge that can be combined with the new material. Artists who have mastered the basics of their discipline, for instance, have a foundation of knowledge onto which improvements and changes can be fused. Their expertise allows this process to operate unconsciously, leaving greater resources available for processing new stimuli. Creative people also have relatively high IQs (see p.166), plus the ability to snap back to alertness when a new idea is hatched and to subject that idea to rigorous scrutiny and criticism. Ideas that survive this second creative thought process are likely to be valuable and therefore judged as genuinely new.

MUSICIANS
Brain-imaging studies of musicians at work show that frontal areas keep attention targeted when they play by rote, but turn off in improvization so ideas can "float."

STARRY NIGHT
The artist Van Gogh worked on the painting *Starry Night* while in an asylum. He may have had temporal lobe epilepsy and/ or bipolar disorder, both of which are associated with high levels of creativity.

CREATIVITY AND MADNESS
Creativity and some types of insanity share certain features, such as intense imagination, a tendency to link things that may seem unconnected to others, and openness to ideas that others may swiftly discount. The difference between highly creative people and those who tip into madness is that creative people maintain insight. They recognize that their imaginings are not real and remain able to control any bizarre symptoms and channel them into their work.

MENTAL-DISORDER TESTING
Very creative people score highly on tests for mental disorders but rarely fulfill the diagnostic criteria for these conditions, so their mental states can be seen as being somewhere between normal and insane.

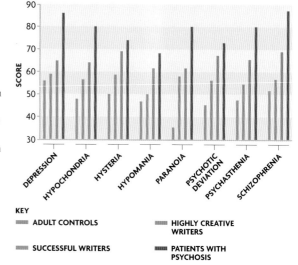

SCORE

90
80
70
60
50
40
30

DEPRESSION
HYPOCHONDRIA
HYSTERIA
HYPOMANIA
PARANOIA
PSYCHOTIC DEVIATION
PSYCHASTHENIA
SCHIZOPHRENIA

KEY
- ADULT CONTROLS
- SUCCESSFUL WRITERS
- HIGHLY CREATIVE WRITERS
- PATIENTS WITH PSYCHOSIS

HUMOR

A lot of humor arises from the juxtaposition of apparently unconnected ideas, which is similar to the process underlying creativity. Studies looking at how humorous interplay between coworkers affects workplace innovation suggest that keeping workers laughing may "jump-start" their creative faculties, perhaps because humor forces people to attend to "distractions," making them more open to new information. Brain-imaging studies have shown that humor stimulates the brain's "reward" circuit and elevates circulating levels of dopamine, which is linked to motivation and pleasurable anticipation.

EXPECTATION OF INTENTION

INCONGRUITY

BRAIN AREAS LINKED TO HUMOR
The first frame sparks activity in brain areas linked to predicting intention—here, the cartoon character's. The next frame activates areas linked to surprise and emotion, suggesting that such incongruity is central to humor.

EXPECTATION OF INTENTION

APPRECIATION

BRAIN IMAGING DURING CARTOON READING
The top row of fMRI scans show brain areas activated by the first frame of the cartoon above, including the temporal and parietal areas and the cerebellum. These become active when, by observing a person's actions, we "know" what their intentions are. When the expectation is subverted, as in the second frame, it creates activity in the left amygdala (bottom row, circled). The amygdala is active in emotion, and the left side is particularly linked to pleasant feelings.

TURNING ON CREATIVITY

As soon as we can categorize a stimulus we tend not to scrutinize it further, but immediately edit it out. So, when we see a dog, we mentally label it as "dog" and do not stop to take in every detail. The frontal lobes manage this editing process, and there is some evidence to suggest that if activity in this area is inhibited, people "take in" more. Tests using transcranial magnetic stimulation (TMS) to "turn off" the frontal lobes show that creative skills can emerge as frontal-lobe activity decreases.

TMS TEST
Volunteers subjected to TMS displayed new creative drawing skills when frontal-lobe activity was turned off.

PRACTICE

BEFORE

DURING

AFTER

BELIEF AND SUPERSTITION

OUR BRAINS ARE CONSTANTLY TRYING TO MAKE SENSE OF THE WORLD IN ORDER TO GUIDE OUR ACTIONS. ONE WAY OF DOING THIS IS BY CREATING EXPLANATORY STORIES OR IDEAS INTO WHICH WE FIT OUR EXPERIENCES. SUCH FRAMEWORKS ARE OFTEN USEFUL, BUT MAY NOT ALWAYS BE CORRECT.

BELIEVING IS SEEING

Most people have some kind of belief system, which forms a framework for their experience. Some were taught their beliefs, while others arrived at them by examining their experience and working out their own interpretation. Once a belief system has been formed, it acts both as an explanation for what has happened in the past and also a "working hypothesis" that is projected onto the world. For example, if a person believes that the world is governed by a benign supernatural being, they will "see" events such as coincidences or strokes of good fortune as evidence of this, while a person with a materialist belief system would interpret them merely as chance happenings. People who are quick to see meaningful connections between, for example, random events are more inclined than others to have a magical or superstitious belief system.

HOLY TOAST
People with a tendency toward magical thinking are quicker to see patterns like the "face" in this piece of toast. They are also more likely to see such things as "meaningful"—perhaps even as signs from God.

PATTERN-MAKING
The ability to "see" patterns helps us make sense of the world and respond appropriately. But we can be both too good and too poor at it.

Autism
Autistic people do not see patterns that are obvious to most of us, so get swamped by information, all of which seems equally important.

Literal-mindedness
Failure to recognize subtle patterns leads to concrete-mindedness, such as failure to understand metaphors (as seen in Asperger's syndrome).

Superstition
Too much pattern-making may lead people to "see" things that are not there, or make links between events that are not actually connected.

FLYING PIG
The human brain has evolved to pick up very quickly on visual stimuli that might signal danger or opportunity. Hence faces, human bodies, and animal forms are among the most likely things to be "seen" in clouds.

RELIGION IN THE BRAIN

Religious practice is largely determined by cultural factors. However, studies of identical twins who have been brought up separately suggest that the likelihood of a person experiencing a religious conversion or spiritual transcendence may be due more to genes than to upbringing. Spiritual transcendence shares some features with other "weird" experiences, such as out-of-body experiences, auras, and "the sensed presence" (see opposite page). These are associated with flurries of unusually high activity in the temporal lobes. The areas involved in intense religious experiences seem to be more widespread, however. For example, a study of nuns from a meditative order showed that, as they recalled an intense religious experience, many different areas were activated. So there does not seem to be a single "God-spot."

SALEM WITCH TRIALS
Rigid belief systems can lead people to "see" things that do not exist. During the Salem witch trials of 1692, for example, religious bigots "saw" evidence of the devil in the behavior of entirely ordinary people.

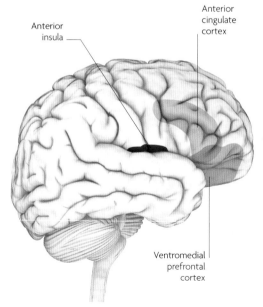

Anterior cingulate cortex

Anterior insula

Ventromedial prefrontal cortex

THE BASIS OF BELIEF
Belief and disbelief are driven by parts of the brain to do with emotions, not reasoning. Belief activates the ventromedial prefrontal cortex, which processes reward, emotion, and taste, while disbelief is registered by the insula, which generates feelings of disgust.

BRAIN CHEMISTRY

High natural levels of the neurotransmitter dopamine may explain why some people are unusually quick to pick out patterns. Believers are known to be more likely than sceptics to see a word or face in nonsense images, and sceptics more likely to miss real faces or words that are partly hidden by visual "noise." One study found that sceptics' tendency to see hidden patterns increased when they were given L-dopa, a drug that increases dopamine levels.

SCRAMBLED FACE   **REAL FACE**   **SCRAMBLED FACE**

SCRAMBLED FACES STUDY
Believers are more likely than sceptics to see "real" faces when presented with a rapid sequence of "scrambled" faces. Sceptics, by contrast, are more likely to fail to spot "real" faces mixed in with the scrambled ones.

SEEING LITTLE PEOPLE

The content of supernatural "sightings" varies according to culture. Fairies were once commonly seen, while today it is more usual for people to report seeing alien beings. Claims of being abducted by aliens seem to be more common at times when the magnetic effects of solar radiation are high. One theory is that the radiation causes tiny temporal-lobe seizures in susceptible people, creating hallucinations.

THE COTTINGLEY FAIRIES
This faked photograph (part of a series) was made by two mischievous children in 1917. Many adults believed that the fairies were real.

THE HAUNTED BRAIN

Apparently "supernatural" experiences may be due to disturbances in various parts of the brain. Tiny seizures in the temporal lobes are thought to be responsible for many of the emotional effects reported in such events, such as feelings of ecstasy or intense fear. Temporal-lobe disturbance is also associated with the sense of an invisible presence that often accompanies perceiving ghosts. Distortions of space and embodiment, such as the illusion of looking down at oneself, known as an "out-of-body" experience, are linked to reduced activity in the parietal lobes, which normally maintain a relatively stable sense of space and time. Hallucinations may result from faulty visual or auditory processing or failure to interpret sights and sounds normally.

KEY
- ● **TEMPORO-PARIETAL JUNCTION (TPJ)**
- ● **MOTOR CORTEX**
- ● **SOMATOSENSORY CORTEX**
- ● **AUDITORY CORTEX**
- ● **FOCUS OF EPILEPTIC ACTIVITY IN TEMPORAL LOBE**

OUT-OF-BODY EXPERIENCES (OBEs)
This diagram shows areas where electrodes were implanted in the brain of an epileptic person to evoke responses. Stimulation of the TPJ (blue dots) was found to induce OBEs.

WHITE LADY
Expectation has a strong effect on what a person sees. Many "hauntings" arise because people have been led to expect to see a ghost in a certain place. Any unusual sensory effect is then interpreted as a specter.

MAKING GHOSTS

Direct stimulation of the temporal lobes can give a sense of an invisible or divine "presence." Dr. Michael Persinger, of the Laurentian University in Canada, has made a helmet that, he claims, creates "spiritual" experiences in 80 percent of those who try it. Other researchers, however, have failed to reproduce his results and suggest that the effects are due to sensory deprivation and suggestion.

GOD HELMET
The helmet alters brain activity by weak magnetic stimulation. It may produce spiritual experiences in sensitive people.

COGNITIVE ILLUSIONS

ILLUSIONS OCCUR WHEN SENSORY DATA CLASHES WITH OUR ASSUMPTIONS ABOUT THE WAY THINGS ARE. THE BRAIN ATTEMPTS TO MAKE THE INFORMATION "FIT." THE RESULTING CONFUSION GIVES US A GLIMPSE OF HOW THE BRAIN WORKS.

EIGHT-YEAR-OLD CHILD　　**FIVE-YEAR-OLD AUTIST**　　**LEONARDO DA VINCI**

TYPES OF COGNITIVE ILLUSION

The brain has certain rules that it applies to incoming information in order to make sense of it quickly. If we hear a voice and at the same time see a mouth moving, for example, we assume the voice comes from the mouth. Like all such rules, though, this is only a best guess and can be wrong. Hence it leaves us open to the illusion of ventriloquy. Low-level illusions–those created in the early stages of perception–are unavoidable, but those that arise due to higher-level cognition are less robust. It is impossible not to see the after-image that occurs when you have been looking at a bright light, for example, because this is created by low-level nerve activity, which cannot be affected by conscious thought. However, once you know the voice comes from the ventriloquist rather than the dummy, a result of higher-level cognition, the illusion is less convincing. Illusions may be generated by both conscious and unconscious assumptions. A child's concept of how a horse looks, for example, includes four distinct legs (top left), which governs how the horse is visualized. An "expert" viewer of horses–such as the artist Leonardo Da Vinci (top right)–has a more realistic concept.

ARTIST'S EYE
The middle drawing is by a five-year-old autistic savant, who probably had no concept of a horse at all. Unlike the normal child, her concepts do not mislead her.

CANALS ON MARS

Until the early 20th century, some astronomers believed that Mars was crossed by canals. Maps were made, and for nearly a decade the canals seemed to be visible to people with fairly strong telescopes. The canals did not "vanish" until analysis of the Martian atmosphere proved that life there was not possible. Acceptance that the canals could not exist stopped people from seeing them.

MARTIAN MAP

DISTORTING MIRRORS

Information from the outside world, including sensations from the rest of the body, is constantly compared to a "virtual" world within the brain, which includes a conceptual map of the body. When the two fail to match up, the brain assumes that something outside has changed. It can even be fooled that the body has shrunk. The shrinking-body illusion involves stimulating the arm muscles with vibrators, to create the feeling that the limbs are moving in, beyond the sides of the body. The brain decides that the body has shrunk.

IMPOSED TRIANGLE
The brain imposes things that are not there, like this white triangle, when it is the most likely explanation for what we see.

Impulse travels through thalamus to parietal cortex

Impulse travels up to spinal cord

Vibrators strapped to wrists cause sensation of arms moving inward

SHRINKING BODY
The brain's body map is encoded in the parietal cortex, the part of the brain dealing with space. This illusion activates the area as though it is registering an actual change in body shape.

AMBIGUOUS ILLUSIONS

Something strange happens when we look at ambiguous figures. The input to the brain stays the same, but what we see flips from one thing to another. This demonstrates that perception is an active process, driven by information that is already in our brains as well as information from the outside world. The switching occurs because the brain is searching for the most meaningful interpretation of the image. Normally, the brain settles quickly on a solution by using basic rules such as, "if one thing surrounds another, the surrounded shape is the object and the other thing is the ground." Ambiguous figures confound such rules. For instance, in the vase illusion (left) it is impossible to see which shape is on top, so the brain tries one way of seeing it, then another. You see both images, but you can never see both of them simultaneously.

SHAPE SHIFTERS
In the vase illusion (top), the figures switch between two facing profiles and the outline of a vase. The bottom figure can be seen as either a rabbit or a duck.

MY WIFE AND MY MOTHER-IN-LAW
In this illusion, the figure of either a young woman or an old hag may dominate at first, but once you have "seen" the alternative, the brain finds it again easily.

DISTORTING ILLUSIONS

Distorting illusions are characterized by visual images that generate a false impression of an object's size, length, or curvature. They generally exploit the "allowances" the brain normally makes in order to make sense of what it sees. For example, the brain "allows" that objects of the same size will look smaller if they are farther away, and that larger objects in an array should command greater attention than small ones. Like other illusions, distortions may occur at low or high levels of perception (see opposite page). Those that happen in the earliest stages, before the brain "recognizes" what it is looking at, are the most robust because they cannot be influenced by conscious thought.

LEANING TOWERS
These images of the Leaning Tower of Pisa are identical, but the one on the right seems to lean more. This is because the brain treats them as a single scene. Usually, if two adjacent towers rise in parallel their outlines converge due to perspective. When seeing two towers with parallel outlines, the brain assumes the towers are diverging.

PERSPECTIVE ILLUSION
Even though the figures walking along the road are the same height, the brain insists that the one farthest away looks taller. This is because the rule of perspective—things shrink with distance—is applied at an early stage of perception.

EBBINGHAUS ILLUSION
The central circle is the same size in both images, but we see it as bigger when compared to smaller circles, rather than larger ones.

PARADOX ILLUSIONS

It is possible to represent objects in two dimensions that cannot actually exist in the real, three-dimensional world. Paradox illusions are generated by such images, which are often dependent on the brain's erroneous assumption that adjacent edges must join. Although impossible, the best examples are oddly convincing, and the conscious brain is teased and intrigued by them. As with ambiguous illusions, the brain tries first one interpretation and then another, but is unable to settle because none of the available views make sense. Brain-imaging scans show that impossible images are recognized by the brain very early in the process of perception, well before conscious recognition. Unlike the conscious brain, the unconscious part is not very concerned with such images, and spends less time trying to process them than it spends on "real" objects.

THE TRIBAR
The Penrose triangle, also known as the tribar, is a perspective drawing that comprises three three-dimensional bars that appear to be connected, but in reality could not be.

THE IMPOSSIBLE ELEPHANT
Although it is impossible to determine how many legs this elephant has, the brain keeps trying to match up the shaded areas of "legs" with the apparently detached feet.

M.C. ESCHER

"Mauk" Escher, a Dutch graphic artist, started drawing elaborate impossible realities in the 1930s and produced a huge quantity of now famous illusions. He created the images from imagination rather than by reference to observation, and incorporated many sophisticated mathematical concepts into his artworks. His images are both tantalizing and emotionally charged—some of his landscapes are witty, while others have a dark, surreal quality. Several of his works show buildings that could never actually be constructed.

RELATIVITY
The scene shown here is impossible in that it could exist only in a world in which gravity worked in three directions rather than one.

HOW DOES THE ELECTRICAL FIRING OF CELLS IN OUR BRAIN
PRODUCE OUR CONSCIOUS EXPERIENCE OF THE WORLD,
AND WITH IT SUCH THINGS AS OUR SENSE OF A PRIVATE
SELF AND OUR ABILITY FOR ABSTRACT THOUGHT AND
REFLECTION? THIS IS A FAMOUSLY DIFFICULT QUESTION.
ANSWERING IT INVOLVES BUILDING A BRIDGE BETWEEN
THE PHYSICAL AND MENTAL WORLDS. AS NEUROSCIENCE
ADVANCES, WE ARE GETTING CLOSER TO UNDERSTANDING
WHAT CONSCIOUSNESS IS AND HOW IT COMES ABOUT.
FOR EXAMPLE, DIFFERENT CONSCIOUS STATES CAN NOW
BE CORRELATED WITH ACTIVITY IN SPECIFIC BRAIN AREAS.

CONSCIOUSNESS

WHAT IS CONSCIOUSNESS?

CONSCIOUSNESS IS ESSENTIAL—WITHOUT IT, LIFE WOULD HAVE NO MEANING. WE CAN IDENTIFY THE SORT OF BRAIN ACTIVITY THAT GENERATES CONSCIOUS AWARENESS, BUT HOW THIS APPARENTLY INTANGIBLE PHENOMENON ARISES FROM A PHYSICAL ORGAN REMAINS A MYSTERY.

SPANDRELS
This is the name given to the spaces between arches. Although we talk of them as objects, without the arch they cease to exist. Consciousness may have appeared in the same way, as a result of other evolved features.

THE NATURE OF CONSCIOUSNESS

Consciousness is like nothing else. A thought, feeling, or idea seems to be a different kind of thing from the physical objects that make up the rest of the universe. The contents of our minds cannot be located in space or time. Although they appear to be produced by particular types of physical activity in the brain, it is not known if this activity itself forms consciousness (the Monist/materialist view) or if brain activity correlates with a different thing altogether that we call "the mind" or consciousness (the dualist view). If consciousness is not simply brain activity, this suggests that the material universe is just one aspect of reality and that consciousness is part of a parallel reality in which entirely different rules apply.

2 Data generates brain activity that itself is the conscious perception

1 Data about visual stimuli from eyes enters brain

MONISM
According to this theory, consciousness is part of the material universe. It is identical to the brain activity that correlates with it. It developed when cognitive mechanisms evolved, but only as a result of them, rather than for any purpose of its own.

2 Data generates brain activity

3 Brain activity allows mind to make conscious perception

1 Data about visual stimuli from eyes enters brain

DUALISM
Consciousness is not physical but exists in another dimension to the material universe. Certain brain processes are associated with it, but are not identical to it. Some dualists believe consciousness may exist without the brain processes associated with it.

RENÉ DESCARTES AND DUALISM

The French philosopher René Descartes (1596–1650) is regarded as the founder of modern dualism. He proposed that the material world is separate from the realm of the mind, which includes thoughts, emotions, pleasure, and pain. "Mind" things have no size, shape, or motion, but they can interact with the material world, so that thoughts can cause actions and material stimuli can cause thoughts. He postulated that this interaction takes place in the pineal gland, a small brain nucleus that was not at the time thought to have any other function.

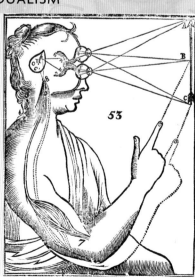

REM SLEEP

DAYDREAMING NARRATIVE

DROWSY

NON-REM SLEEP

NEURAL ACTIVITY

High

Low

Inward (own thoughts)

DIRECTION OF FOCUS

VISUALIZING THE MIND
This diagram is a representation of different states of mind, or modes of consciousness, framed within a box that represents the mind itself. The states of mind are positioned within the box according to the degree of neural activity that correlates with each, the direction of the focus of its attention (toward the outer world or inward toward thoughts themselves), and the level of concentration each state of mind commands.

TYPES AND LEVELS OF CONSCIOUSNESS

Consciousness has different modes, such as emotions, sensations, thoughts, and perceptions, which are all experienced at different levels of neural activity, focus, and concentration. The level of neural activity determines the intensity of consciousness. The direction of focus can be towards the outside world or the inner world (thinking about thoughts). Concentration can be loosely targeted, involving a range of objects or fixed, involving just one particular aspect. Consciousness also divides into three types of awareness: awareness in the moment–the brain registers and reacts to moment-by-moment events but does not encode them in memory; conscious awareness–events are registered and encoded in memory; and self-consciousness–events are registered and remembered, and the person is conscious of doing this.

INTROSPECTION

FOCUSED ATTENTION, SUCH AS WORK

RELAXED ALERT

RELAXED SOCIALIZING

RELAXED OBSERVING

RELAXED GENERAL

High (targeted attention)

CONCENTRATION

Low (diffuse attention)

KEY

SLEEP

RELAXED

FOCUSED

THE THINKER

Most conscious thinking is couched in language. Words function as symbolic "handles," used to grasp the objects they represent. However, about 25 percent of thoughts are experienced as sensations or perceptions.

FIXED CONCENTRATION

When focusing on an object, attention narrows. Other potential focal points are neglected. This can be useful—this child notices less of a potentially traumatizing medical procedure when focused on a toy.

THE CHINESE ROOM

Is consciousness needed for "understanding"? Philosopher John Searle invented the idea of a room in which every dictionary and rule relating to the Chinese language was stored. Inside is a man who is able to translate and respond to questions written in Chinese by manipulating these resources, despite not being able to speak a word of Chinese. Hence, someone posting the words "How does your dog smell?" in Chinese may receive the reply, in Chinese, "Awful!" From outside it looks as though the man inside must have "understood" the question, but Searle argues that merely behaving this way is not the same as understanding. In the same way, a computer could never be described as "having a mind" or "understanding." Other philosophers argue that understanding—and perhaps every other type of consciousness—is merely the process of behaving as though one understands.

Book of Chinese symbols — Room — Non-Chinese speaker

Message in — Message out

LOCATING CONSCIOUSNESS

HUMAN CONSCIOUSNESS ARISES FROM THE INTERACTION OF EVERY PART OF A PERSON WITH THEIR ENVIRONMENT. WE KNOW THAT THE BRAIN PLAYS THE MAJOR ROLE IN PRODUCING CONSCIOUS AWARENESS BUT WE DO NOT KNOW HOW. CERTAIN PROCESSES WITHIN THE BRAIN, AND NEURONAL ACTIVITY IN PARTICULAR AREAS, CORRELATE RELIABLY WITH CONSCIOUS STATES, WHILE OTHERS DO NOT. THESE PROCESSES AND AREAS SEEM TO BE NECESSARY FOR CONSCIOUSNESS, ALTHOUGH THEY MAY NOT BE SUFFICIENT FOR IT.

SIGNIFICANT BRAIN ANATOMY

Different types of neuronal activity in the brain are associated with the emergence of conscious awareness. Neuronal activity in the cortex, and particularly in the frontal lobes, is associated with the arousal of conscious experience. It takes up to half a second for a stimulus to become conscious after it has first been registered in the brain. Initially, the neuronal activity triggered by the stimulus occurs in the "lower" areas of the brain, such as the amygdala and thalamus, and then in the "higher" brain, in the parts of the cortex that process sensations. The frontal cortex is activated usually only when an experience becomes conscious, suggesting that the involvement of this part of the brain may be an essential component of consciousness.

SELF AWARENESS
In order to be conscious, the brain needs to "own" its perceptions—that is, to recognize that those perceptions are occurring within itself. To do this it has to generate a sense of self (as opposed to unconscious awareness). Without this, consciousness may not be possible.

CRUCIAL PARTS OF THE BRAIN
Various areas of the brain are involved in generating conscious experience, even though none of them alone is sufficient to sustain it. If any of these are severely damaged, consciousness is compromised, altered, or lost.

Motor cortex
Body awareness (involving motor cortex) may be crucial to sense of self, which seems necessary for consciousness

Supplementary motor cortex
Deliberate actions are "rehearsed" here, distinguishing them from unconscious reactions

Primary visual cortex
Without this there is no conscious vision, even if other parts of visual cortex are functioning

Dorsolateral prefrontal cortex
Different ideas and perceptions are "bound" together here—a process thought to be necessary for conscious experience

Orbitofrontal cortex
Conscious emotion arises here; if inactive, reactions to stimuli are merely reflexive body actions with no emotion

Temporal lobe
Personal memories and language depend on these; without these faculties, consciousness is severely curtailed

Tempo-parietal junction
Stores the brain's "map" of self in relation to world and pulls information together from many areas

Thalamus
Directs attention and switches sensory input on and off

Hippocampus
Underlies memory encoding, without which consciousness is restricted to a single point in time

Reticular formation
Stimulates cortical activity, without which there is no conscious awareness

THE "BRAIN-IN-A-VAT"

The idea of a conscious but disembodied brain is central to many science fiction and horror films, and is often used as a thought experiment in philosophical debates about the nature of reality. In recent years, the notion has ceased to be entirely theoretical as modern technology edges toward the possibility of inducing in the brain a virtual reality, indistinguishable from the reality experienced through the body. It is even possible that such a thing has been achieved already, and the external world, as we experience it, is not "real" at all.

VIRTUAL REALITY
The idea that we are simply disembodied brains hooked up to a supercomputer that simulates conscious experience is a famous thought experiment.

Computer provides stimulation

Brain experiences virtual world

THE MATRIX
This 1999 film explores the idea of virtual reality being the only "reality" humans experience. People's brains are "plugged" into the Matrix, a huge computer program simulating physical experience.

REQUIREMENTS OF CONSCIOUSNESS

Every state of conscious awareness has a specific pattern of brain activity associated with it. These are commonly referred to as the neural correlates of consciousness. For example, seeing a patch of yellow produces one pattern of brain activity, seeing grandmother, another. If the brain state changes from one pattern to another, so does the experience of consciousness. The processes relevant to consciousness are generally assumed to be found at the level of brain cells rather than at the level of individual molecules or atoms. It is likely that, for consciousness to arise, the factors listed below need to be present. Yet it is also possible that consciousness does arise at the far smaller atomic (quantum) level, and if so it may be subject to very different laws.

VISUAL PHANTOMS

Conscious perception does not rely solely on external stimuli—it can also arise internally. Our brains constantly "fill in" missing data to make sense of the world. For example, you may see phantomlike vertical lines connecting the two blocks in the first column. This "imaginary" perception depends on similar neural-activity patterns as conscious perceptions of "real" stimuli.

NORMAL   **EPILEPTIC SEIZURE**

LEVEL OF COMPLEXITY
Neural activity must be complex for consciousness to occur, but not too complex. If all the neurons are firing, such as in an epileptic seizure, consciousness is lost.

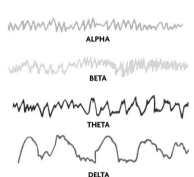

ALPHA

BETA

THETA

DELTA

FIRING THRESHOLDS
Consciousness arises only when brain cells fire at fairly high rates. The high firing rate of Beta waves indicates alertness, while the low rate of Delta waves indicates deep sleep.

SYNCHRONOUS FIRING
Clusters of cells across the brain fire in unison. This seems to "bind" independent perceptions (say, the left and right visual fields) into one conscious perception.

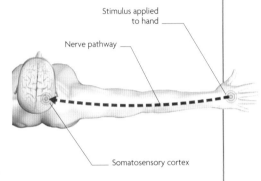

Stimulus applied to hand

Nerve pathway

Somatosensory cortex

TIMING
It takes $\frac{1}{2}$ a second for the unconscious brain to process stimuli into conscious perceptions, but the brain fools us into thinking we experience things immediately.

MEASURING NEURAL ACTIVITY
Every conscious state correlates with a unique pattern of neural activity. These patterns of firing brain cells can be detected by measuring the level of electrical activity in the brain through the skull.

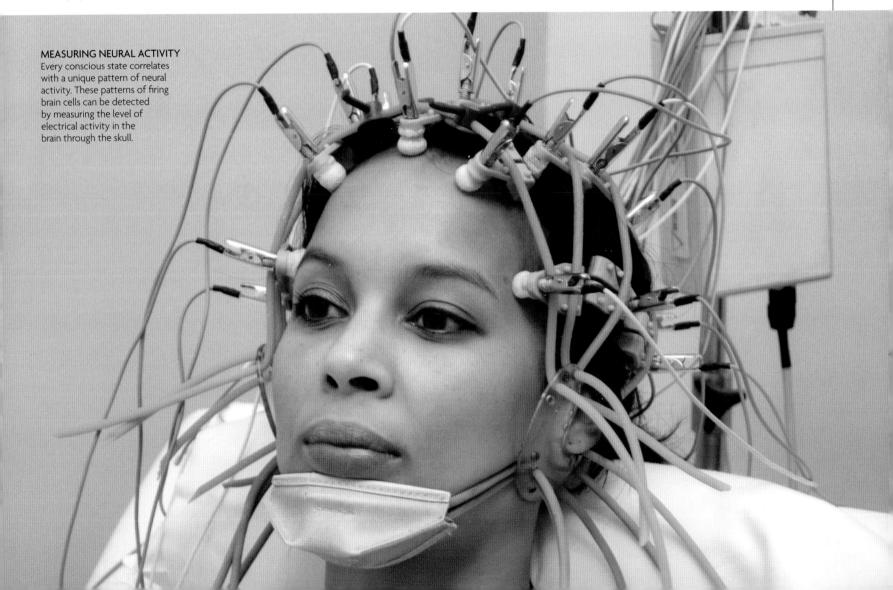

ATTENTION AND CONSCIOUSNESS

ATTENTION CONTROLS AND DIRECTS CONSCIOUSNESS.
IT ACTS LIKE A HIGHLIGHTER THAT MAKES CERTAIN PARTS
OF THE WORLD "JUMP OUT" AND CAUSES THE REST TO
RECEDE. IT SELECTS THE FEATURE THAT IS CURRENTLY
MOST IMPORTANT IN THE ENVIRONMENT AND AMPLIFIES
THE BRAIN'S RESPONSE TO IT.

WHAT IS ATTENTION?

Attention causes you to select one item from the sensory inputs
you are receiving and allows you to become more fully or sharply
conscious of it. Consciousness and attention are so closely linked
that it is almost impossible to attend to something and not be
conscious of it. Overt attention involves consciously directing the
eyes, ears, or other sense organs toward a stimulus and processing
information from it. Covert attention involves switching attention
to a stimulus without directing
the sense organs toward it.
Attention may seem continuous,
but maintaining focused attention
is actually rare and difficult. It is
also hard to switch attention from
one object to another: the more
attentive you are to one stimulus,
the slower you are to turn your
attention away from it. Hence an
event that captures your attention
will "blot out" anything else for
a fraction of a second.

ATTENTION TYPES

TYPE		DESCRIPTION
Focused attention		This is the ability to single out one object in one's environment and respond to it. An example might be an athlete focusing on the starter's gun, while "tuning out" the noise from the crowd.
Sustained attention		Attention naturally tends to wander. Sustained attention is the ability to maintain concentration on a particular object or activity, such as operating heavy machinery for a continuous period of time.
Selective attention		This form is similar to sustained attention, but involves the ability to resist shifting attention from the selected target, for example when focusing on a putt despite other competing stimuli.
Alternating attention		This involves shifting quickly from one stimulus to another, which requires a different sort of cognitive response—for example, when shifting attention from a model you are painting to the actual painting.
Divided attention		Often known as "multitasking," this involves dividing attention between two or more competing tasks. Recent research suggests that apparently divided attention is actually very quick alternating attention.

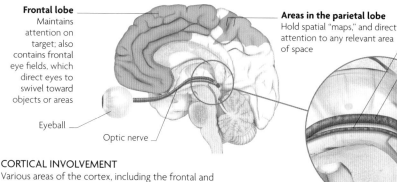

Frontal lobe
Maintains
attention on
target; also
contains frontal
eye fields, which
direct eyes to
swivel toward
objects or areas

Eyeball

Optic nerve

Areas in the parietal lobe
Hold spatial "maps," and direct
attention to any relevant area
of space

Optic
nerve

Lateral geniculate
nucleus

Superior
colliculus

CORTICAL INVOLVEMENT
Various areas of the cortex, including the frontal and
parietal lobes receive input from the sense organs,
and direct attention toward anything striking.

SUPERIOR COLLICULUS
This is part of a network
of brain areas that direct
eye movements. Signals
from the retina arrive
here via the optic nerve;
activity in this area causes
attention to shift in response
to notable stimuli.

INTENSE CONCENTRATION
When you concentrate hard, you filter
out other possible objects of attention
so that maximum cognitive resources
are available for the task in hand.

NEURAL MECHANISMS

If the brain registers an unexpected movement, a loud sound, or some other potentially significant stimulus, it directs the sense organs toward it–for example, by swiveling the eyes in the direction of a sudden movement. This happens automatically, in the lower regions of the brain, and it does not in itself create consciousness of the stimulus. However, attention also increases activity in the neurons that are concerned with the stimulus. If the stimulus is a person, for example, neural activity increases in the visual areas that monitor the place in space where the person is located; the face-recognition area; the amygdala; the temporal-parietal areas, which work out their intentions; and the supplementary motor area, which works out what to do about them. If the neurons are excited beyond a certain point, consciousness "kicks in."

NEURONAL ACTIVITY
When you attend to a thought, emotion, or perception, the brain activity is amplified and becomes more synchronous. This EEG study shows activity while attending to a visual stimulus and ignoring it. Attending to stimuli on the left activates the right hemisphere and vice versa.

ATTENDING TO VISUAL STIMULUS ON RIGHT

ATTENDING TO VISUAL STIMULUS ON LEFT

IGNORING VISUAL STIMULUS ON RIGHT

IGNORING VISUAL STIMULUS ON LEFT

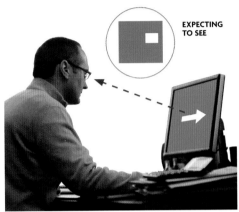

EXPECTING TO SEE

ATTENTION TO LOCATION
In this experiment, an arrow directs the subject's attention to a location where he expects a subsequent target stimulus to appear. While focusing on the location, waiting for something to appear, fMRI scans (below) show sustained activity in the frontal eye fields and parietal cortex—areas concerned with focusing on a particular area in space. Activity in the temporal lobe suggests readiness to identify the target when it appears.

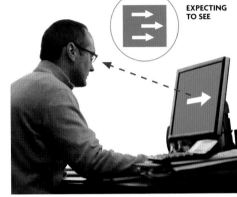

EXPECTING TO SEE

ATTENTION TO DIRECTION
In this experiment, the arrow tells the subject to look out for a moving target that will be traveling from left to right. This directional cue produces sustained signals in the frontal eye fields, as in the location task, but greater activity in the parietal lobes, where calculations are made about spatial direction as well as location. These calculations prime the brain to react to the target when it appears.

Frontal eye fields

Anterior intraparietal area

Posterior intraparietal area

Ventral intraparietal area

Fusiform cortex

Middle temporal complex

Frontal eye fields

Anterior intraparietal area

Posterior intraparietal area

Ventral intraparietal area

Fusiform cortex

Middle temporal complex

INATTENTION BLINDNESS

When we direct attention toward an object or an image, we may have the impression that we are seeing all of it in detail. However, we do not take in nearly as much as information as we think—usually, only relatively large and striking features grab our attention and are subjected to close enough scrutiny to make them memorable. The rest of the image is not attended to and effectively remains unseen.

SPOT THE DIFFERENCE
Changes in images are difficult to spot because we only pick out the major features and fail to see smaller details. Compare the two images here: do you see any differences? Most people have to scan them methodically to see how they differ.

ORIGINAL IMAGE

ALTERED IMAGE

THE IDLING BRAIN

THE BRAIN HAS DISTINCT MODES, EACH OF WHICH USES A DIFFERENT NETWORK OF NEURONS. "RESTING-STATE NETWORKS" BECOME ACTIVATED WHEN WE CEASE TO BE FULLY ENGAGED WITH THE OUTSIDE WORLD.

THE RESTING STATE NETWORK

When the brain is not actively engaged in a task it falls into one of a number of resting states. The most common of these involves the default-mode network (DMN). When the brain is in task mode it responds to sensation by creating action plans, which are then turned into actual actions. In contrast, while in a resting state, the brain creates action plans but does not act them out: they are imagined scenarios. The medial frontal cortex is active in the resting state, indicating social rumination, while the lateral frontal cortex is active in task mode, indicating sequential thought patterns suited to handling objects.

Parietal areas responsible for action plans

Parietal area active in imagining scenarios

LEFT

Medial frontal cortex active in social cognition

RIGHT

KEY

▓ TASK-ORIENTED ACTIVITY

▓ RESTING STATE ACTIVITY

READING THE DEFAULT-MODE NETWORK

Although default mode network activity is recognizably similar in everyone, there are small individual differences, which seem to tally with differences in personality. Researchers at several centers are charting individuals' DMN activity by EEG and correlating the information with those people's personalities. Drawing on this information, it may be possible to produce a brain-activity-related personality test.

TASK AND RESTING STATES
These scans show the brain in two different states—at rest and while performing a task. The green areas show the areas of high activity in the resting state. When a person is actively engaged in a task, the purple areas become active and the green ones calm down.

THE DMN AND SOCIAL AWARENESS

The areas of brain activated in the default-mode network are very similar to those activated when a person is asked to interpret a social situation and, in particular, his or her own situation with regard to other people. This suggests that whenever we are free of immediate mental tasks, we fall back into a state of rumination about our relationships with others, and our place in the social world.

REST

SOCIAL COGNITION

Cingulate cortex

Medial prefrontal cortex

Precuneus

MATCHING STATES
The brain areas that are active when a person is asked to imagine being in a social situation are almost identical to those activated in the resting state— the medial prefrontal cortex and the cingulate cortex.

THE BRAIN'S EGO

The thoughts associated with the default-mode network are mainly self-centered and driven by one's own autobiography and place in the social hierarchy. They often draw on half-forgotten memories and are colored by emotion. These are the concerns that Sigmund Freud identified with the half-submerged mind-state that he called the ego. Some researchers have suggested the DMN is functionally the same as the Freudian ego.

FREUD'S THEORY OF MIND
Freud thought that most brain processes were unconscious. The ego, part of the mind involved in self, was partly conscious. The rest of the conscious mind controlled thoughts and actions, and roughly matches the "task-oriented" mind state.

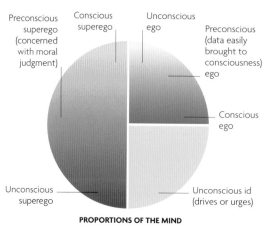

Preconscious superego (concerned with moral judgment)

Conscious superego

Unconscious ego

Preconscious (data easily brought to consciousness) ego

Conscious ego

Unconscious superego

Unconscious id (drives or urges)

PROPORTIONS OF THE MIND

THE WANDERING MIND

People seem to spend about one-third of their waking hours in a resting state mode, and if they are doing something untaxing, such as driving down a straight, empty road, the proportion is even higher. In one experiment, people were invited to sit in a laboratory and do nothing except read a novel and report whenever their mind wandered. Over the course of half an hour, they typically reported one to three episodes of mind-wandering.

RESTING STATE AND CREATIVITY

Most people switch very cleanly from default mode to task mode if they are suddenly called upon to engage with the outside world. In some people, though, the two modes run concurrently. This may make them more creative, because the free-floating, discursive nature of thinking in the default mode may drift toward a solution to a problem that would escape the more targeted, constrained thinking associated with task-oriented cognition. However, overlap between the two modes is also associated with schizophrenia and depression. This may account for some of the unconventional thinking associated with schizophrenia and the lack of concentration displayed by many depressed people.

FIRING THE DMN
The connections between areas involved in the DMN are tighter in schizophrenics and their relatives. This means that if one of the areas is triggered, it is more likely to fire up the whole network.

CONTROL

RELATIVE OF SCHIZOPHRENIC

SCHIZOPHRENIC

DMN IN ANIMALS

The default-mode network has been observed in animals other than humans. In fact, researchers have found it in all animal species tested so far, including dogs and rats. The regions of the brain most active in the DMN appear to be more highly developed the more social the animal species is—with humans forming the largest social groups of any animal and having correspondingly large "social brain" areas. One theory is that the DMN may allow all social animals to keep themselves secure and "up to speed" in their societies.

ON AUTOPILOT
The brain flips into resting state when we are not actively engaged in a task. This includes carrying out actions that are second nature—the moment-by-moment activity is carried out on autopilot while the conscious brain ruminates.

ALTERING CONSCIOUSNESS

THE BRAIN IS CAPABLE OF GENERATING A WIDE RANGE OF CONSCIOUS EXPERIENCES, INCLUDING SOME STATES THAT ALTER OUR PERCEPTIONS AND EMOTIONS TO SUCH AN EXTENT THAT THE ENTIRE WORLD SEEMS DRAMATICALLY DIFFERENT. SUCH "ALTERED STATES" ARE NOW THE SUBJECT OF INTENSE NEUROSCIENTIFIC RESEARCH.

ALTERED BRAIN STATES

Our normal waking state varies from daydreaming, through relaxed awareness, to sharply focused. The brain is capable of generating a much wider range of conscious experiences than this, though. Sometimes we slip outside the normal range spontaneously, when feverish or exhausted, for instance, or during or after an emotionally overwhelming event. We may also deliberately seek to get out of our normal state by engaging in rituals such as prolonged dancing, or through meditation, or by taking drugs.

TRANCE STATE
A trance is an altered state of consciousness that may be induced by hypnosis, drugs, or ritual. It can be pleasurable or frightening.

Frontal lobe
May go "offline" in altered states, reducing critical thinking; can be hyperactive during meditation, indicating increased attention

Parietal lobe
Altered activity here may create out-of-body feeling or distorted experience of space and time

Corpus callosum
Allows the two hemispheres to communicate; blissful states are linked with greater synchrony between hemispheres and sudden switches of activity from one hemisphere to another

Temporal lobe
Flurries of activity here are associated with unexplainable experiences including hallucinations and sensing auras or an invisible presence

Thalamus
May shut off incoming information, sending a person into "a world of their own"

Reticular formation
Alerting signals from reticular formation to cerebral cortex may be reduced, causing increased relaxation and sense of wellbeing

BRAIN AREAS INVOLVED IN ALTERED STATES
Altered states may range from blissful to terrible, and they are generated by correspondingly varied changes in neural activity in the brain, particularly involving the areas shown here.

DISSOCIATION

Dissociation refers to instances when elements of consciousness (the sensations, thoughts, and emotions of the moment) that are sometimes bound together as a whole are, instead, experienced separately or are cut out of conscious awareness. Many altered states fall into this category. Usually, dissociation is referred to as a mental or behavioral disorder, but some "normal" conscious states, such as daydreaming or concentrating, are dissociative. It is more accurate to look at these conscious states as a spectrum (see below), with highly unified or "bound" experience at one end and "fractured" consciousness at the other.

HYPNOSIS

Hypnosis is a form of dissociation in which a person's field of attention is narrowed to a single thought, feeling, or idea. When experiencing this state of mind, normal distractions and preoccupations may be kept out of mind. People undergoing hypnosis voluntarily may become very suggestible to the hypnotist's ideas, so it is often used therapeutically, for instance, to break a habit such as smoking.

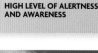

BOUND TOGETHER   **NORMAL**   **FRACTURED**

| FEELING OF ONENESS OR "MEANINGFULNESS" | STATE OF EXTREME RELAXATION WITH FEWER INTROSPECTIVE THOUGHTS | DAYDREAMING; CAN SPRING BACK TO ALERT IMMEDIATELY | HIGH LEVEL OF ALERTNESS AND AWARENESS | SEPARATION FROM SELF OR SENSE OF BEING DISTANCED FROM REALITY |

BRAIN ACTIVITY DURING MEDITATION

These SPECT scans show contrasting activity in Buddhist monks when resting and when meditating. The top row shows increased activity in the frontal lobe of a meditating monk (red areas at the top of the scan), the bottom row shows decreased activity in parietal areas (yellow areas at the bottom). Both these indicators suggest a state of intense concentration and also a loss of normal spatial awareness. The reduced activation found in meditating brains is also found in the brains of people who have been injected with psilocybin, the psychoactive component of "magic mushrooms." The drug seems to provide a short cut to the state of calm otherworldliness associated with meditation.

AT REST (FRONTAL LOBE)

MEDITATION (FRONTAL LOBE)

AT REST (PARIETAL LOBE)

MEDITATION (PARIETAL LOBE)

MEDITATING MONK
During meditation, practiced Buddhist monks produce synchronous gamma waves—a sign of higher mental function. They also show greater gamma activity than others, even when not meditating.

SLEEP AND DREAMS

ABOUT A THIRD OF LIFE IS SPENT ASLEEP, DURING WHICH TIME THE BRAIN REMAINS ACTIVE, FULFILLING A RANGE OF IMPORTANT FUNCTIONS. DURING SLEEP, THE BRAIN GENERATES DREAMS, WHICH PROVIDE US WITH SOME OF THE MOST INTENSE AND STRANGE EXPERIENCES THAT WE HAVE.

THE SLEEPING BRAIN

No one is quite sure what it is about sleep that makes it so important. One theory is that it allows "down time" for the body to repair itself. Another is that it simply keeps the person out of danger for a period of time during each day, by keeping him or her still. A third is that the brain needs to switch off from the outside world in order to sort, process, and memorize information. Certainly, important memory functions do occur during sleep, but whether or not this is the primary purpose of sleep remains unclear. Sleep-wake cycles are controlled by neurotransmitters that act on different parts of the brain to induce sleep or waking up. Research also suggests that a chemical called adenosine builds up in the blood while we are awake and causes drowsiness; while we sleep, the chemical is gradually broken down.

SLEEP PROBLEMS

About one in five people suffer problems with sleep. The most common complaint is insomnia—the inability to fall or stay asleep. Insomnia is treated with drugs that bind to receptors for GABA (the brain's inhibitory neurotransmitter). Narcolepsy is a sleep disorder that causes people to fall asleep suddenly and inappropriately, or to feel exhausted throughout the day. Narcoleptics cannot experience the amount of restorative deep sleep that healthy people have and live in a state of sleep deprivation. When they fall asleep—which may occur with little warning—they enter REM sleep almost immediately and have vivid dreams. Sleepwalking occurs in deep sleep when a block that stops motor impulses is lifted but other sleep mechanisms remain. Sleepwalkers do complex things, such as driving cars, but perform actions robotically because they are following automatic action plans stored in the unconscious brain.

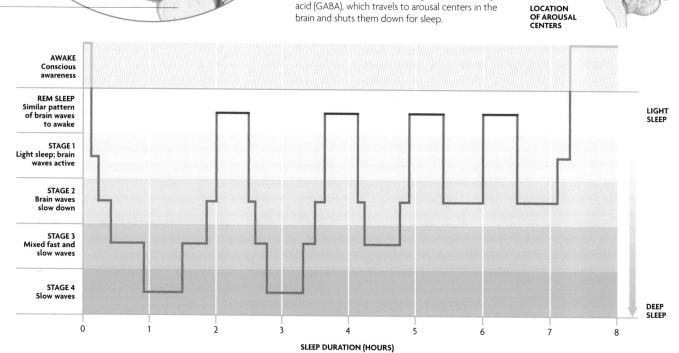

Thalamus
Ventrolateral preoptic nucleus
Arousal centers
Cerebellum
Pons
Medulla

SHUTTING DOWN AROUSAL SIGNALS
The ventrolateral preoptic nucleus in the hypothalamus produces the neurotransmitter gamma aminobutyric acid (GABA), which travels to arousal centers in the brain and shuts them down for sleep.

LOCATION OF AROUSAL CENTERS

KEY
— AWAKE
— REM SLEEP
— NON-REM SLEEP

THE SLEEP CYCLE
Although sleep may seem like a constant state, it actually occurs in cycles. Brief, dream-like fragments mark stage one, while stage two involves total loss of consciousness and muscle paralysis. Deep sleep occurs in stages three and four, where brain activity is low. Rapid eye movement (REM) sleep signals vivid dreaming.

AWAKE Conscious awareness
REM SLEEP Similar pattern of brain waves to awake
STAGE 1 Light sleep; brain waves active
STAGE 2 Brain waves slow down
STAGE 3 Mixed fast and slow waves
STAGE 4 Slow waves

LIGHT SLEEP
DEEP SLEEP

SLEEP DURATION (HOURS)

THE DREAMING BRAIN

There are two types of dreaming. During deep sleep we have vague, often emotionally charged and nonsensical dreams that are often forgotten immediately. The brain is not very active, but seems to be gently processing information in order to lay it down in memory. In REM sleep the brain becomes very active and produces vivid, intense "virtual realities," typically with a narrative. The part of the brain that processes sensations is very active during REM dreaming. The frontal lobes, which include areas that apply critical analysis to our experience, are effectively turned off, so when crazy events happen in our dreams, we just accept them.

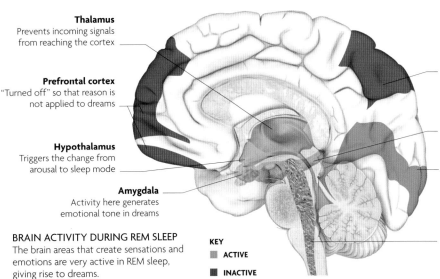

Thalamus
Prevents incoming signals from reaching the cortex

Prefrontal cortex
"Turned off" so that reason is not applied to dreams

Hypothalamus
Triggers the change from arousal to sleep mode

Amygdala
Activity here generates emotional tone in dreams

Parietal cortex
Spatial awareness and movement control are blocked

Hippocampus
Relays new memories to cortex for storage

Visual cortex
Generates internal imagery, without input from eyes

Reticular formation
Switches between sleep and arousal

BRAIN ACTIVITY DURING REM SLEEP
The brain areas that create sensations and emotions are very active in REM sleep, giving rise to dreams.

KEY
■ ACTIVE
■ INACTIVE

AWAKE
This PET scan shows the areas that are active when a person is awake (shown in red and yellow). The green and blue areas are less active.

DEEP SLEEP
This PET scan shows that activity quiets down in many areas of the brain during deep sleep. The purple areas are the least active.

DRUGGED SLEEP
Most sleeping drugs induce a deeper sleep than normal. The purple areas on this PET scan show that much of the brain is inactive.

REM SLEEP
This fMRI scan shows activity (yellow most active, then red) during REM sleep, spanning areas involved with generating sensations.

WAKING AND LUCID DREAMS

Usually, when shifting from dreaming to waking, several changes occur together in the brain. The block on incoming stimuli is lifted, so external sensory inputs enter the brain again, which overrides and turns off the internally generated sensations that comprise dreams. The block on outgoing signals from the motor cortex is also lifted, so that it becomes possible to move again. Additionally, the frontal lobes are reactivated, shifting us back into a normal state of consciousness in which we know who and where we are, and can tell the difference between fantasy and reality. Lucid dreams occur when the frontal lobes "wake up" during sleep, but the block on incoming and outgoing signals continues. Because the frontal lobes are active, the dreamer is able to deduce that he or she is actually dreaming and experience events in a normal state of mind.

ANYTHING IS POSSIBLE
In lucid dreams you can control the action just as in a waking daydream, but the experience is more intense and seems real.

SLEEP PARALYSIS
Waking up while the motor-impulse blockade is still operating is known as sleep paralysis. This frightening sensation feels like being weighed down, which may be the origin of the myth of the incubi and succubi, evil spirits that were thought to squat on sleepers.

FREUD AND PSYCHOANALYSIS

Sigmund Freud was an Austrian psychiatrist, who founded the study of psychoanalysis. He called dreaming the "royal route to the unconscious," because he thought that dreams revealed the emotions and desires that we suppress when we are awake. He postulated that these suppressed desires are often too shocking to be consciously admitted, and even in dreams they have to be disguised in symbols. Freudian dream analysis aimed to decode the symbols to reveal the true nature of the desires of the dreamer.

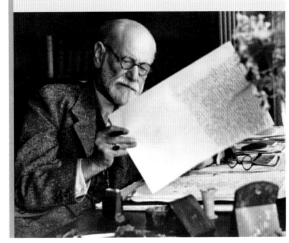

TIME

TIME IS NOT A CONSTANT IN THE BRAIN—IT SPEEDS UP AND SLOWS DOWN ACCORDING TO WHAT IS BEING EXPERIENCED. THE BRAIN HAS MANY DIFFERENT WAYS OF MEASURING TIME. LONGER DURATIONS, SUCH AS DAY LENGTH, ARE MEASURED BY THE EBB AND FLOW OF HORMONES, WHILE THE MILLISECOND INTERVALS INVOLVED IN MANY BRAIN PROCESSES ARE MARKED BY THE OSCILLATION OF NEURONS.

SUBJECTIVE TIME

The passage of time as we experience it (known as subjective time) is not the same as the regular passage of time as measured by our clocks (objective time). The crucial difference is that subjective time can speed up and slow down, according to what we are experiencing. On a moment-by-moment scale, the rate at which time seems to pass is dictated by the rate of firing, or oscillation, of clusters of neurons. The faster they fire, the more events we register in any given second, giving us the impression that time lasts longer. Neuronal firing is controlled by neurotransmitters—excitatory ones speed it up, and inhibitory ones slow it down. Young people have more excitatory neurotransmitters and, therefore, are able to cope with faster external events.

TIME PASSING SLOWLY
Stimulants like caffeine speed up the brain, allowing more external events to be registered. This produces a sense of time stretching out.

THE BRAIN CLOCK
The brain has different "clocks" for different time scales. One is formed by a dopamine-generated neuronal circuit that runs between the substantia nigra, the basal ganglia, and the prefrontal cortex. Each "cycle" of the clock creates a single "packet" of subjective time.

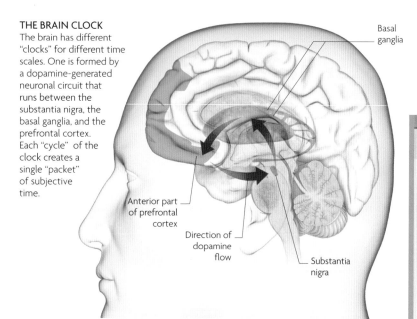

Basal ganglia

Anterior part of prefrontal cortex

Direction of dopamine flow

Substantia nigra

TIME RUSHING BY
Severe depletion of dopamine, as in Parkinson's disease, may slow the brain down so much that the external world seems to be rushing by.

CATATONIA

Catatonia is a state most commonly observed in people with certain types of schizophrenia. The sufferer becomes motionless and stops reacting to external stimuli. They may remain mute, or rigid, for days on end, sometimes striking bizarre poses, which would normally be impossible to maintain. The state seems to come about when the flow of dopamine slows down, and people who have experienced this condition report that they lose all sense of time.

PACKETS OF TIME

The brain divides time into "packets" (a cycle of neural activity), each of which registers a single event. The size of the packet depends on how fast the relevant neurons are firing, but regardless of the size of the packet, the brain will only be able to take in one event from that packet. If two events happen, the brain will miss the second one. Some events will always appear blurred to us, such as the beating of a dragonfly's wings, because several flaps occur in each packet.

EXPERIENCING EVENTS

If the "clock" neurons fire only once in $^1/_{10}$ of a second, only one event will be registered in that time, although many more may actually occur. If the neural clock doubles its speed, both events will be registered because the neural clock will have created two "packets" of subjective time.

Experienced as one event
Frames 1 and 2 fall within one "packet" of time and so are experienced as only one event

Cycle speeds up
The dopamine cycle doubles its speed, so more events will be registered by the brain

Experienced as two events
With the increase in cycle speed, frames 3 and 4 are registered as two events.

Beginning of cycle

0.1 SEC   0.2 SEC   0.25 SEC   0.3 SEC

TIME

PLASTIC CONCEPT OF TIME
Salvador Dali's painting *The Persistence of Memory* illustrates the point that our notion of time is flexible—it can feel like it speeds up or even stops.

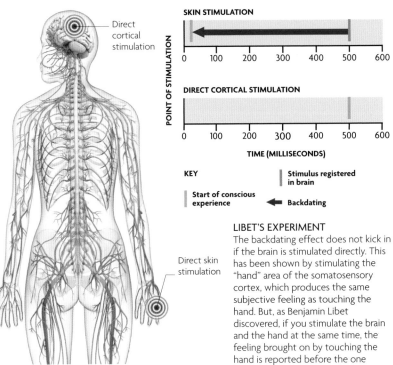

SKIN STIMULATION

POINT OF STIMULATION

0 100 200 300 400 500 600

DIRECT CORTICAL STIMULATION

0 100 200 300 400 500 600

TIME (MILLISECONDS)

KEY

Stimulus registered in brain

Start of conscious experience

Backdating

Direct cortical stimulation

Direct skin stimulation

LIBET'S EXPERIMENT
The backdating effect does not kick in if the brain is stimulated directly. This has been shown by stimulating the "hand" area of the somatosensory cortex, which produces the same subjective feeling as touching the hand. But, as Benjamin Libet discovered, if you stimulate the brain and the hand at the same time, the feeling brought on by touching the hand is reported before the one produced by stimulating the brain.

BACKDATING TIME
It takes on average half a second for the unconscious mind to process incoming sensory stimuli into conscious perceptions. Yet we are not aware of this time lag—you think you see things move as they move, and when you stub your toe you get the impression of knowing about it right away. This illusion of immediacy is created by an ingenious mechanism, which backdates conscious perceptions to the time when the stimulus first entered the brain. On the face of it, this seems impossible because cortical signals take the same "real" time to process to consciousness, but somehow we are tricked into thinking we feel things earlier. One way it might be explained is that consciousness consists of many parallel streams and that the brain jumps from one to another, revising them and redrafting them.

HALF A SECOND LATE
We become conscious of events around us nearly half a second after they occur, but we do not notice this time lag.

THE SELF AND CONSIOUSNESS

THE HUMAN BRAIN GENERATES AN IDEA OF "SELF" THAT ALLOWS US TO "OWN" OUR EXPERIENCES AND FORGES A CONNECTION BETWEEN OUR THOUGHTS AND INTENTIONS, OUR BODIES, AND OUR ACTIONS. OUR SENSE OF SELF ALSO ALLOWS US TO EXAMINE OUR OWN MINDS AND TO USE WHAT WE SEE TO GUIDE OUR BEHAVIOR.

WHAT IS THE SELF?

We divide the world into that which is subjective and internal and that which is objective and external. The boundary between the two acts like a container, which holds the former and places the latter outside. This container is what we know as the "self". Among other things, it includes our thoughts, intentions, and habits, as well as our actual bodies. Except in altered states (see p.186), all experiences we report include a sense of self, but most of the time the sense is unconscious. This "consciousness-with-self" is what we generally call "consciousness". When the sense of self becomes conscious, we talk of being "self-conscious".

LEVELS OF CONSCIOUSNESS

The sense of self lies at the heart of our experiences. It takes various forms and operates at different levels of our consciousness.

Introspection	You think about your own thoughts or action; one form is being "self-conscious" about your performance of an act.
Normal Consciousness	You feel that your thoughts are your own, and your actions are the result of your decisions; you can report experiences.
Knowledge	You react to the environment, perhaps by doing complex actions (such as driving), but if asked you can't recall doing it.
Unconsciousness	In deepest sleep, your brain does not perceive the outside world or generate a sense of self to experience anything.

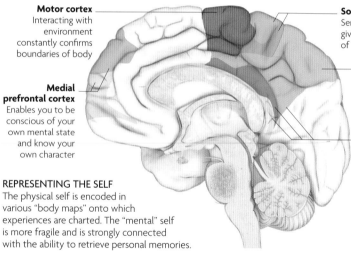

Motor cortex
Interacting with environment constantly confirms boundaries of body

Medial prefrontal cortex
Enables you to be conscious of your own mental state and know your own character

Somatosensory cortex
Sensations from body give repeated reminders of physical embodiment

Parietal cortex
This "maps" the body and its relationship to outside world

Cingulate cortex
Enables you to think about your position in relation to other people

REPRESENTING THE SELF
The physical self is encoded in various "body maps" onto which experiences are charted. The "mental" self is more fragile and is strongly connected with the ability to retrieve personal memories.

SELF-REFLECTIVE THOUGHT
This kind of thought creates activity in several areas of the brain. The areas towards the top and back are mainly concerned with body "maps," while those at the front are concerned with the mental self.

EXAMINING THE "I"
Trying to examine the "I" is like trying to look at your own eye—it is impossible because you are trying to see the thing you are using to see with. In effect, a shadow self arises, observing the "I."

AGENCY AND INTENTION

Agency is our sense of control over our actions. We feel that our conscious thoughts dictate what we do, but this appears to be incorrect. A famous experiment by Benjamin Libet (see p.191) revealed that a person's brain starts to plan and execute a movement unconsciously, before the person has consciously decided to do it. This is often interpreted to show that our sense of agency and of making "decisions" is illusory. The sense of agency we experience may actually have evolved primarily to give us early warning not of our own actions, but of the actions of others. Because we feel ourselves to be agents, we also intuit agency in others, and thus think we know their intentions and can predict what they will do.

THE EVOLUTION OF AGENCY
Awareness of what we are about to do may have arisen late in our evolution, once the action-planning part of our brain had connected to the areas that support consciousness.

SCHIZOPHRENIA AND AGENCY

People with schizophrenia may have a disturbed sense of agency. Some attribute their own actions to the intentions of others, claiming they are being "controlled" by outside forces; others, that they "cause" events unconnected with their own actions, such as moving the sun. Studies have suggested that these disturbances of the sense of agency are the result of misperceiving the time gap between action and consequence.

UNCONSCIOUS REFLEX
We have no sense of agency about a knee-jerk reaction because it occurs without us consciously "willing" it.

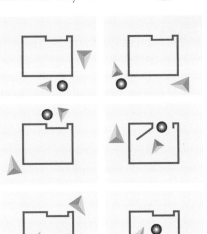

SEEING INTENTION BEHIND ACTIONS
Our tendency to see intention leads us to visualize it even in the behavior of nonsentient objects. Read as a cartoon strip, the pictures on the left suggest a chase in which the smaller objects "hide" and "escape" from the largest one.

AUDITORY HALLUCINATION
This fMRI scan shows brain activity in a hallucinating schizophrenic. The lit-up right hemisphere speech areas may elicit sounds that could be imagined as an external voice, distorting the sense of agency.

DISLOCATED SELF

The brain holds various "body maps" – internal representations of the physical self. The earliest, most basic map to emerge tells us where our body ends and the rest of the world begins. A more developed body "atlas" enables us to know our spatial location in the world. Normally, the internal maps and the body itself are closely matched, but it is possible for them to be askew. If a person loses a limb, for example, they may develop what is known as a phantom limb—a feeling that they have a limb that, in fact, no longer exists (see p.104). People can also be tricked into "owning" a limb or even a body that is not actually theirs.

INFANT BODY MAPS
Babies probably do not distinguish between their body and external objects until their body maps start to take in information from the world.

OUT-OF-BODY EXPERIENCES

Out-of-body experiences (OBEs) occur when the internal representation of the body is out of kilter with the real body. This happens all the time in dreams, but when it happens during wakefulness it may be interpreted as a supernatural event. OBEs typically occur as you wake up, before the brain has properly reconnected with the external world (see p.173).

NEAR-DEATH EXPERIENCES

OBEs are often accompanied by feelings of ecstasy, and they are a central feature of many so-called "near-death experiences."

VIRTUAL BODY
Volunteers were given goggles, through which they could see a camera view of their own back sitting in front of them. Touching this virtual back with a pen led to reports that they could actually feel this sensation, making them feel the virtual body was their own.

THE COLLECTIVE UNCONSCIOUS

Carl Jung (1875–1961) was a Swiss psychiatrist who developed the idea of the collective unconscious—a part of the unconscious mind shared by everyone as a product of ancestry. He thought it included "archetypes" (innate, universal concepts) such as the mother, God, hero and so on, and that we detect their influences in the form of myths, symbols, and instinct. Presumably he saw the collective unconscious as a sort of "folk memory", embodied in the structure of the brain.

NO TWO BRAINS ARE EXACTLY ALIKE. ALTHOUGH THEY ARE BUILT ACCORDING TO THE SAME BASIC PLAN, EACH ONE IS PRODUCED FROM INSTRUCTIONS ENCODED IN A UNIQUE SET OF GENES, WHICH ARE ENGAGED IN COMPLEX INTERACTION WITH THE ENVIRONMENT. WE OFTEN THINK THAT OUR INDIVIDUALITY IS EXPRESSED THROUGH OUR PERSONALITY, BUT RECENT STUDIES SUGGEST THAT PERSONALITY IS A MUTABLE PHENOMENON. WE ALL HAVE SUBTLY DIFFERENT PERSONALITIES THAT WE EXHIBIT IN DIFFERENT SITUATIONS.

THE INDIVIDUAL BRAIN

NATURE AND NURTURE

NATURE AND NURTURE ARE THE TWO FACTORS SHAPING THE WAY THE BRAIN FUNCTIONS. NATURE REFERS TO AN INDIVIDUAL'S GENOTYPE—THAT IS, THE PARTICULAR SET OF GENES INHERITED FROM THE PARENTS. THE BRAIN IS ALSO ALTERED BY NURTURE, WHICH IS ALL THE ENVIRONMENTAL FACTORS AN INDIVIDUAL IS EXPOSED TO THROUGHOUT LIFE.

GENES AND THE ENVIRONMENT

A gene is a unit of hereditary information linked to one or more physical traits (such as eye color). Genes are made of DNA (see panel, below) and some genes achieve their effects by the production of proteins. Genes are like dimmer switches–they can turn their activity (expression) on, off, up, or down. In the brain, gene expression affects the levels of neurotransmitters, which, in turn, influences complex functions like personality, memory, and intelligence. However, neurotransmitters also affect gene expression. Environmental influences affect patterns of gene expression, so that brain function also depends upon factors such as diet, geographical surroundings, social networks, and even stress levels. Chemical tags attach to DNA and alter gene expression, a process known as epigenetic alteration. They sometimes occur in response to stress and alter genes involved in behavior. For example, lack of maternal care has been found to produce epigentic changes in mammals, which makes them poor mothers. These changes pass through the gene line to future generations, so events that affect one person may also affect their grandchildren.

MUSICAL BRAIN
Having a "musical brain" may be the result of being raised in a family that values music and/or genetic influences.

THE DNA MOLECULE

Found in the nuclei of all cells in the human body except red blood cells, the DNA molecule is shaped like a twisted ladder—the famous double helix. The two strands of the helix are held together by chemicals called bases, which are arranged in pairs. There are four bases, known by the letters A, C, G, and T, and they always pair in the same combinations (A pairs with T, and C pairs with G). The sequence of base pairs can be read by the cell as the instructions for making proteins.

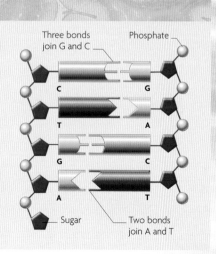

Three bonds join G and C

Phosphate

C — G

T — A

G — C

A — T

Sugar

Two bonds join A and T

BUILT FOR SPEED
Like many aspects of physical performance, sprinting is genetically influenced. For example, a gene for insulin-like growth factor (IGF) influences an athlete's muscle mass. Although most successful sprinters share a genetic advantage, the right genes alone are not enough. Athletes have to train hard and have a desire to win if they are to become champions.

GENETICS AND THE BRAIN

Proteins have many roles in the body. Some form structures, such as hair, while others, such as enzymes, regulate processes. Several genes in the genome may code for the protein molecules that make serotonin, one of the neurotransmitters involved in mood. Each variant of this gene makes a slightly different protein molecule, which may carry out its job more, or maybe less, efficiently. Thus, gene variants may result in one person having more serotonin, and another person less serotonin. Less serotonin may mean a predisposition to depression or a tendency to overeat. This is also true of other neurotransmitters, such as dopamine –a lack of dopamine has been linked to increased risk-taking behavior. Therefore, your genotype can affect the structure and functioning of your brain, which, in turn, will influence behavior.

MICROARRAY
Gene expression in brain cells can be monitored using a microarray, in which each dot is a different gene.

TWINS

Studies of twins who were separated at birth and brought up in different families have shown that an identical twin reared away from his or her co-twin is still very similar in terms of interests, personality, and attitudes. Therefore, genes would seem to exert a powerful influence on the shaping of the brain throughout life. A classic example is the two "Jims," who were adopted at the age of four. The adoptive parents—unknown to one another—both named the boys James, and both were known as Jim. Both twins began suffering from tension headaches aged 18. Both were poor spellers but good at math, and as adults, both followed a similar career path in law enforcement.

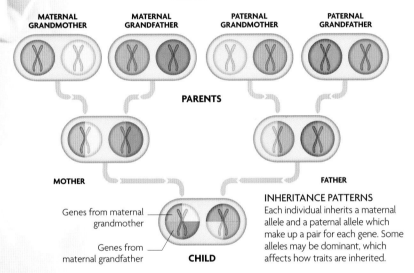

GRANDPARENTS

MATERNAL GRANDMOTHER   MATERNAL GRANDFATHER   PATERNAL GRANDMOTHER   PATERNAL GRANDFATHER

PARENTS

MOTHER   FATHER

Genes from maternal grandmother

Genes from maternal grandfather   **CHILD**

INHERITANCE PATTERNS
Each individual inherits a maternal allele and a paternal allele which make up a pair for each gene. Some alleles may be dominant, which affects how traits are inherited.

THE PLASTIC BRAIN

The brain was once believed to be immutable from birth, with a certain number of brain cells and fixed neuronal circuits. The only changes thought to occur were the loss of brain cells and a reduction in brain volume. But researchers have shown that experience and learning remodel brain circuits. Examples of such neuronal plasticity include long-term potentiation, where memory and learning generate new circuits (see p.158); the remodeling of the brain after a stroke or in drug addiction to strengthen pathways or create new ones; and the formation of new brain cells (neurogenesis). The brain, it seems, has a certain ability to repair itself and continue to grow and develop throughout life.

BIRTH OF NEURONS
This colored electron micrograph shows neural progenitor cells. These cells lie between stem cells and fully differentiated cells. They are capable of developing into neurons and other neural cells.

FIRED UP
This micrograph shows brain tissue stained with antibodies that "light up" changes in synapses and brain proteins linked to the formation of memory through long-term potentiation.

INFLUENCING THE BRAIN

EVERYONE'S BRAIN IS DIFFERENT—GENDER AND SEXUAL ORIENTATION ARE REFLECTED BY CHANGES IN THE BRAIN'S ANATOMY AND FUNCTIONING, THE BRAINS OF RIGHT-HANDED AND LEFT-HANDED PEOPLE ARE ORGANIZED DIFFERENTLY, AND EVEN SOCIAL AND CULTURAL INFLUENCES CAN SHAPE THE WAY THE BRAIN CARRIES OUT CERTAIN TASKS.

THE GENDERED BRAIN

A number of structural and functional differences have been found between male and female brains. Both the corpus callosum and the anterior commissure (a more primitive connection between the two hemispheres that links the unconscious areas) are larger in women than in men. This may be why women are more emotionally aware–the more emotional right side is better connected to the more analytical left side of the brain. It may also allow emotion to be incorporated more readily into thought and speech. When doing complex tasks, women use both sides of their brain, while men use the side more obviously suited to the task.

ONE OF THE CROWD
Just as each individual's face in this crowd is different and unique, so too are their brains. Genetic differences at birth are just one factor—cultural and environmental influences during life can also have a profound effect.

MALE   **FEMALE**

RESPONDING TO LANGUAGE
These fMRI scans reveal that women show activity on both sides of the brain when responding to language. In men, however, the activity is restricted more to the left hemisphere (shown on the right side of the scan).

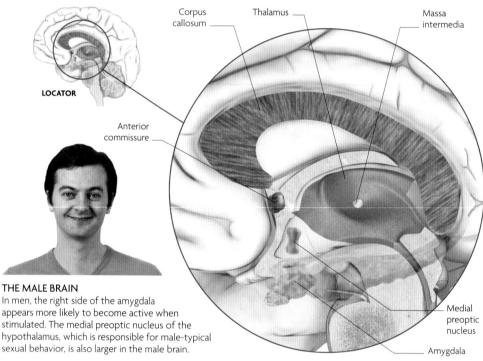

Corpus callosum · Thalamus · Massa intermedia · Anterior commissure · Medial preoptic nucleus · Amygdala

THE MALE BRAIN
In men, the right side of the amygdala appears more likely to become active when stimulated. The medial preoptic nucleus of the hypothalamus, which is responsible for male-typical sexual behavior, is also larger in the male brain.

LOCATOR

THE GAY BRAIN

Brain scans show how, in homosexual people, important brain structures involved in mood, emotion, anxiety, and aggression tend to resemble those of heterosexuals of the opposite sex. Heterosexual men tend to have asymmetric brains, with the right hemisphere slightly larger than the left, a characteristic shared by gay women. Patterns of brain connectivity are similar between heterosexual women and gay men, particularly in areas involved with anxiety.

HETEROSEXUAL MEN   **HETEROSEXUAL WOMEN**

HOMOSEXUAL MEN   **HOMOSEXUAL WOMEN**

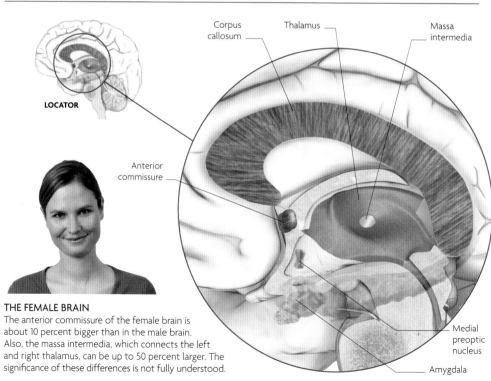

Corpus callosum · Thalamus · Massa intermedia · Anterior commissure · Medial preoptic nucleus · Amygdala

LOCATOR

THE FEMALE BRAIN
The anterior commissure of the female brain is about 10 percent bigger than in the male brain. Also, the massa intermedia, which connects the left and right thalamus, can be up to 50 percent larger. The significance of these differences is not fully understood.

LEFT OR RIGHT HAND?

Around 90 percent of people are right-handed–that is, they use the right hand rather than the left for tasks requiring fine motor control, such as signing their name. Analysis of tools and other archaeological evidence reveals this has been the case since the Stone Age. Right-handedness may be linked to left-hemisphere dominance for language. About 70 percent of left-handed people have language dominance in the left side of the brain, but 30 percent perform language functions using both sides equally. There is also a hypothesis that left-handed people are more likely to be better at visual perception and thinking. About 26 percent of children from two left-handed parents will be left-handed. Only around nine percent of children from two right-handed parents will be left-handed, and there is a high tendency among twins for one to be left-handed.

THE WRONG HAND?

It is not known why a minority of the population is left-handed. Handedness is set in the womb, and the cause is likely to be genetic. Left-handedness has a negative image in some cultures—parents may encourage their children to switch hands to appear "normal," and numerous languages refer to the left hand as being clumsy or sinister. Stuttering and dyslexia are more common among left-handers, but they are often good at sports like swimming and basketball.

LEFT-HANDED LEADERS
Both Barack Obama and John McCain, his rival in the 2008 US presidential election, are left-handed. Obama makes it five left-handers out of the last seven US Presidents—a much higher percentage than among the general population.

WHAT DO YOU SEE?
There is a spotted Dalmatian hidden in this picture. The idea that left-handed people think visually has led to claims that they will spot the dog more quickly than right-handed people.

CULTURAL INFLUENCES

Researchers have shown that culture influences the way the brain works. They carried out tests during fMRI scans on people raised in the US and people raised in East Asia, in which participants did puzzles involving lines in a square (see below). US culture is perceived to be focused upon the individual, while East Asian culture tends to be more focused on family and community. The brains of the US participants had to work harder when they were doing tasks involving context, while those of the East Asians worked harder when they had to judge individual lines. Brain activity lessened when participants undertook tasks related to their culture's comfort zone. Participants were also asked how closely they identified with their culture, and the brains of those who identified most strongly had to work the hardest when doing tasks related to the "opposite" culture.

RELATIVE TASK	ABSOLUTE TASK

PERCEPTUAL TEST
The length of the line in this square may be perceived differently if it is compared to another line. Whether the brain is comfortable judging its length depends on the context of the test and cultural background.

COMPARISON SQUARE

ABSOLUTE

RELATIVE

ABSOLUTE AND RELATIVE TASKS
In an absolute task, the line's length is compared to that of the line in the comparison square. In the relative task, the length of the line and its relation to the size of the square is compared to the same relationship in the first square.

BRAIN ACTIVATION PATTERNS
East Asian brains have to work less at the relative line perception task, whereas Americans are the opposite, with the absolute task being less demanding of their brains. This is because these tests are "easier" when the tasks are more in line with cultural norms.

PERSONALITY

PERSONALITY IS GENERALLY AGREED TO BE A GROUP OF BEHAVIORAL CHARACTERISTICS TYPICALLY EXHIBITED BY AN INDIVIDUAL. SOME PEOPLE DISPLAY THE SAME BEHAVIOR IN DIFFERENT SITUATIONS AND AT DIFFERENT TIMES, WHILE OTHERS ARE MUCH MORE CHANGEABLE.

LEARNING TO BE YOU

Each one of us has a genetic blueprint that predisposes us to characteristics such as aggression or extroversion. Although genes contribute greatly to personality development, the way we turn out also depends on how we learn to behave. Personality can be seen as a bundle of habitual responses. These may be learned by copying behavior from caregivers or even from television. If a response is repeated frequently, it is encoded as a memory. Thereafter, it is as much a "part" of the person as a genetic inclination.

MIMICKING BEHAVIOR
Many of the mind habits that make up personality are initially learned by mimicking the adults that care for us as infants.

PERSONALITY AND THE BRAIN

Many different personality traits have been linked to specific patterns of activity in the brain, some of which are linked to the expression of certain genes or particular genetic mutations. For example, a person who produces more excitatory neurotransmitters is less likely to feel the need to seek thrills than someone who needs a lot of stimulation to experience the same level of excitement.

PERSONALITY MARKERS IN THE BRAIN

Extroversion	Extroverts have reduced activity, in response to stimuli, in the neural circuit that keeps the brain aroused (shown here). As a result, they need more environmental stimuli to keep them feeling energized.	Dorsolateral prefrontal cortex / Anterior cingulate cortex / Thalamus
Aggression	People with a version of a gene previously linked to impulsive violence show abnormally reduced volume and unusually low activity in the cingulate cortex—an area concerned with monitoring and guiding behavior.	Cingulate cortex
Social behavior	Socially secure people have a stronger response to friendly looking people in the striatum—an area concerned with reward—than shy people. Avoidant types show a stronger reaction in the amygdala to unfriendly looking people.	Striatum / Amygdala
Novelty seeking	People who like novelty may have better connections between areas shown here. The hippocampus sends signals to the striatum—which registers pleasure—when it identifies an experience as new.	Striatum / Hippocampus
Cooperation	Cooperative people show increased activity in the insula if they think their treatment is unfair. Uncooperative people do not register unfairness to the same extent, suggesting an underdeveloped sense of trust.	Insula
Optimism	Optimism is linked to enhanced activation in the amygdala and in the anterior cingulate cortex when imagining positive future events relative to negative ones.	Cingulate cortex / Amygdala

Param
"D

AVEC

FREDRIC MARCH

MIRIAM HOPKINS
ET
ROSE HOBART

REALISATION DE
ROUBEN MAMOULIAN

PERSONALITY ASSESSMENT

Personality testing is used for many reasons, such as for determining a person's suitability for a job or promotion. Some tests are standardized assessments that require people to answer questions about their typical behavior. The results are used to determine the individual's personality profile. Type tests place people in a particular category. Myers–Briggs, for example (below, right) sorts people into categories based on the predominance of certain attributes. Trait tests do not fit people into types, but draw up a profile based on where they lie along a number of dimensions. Projective tests, such as the Rorschach inkblot test, invite people to "reveal" aspects of their personality when responding to ambiguous stimuli.

PROJECTIVE TESTS
By "seeing" meaning in random shapes, such as inkblots, people "project" aspects of their personality.

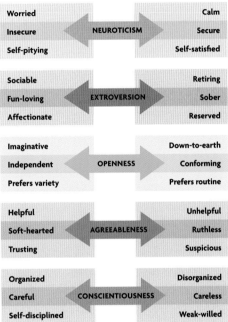

THE BIG FIVE
According to this trait test model, basic differences in personality can be "boiled down" to five dimensions. People may fall anywhere on each dimension.

Worried — NEUROTICISM — Calm
Insecure — Secure
Self-pitying — Self-satisfied

Sociable — EXTROVERSION — Retiring
Fun-loving — Sober
Affectionate — Reserved

Imaginative — OPENNESS — Down-to-earth
Independent — Conforming
Prefers variety — Prefers routine

Helpful — AGREEABLENESS — Unhelpful
Soft-hearted — Ruthless
Trusting — Suspicious

Organized — CONSCIENTIOUSNESS — Disorganized
Careful — Careless
Self-disciplined — Weak-willed

MYERS–BRIGGS INDICATORS
The Myers–Briggs test asks a wide range of questions and places the person in one of 16 types. Despite criticisms of its lack of validity, it is the most widely used personality test used by businesses.

	SENSING		INTUITIVE	
JUDGING	ISTJ	ISFJ	INFJ	INTJ
PERCEIVING	ISTP	ISFP	INFP	INTP
PERCEIVING	ESTP	ESFP	ENFP	ENTP
JUDGING	ESTJ	ESFJ	ENFJ	ENTJ
	THINKING	FEELING		THINKING

(INTROVERT / EXTROVERT)

MANY PERSONALITIES?

Type tests like the Myers–Briggs (above) have been found to give different results according to the situation in which the person is tested. Trait tests allow for people to be different at different times, but still assume they have a "major" personality that is more real than others. Some evidence suggests, however, that practically everyone has more than one personality, and that many people have a large number of them. Memories that are available to a person in one situation may not be accessible in another. In extreme cases, this results in dissociative identity disorder (DID), but in normal people it merely shows up as mood changes, memory "glitches," and the coming and going of different skills, behaviors, and ways of seeing the world.

DR. JEKYLL AND MR. HYDE
Dramatic personality changes, such as a "split personality," are a staple of horror films and ghost stories. They reflect a distrust of people who appear not to have stable personalities.

DISSOCIATIVE IDENTITY DISORDER

Extreme multiplicity, in which personalities are completely compartmentalized, results in people switching from one personality to another without retaining any memory of the previous state. They may behave differently according to which personality they are, and may even adopt a different name and history for each one. Because they have no memory of the others, each of them is likely to have memory gaps. Some people with DID find, for example, that they do things of which, in another personality, they disapprove.

BRAIN MONITORING AND STIMULATION

IT IS NOW POSSIBLE TO WATCH THE BRAIN'S ACTIVITY TAKING PLACE ON AN EXTERNAL DISPLAY AND DELIBERATELY CHANGE IT. THIS IS KNOWN AS NEUROFEEDBACK. MORE DIRECTLY, ACTIVITY CAN BE STIMULATED BY ELECTRICAL INPUT SENT THROUGH THE SKULL OR FROM ELECTRODES IMPLANTED INTO THE BRAIN ITSELF.

NEUROFEEDBACK

Brain activity is constantly altered by what an individual feels, thinks, or senses. The neurofeedback process works by turning the brain's activity itself into an external stimulus, which the person then responds to. For instance, EEG sensors may be used to pick up a person's brainwaves. Different mind-states, such as relaxation or anxiety, have characteristic wave-forms that are translated into a dynamic visual display. The activity registered by the EEG is then sent to a device that turns them into a form that the person can easily understand and manipulate. This may be as simple as a line that moves up or down, or a more complex game. The person tries to change the on-screen information by using the brain. The result of the effort is then displayed, so the person learns what to do in order to achieve the desired effect. Repeatedly doing this makes it increasingly easy to gain a desired state of mind, such as relaxation or focused attention.

MUSICAL MIND
Neurofeedback can help musicians attain a mind-state in which they play better. Students from London's Royal College of Music improved their performances by up to 15 percent after a course of treatment.

Step 1 EEG (or a similar brain "reading" device) charts the neural activity in the person's brain. The information is then transferred to a computer.

Step 2 The computer turns the neural patterns into a dynamic visual display, such as an interactive game with a clear goal like making an on-screen object move.

Step 4 The player associates the "wins" in the game with certain brain states. The process then begins again, and through repetition the player learns to achieve them more easily.

Step 3 The person plays the game just by altering his or her brain-state. The machine registers neural changes, such as those marking relaxation, and "rewards" them with wins.

FEEDBACK LOOP
The neurofeedback process teaches people to change their brain-state. Once people have learned to do this with the equipment, they find it easier to do so at will.

MIND CONTROL
EEG is the usual brain "reading" process used for neurofeedback. Dozens of scalp-mounted electrodes pick up oscillations of underlying neurons and convert them into waves.

ECT

Electroconvulsive therapy (ECT) involves sending an electric current through the brain until the neurons are so stimulated that they produce a seizure (see p.226). It is used as a treatment of last resort for chronic depression, and it often works when drugs and psychotherapy have no effect. The way that it works is not fully understood, but it is thought that the seizure resets certain neurons' potential to fire, making them more or less sensitive. The seizure induced by ECT is short-lasting and harmless, and muscle relaxants are used to prevent convulsions. However, patients often complain of memory problems following the treatment.

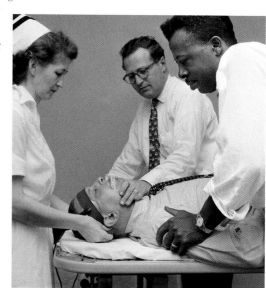

HISTORIC ECT
ECT was widely used in the 1950s in mental institutions. At that time it was a crude technique, which involved creating a whole-brain seizure that caused the patient to thrash about.

TMS

Transcranial magnetic stimulation (TMS) sends a magnetic pulse through the skull and into the brain. The pulse temporarily disrupts normal activity in the part of the brain beneath it. Repeated stimulation of a particular area causes long-term changes in the way it functions. For example, it can increase activity in parts of the brain that are known to be underactive in people with depression, or decrease it in areas known to be overactive in those with obsessive compulsive disorder. Repeated sessions of TMS are increasingly used as treatment for these and other conditions.

magnetic pulse travels through the skull

area of brain activity disrupted

TMS WAND

A TMS wand induces electric currents by electromagnetic induction. It is usually held in the therapist's hand and placed close to—but not touching—the head, over the target area of the brain.

DEEP BRAIN STIMULATION

In deep brain stimulation, tiny electrodes are placed surgically in the brain. They radiate current to nearby target areas, activating otherwise sluggish neurons, which in turn create local changes in brain chemistry. The electrodes are attached to very fine wires, which are inserted deep into the brain through small holes in the skull. They are situated in different brain areas according to the condition being treated and may be sited quite differently in each patient. In some cases, the wires are connected to an external switch that allows the patient to turn the current on and off as required.

BRAIN SURGERY

Patients are operated on while conscious so that they are able to communicate. Their reactions guide the surgical team to implant the electrodes in the right spot.

TREATING STROKE

Neurostimulation may be used to help people recover from the effects of stroke. The damaged area of the brain is stimulated in order to help neighboring neurons grow and take over the work of the cells that have been killed off. Conversely, inhibitory stimulation may be applied to the brain cells corresponding to the damaged area on the opposite side of the brain. This prevents the opposite side of the brain from compensating for the damaged area and interfering with its recovery.

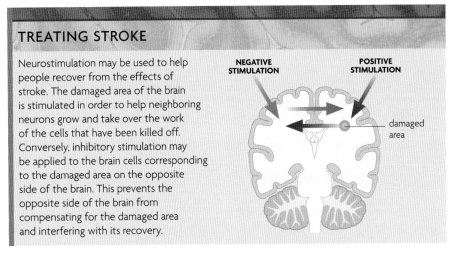

NEGATIVE STIMULATION

POSITIVE STIMULATION

damaged area

TDCS

Transcranial direct current stimulation (tDCS) is a way of stimulating (or inhibiting) selected neurons by sending a minute charge of electricity through the cortex via scalp-mounted electrodes. The current used is less than 2 milliAmps, so small that most people can barely feel it. Thousands of studies show that it is safe and that it may reduce symptoms of mood disorders, chronic pain, tinnitus, motor and speech disorders, especially after stroke, and possibly schizophrenia and dementia. It also enhances brain function in healthy people; for example, it can be used to improve math skills and creativity, and lead to swifter learning.

headset

electrode

control unit

TDCS UNIT

A tDCS device uses a battery-driven current stimulator that sends electricity through wires to electrodes clamped to the skull using elasticated bands or a lightweight plastic headset.

Depression: prefrontal cortex

Creativity: prefrontal area (studies have also found negative stimulation to be effective)

Speech fluency, and verbal memory enhancement: Broca's area

LEFT

Math enhancement: parietal cortex

BRAIN AREAS

Stimulating (or inhibiting) different brain areas with tDCS has different effects. These are some of the areas where anode stimulation (red) or cathode inhibition (blue) has been shown to alter experience or enhance a particular skill.

KEY

● ANODE STIMULATION

● CATHODE INHIBITION

RIGHT

STRANGE BRAINS

ON THE WHOLE, ONE BRAIN LOOKS VERY MUCH LIKE ANOTHER, GIVE OR TAKE A SMALL VARIATION IN SIZE. SOME BRAINS, HOWEVER, ARE DRAMATICALLY DIFFERENT FROM NORMAL, AND IN MANY CASES PHYSICAL ECCENTRICITY PRODUCES UNUSUAL WAYS OF BEHAVING AND SEEING THE WORLD.

THE SPLIT BRAIN

The corpus callosum carries signals between the two hemispheres. Rarely, this tissue is surgically severed in people with epilepsy, in order to prevent the spread of seizures. Researchers projected images separately to each hemisphere (see split-brain experiment, below) of split-brain patients. Normally the two sides would share the information via the corpus callosum, but without it each side recognized only its own image. The patients could identify the picture known by the language-dominant left brain, but denied seeing anything else. Yet they were able to select the object seen by the right brain, using the left hand (which is controlled by the right hemisphere). Asked why they selected that object, however, they were unable to say. This suggests that the right hemisphere (in right-handers) is unconscious—even though the information it holds affects behavior.

CONNECTING THE HEMISPHERES
This diffusion tensor image clearly shows the wide band of fibers that forms the corpus callosum, which connects the left and right hemispheres of the brain.

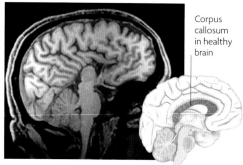

Corpus callosum in healthy brain

NO CONNECTION
Occasionally the corpus callosum fails to develop, in a condition known as agenesis of the corpus callosum (shown here in an MRI scan). This leaves the two hemispheres of the brain unconnected.

TESTING YOUR CORPUS CALLOSUM

Close your eyes and spread out your hands, palms facing upward. Get someone to touch one of your fingertips, and with your opposite hand try to touch the corresponding finger with thumb of the same hand (see below). If information is flowing properly between the hemispheres, you should be able to do this without opening your eyes.

Touch thumb to finger on left hand

Sensation experienced on right hand

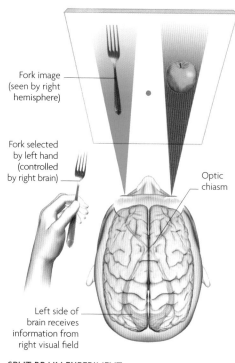

Fork image (seen by right hemisphere)

Fork selected by left hand (controlled by right brain)

Optic chiasm

Left side of brain receives information from right visual field

SPLIT-BRAIN EXPERIMENT
In a split-brain experiment, the image shown to the right side of the brain can guide the actions of the left hand to select an object, even though the person is not conscious of seeing the image and is only aware of seeing the apple.

WEIRD BRAINS

Brain scans have revealed some astonishing physical abnormalities, such as brains that are missing an entire hemisphere. The effect of losing half a brain would be catastrophic if it happened in later life. However, several cases have come to light in which brain growth has been severely restricted in infancy and yet the person has gone on to live a near normal life with few, if any, adverse symptoms.

Left hemisphere missing

HALF A BRAIN
Despite having one side of her brain removed, this girl learned to be fluent in two languages.

SIZE DOESN'T MATTER

Brains do not, generally, vary greatly in size, and there is little evidence to suggest that bigger brains produce greater intelligence. At one extreme, Irish writer Jonathan Swift (1667–1754) had a brain that, at the time of his death, weighed a relatively enormous 70oz (2,000g). In 1928, the Moscow Brain Research Institute started collecting and mapping the brains of famous Russians, including that of the physiologist Ivan Pavlov (1849–1936). His brain was at the other end of the size scale, weighing a mere 53½oz (1,517g).

JONATHAN SWIFT **IVAN PAVLOV**

VARYING SIZES
The brains of famous intellectuals vary greatly in size, so the connection between IQ and size is unclear.

THE TERRORIST'S BRAIN

Ulrike Meinhof (1934–76) was a member of the infamous Baader-Meinhof Gang, responsible for a number of killings, bombings, and kidnappings in Germany during the 1970s. She was captured and committed suicide in prison. After her death, studies suggested that brain damage resulting from an operation on a swollen blood vessel might have accounted for her violent behavior.

FACE OF A KILLER
This rare image of Meinhof was taken when she was arrested in 1972. In 1962, she had a metal clip inserted in her brain during surgery, which helped police identify her.

EINSTEIN'S BRAIN

Albert Einstein's brain was removed after his death. Many years later, it was examined by Dr. Sandra Witelson and compared with other brains in a brain bank. It was found to be wider than normal, and part of a deep groove that normally runs through the parietal lobe was missing. The area affected is concerned with mathematics and spatial reasoning, and it is possible that the missing groove allowed neurons in that area to communicate more easily, giving him his extraordinary talent for describing the universe mathematically.

Parietal lobe

TOP VIEW

Lateral sulcus

LATERAL VIEW

A MATHEMATICAL BRAIN?
Einstein's brain was wider than normal (top) and the part of the lateral sulcus normally found in the parietal cortex was apparently missing.

OUR BRAIN CHANGES OVER THE COURSE OF OUR LIFE, AND
THIS HAS FAR-REACHING EFFECTS ON WHAT WE CAN DO
AND HOW WE BEHAVE. DEVELOPMENT STARTS A FEW WEEKS
AFTER CONCEPTION, AND TO BEGIN WITH IS INCREDIBLY

DEVELOPMENT
AND AGING

THE INFANT BRAIN

THE HUMAN BRAIN FORMS FROM THE OUTERMOST LAYER OF TISSUE IN A DEVELOPING
EMBRYO, AND IT UNDERGOES SEVERAL TRANSFORMATIONS BEFORE EMERGING AS THE
RECOGNIZABLE ORGAN. AFTER A PERIOD OF RAPID CELL GROWTH, NEWLY GENERATED
NEURONS MOVE AROUND TO FORM THE VARIOUS PARTS OF THE BRAIN. IT TAKES MORE
THAN 20 YEARS FOR THE BRAIN TO BECOME FULLY MATURE.

CONCEPTION TO BIRTH

In the days after conception, the embryo
is just a minute ball of cells. Development
of the brain and nervous system starts
at about three weeks as the cells
differentiate into layers, the outermost
of which thickens and flattens to form a
feature called the neural plate (see below)
along the back of the embryo. This
broadens and folds to form the liquid-
filled neural tube, which will become
the brain and spinal cord. The brain
starts to develop at about four weeks
as a bulb at the upper end of the neural
tube, while the lower part begins to form
the spinal cord. The main sections of the
brain, including the cerebral cortex, are
visible within seven weeks. Over the
next weeks, the brain grows, develops,
and becomes more complex.

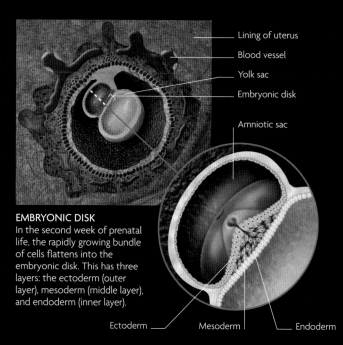

- Lining of uterus
- Blood vessel
- Yolk sac
- Embryonic disk
- Amniotic sac

EMBRYONIC DISK
In the second week of prenatal
life, the rapidly growing bundle
of cells flattens into the
embryonic disk. This has three
layers: the ectoderm (outer
layer), mesoderm (middle layer),
and endoderm (inner layer).

Ectoderm — Mesoderm — Endoderm

DEVELOPMENT OF THE CORTEX
The cerebral cortex develops from the
forebrain, one of three vesicles formed from
the neural tube. The frontal lobes form first,
followed by the parietal, then temporal and
occipital lobes.

KEY FOR EMBRYO DEVELOPMENT
- FOREBRAIN (PROSENCEPHALON)
- MIDBRAIN (MESENCEPHALON)
- HINDBRAIN (RHOMBENCEPHALON)
- SPINAL CORD

Cerebellum — Cerebrum
Brainstem

3 WEEKS
Neural tube forms
Forebrain prominence
Neural tube

Within three weeks of conception,
the neural tube is well developed
along the back of the embryo and
the prominence that will develop
into the forebrain is clearly defined.

5 WEEKS
Ear bud
Eye bud
Neural tube

The future forebrain, midbrain, and
hindbrain can be seen clearly by five
weeks, and rudimentary eye and ear
buds emerge. The optic nerve, retina,
and iris start to form.

7 WEEKS
Cranial nerves
Ear bud
Eye bud

The embryo is around ¾in (2cm) long,
and the bulges that will become the
brainstem, cerebellum, and cerebrum
are now clearly visible. The cranial and
sensory nerves also start to develop.

11 WEEKS
The cerebrum enlarges, and the eyes
and ears mature, moving into position.
The fetus's head is still large relative
to the body. The hindbrain divides into
the cerebellum and the brainstem.

FORMATION OF THE NEURAL TUBE

The key event in the development of
the nervous system is the formation
of the neural tube. This process is
known as neurulation, and begins
when the primitive spinal cord
(notochord) sends a signal to the
tissue above it to thicken, forming the
neural plate. The neural plate turns
inward and forms a depression,
known as the neural groove. Folds
within the groove fuse together and
then close in on themselves to form
the neural tube. Some neural-fold
tissue is pinched off to form the
neural crest, which will become
the peripheral nervous system.

Ectoderm Outermost of tissue layers that thickens to form neural plate

Notochord

Neural groove Neural plate folds inward to form neural groove

Endoderm Innermost of three tissue layers of an embryo

Mesoderm Middle of three tissue layers

FORMATION OF THE NEURAL GROOVE

Ectoderm This part of ectoderm will detach from rest

Neural groove This folds in on itself and starts to close up

Notochord

Mesoderm This layer begins to thicken

CLOSURE OF THE NEURAL GROOVE

Ectoderm Closes up over neural tube

Neural crest Becomes peripheral nervous system

Notochord Becomes spinal cord

Neural tube Becomes brain

THE NEURAL TUBE FORMS

NERVE GROWTH AND PRUNING

Only one-sixth of the brain develops before birth, and the growth rate in the first three years of life is phenomenal. Most of the growth, however, is connective tissue, as pathways are forged between neurons. By the age of three, this dense network of fibers requires "pruning" back, a process known as apoptosis. The pruning allows the preserved connections to work more efficiently. It is similar to the way in which "noise" can be extracted from a radio signal to leave only the intended content without the interference.

BIRTH   **2 YEARS**   **4 YEARS**

NEURAL NETWORKS
A dense network of connecting fibers forms between the brain's neurons during the first few years of life. By the age of four, these connections have been pruned back.

LANGUAGE DEVELOPMENT

Speech, and some other higher faculties, are wired into the human brain but appropriate stimulation is needed to help it develop normally. Babies start babbling at about six months, when a stream of syllables, with simple vowel-and-consonant combinations, is formed. "Motherese" is a universal adult reaction to babbling. It involves uttering repetitive sing-song noises, such as "goo-goo" and simple words. It aids speech development in the child and promotes bonding.

25 WEEKS
The hemispheres are now clearly dissected, and some of the deeper grooves that form the bulges and valleys—gyri and sulci—are becoming visible. The cerebellum is tucked under the cerebrum.

BIRTH
The cerebrum develops, and the ridges (gyri) and fissures (sulci) increase in complexity. At birth, a baby has as many neurons as an adult: 100 billion. Most are formed in the first six months of gestation but are not yet mature.

3 YEARS
The basic structure of the child's brain is complete, but parts of it remain "offline," including regions of the prefrontal cortex. Due to development of the hippocampus and amygdala, memories can now be retained.

CRITICAL PERIOD OF DEVELOPMENT
This chart shows that a crucial period of development occurs in the first few years of life. Early motor skills develop within the womb, where the fetus is also able to register sounds. For the first few months after birth, a baby will not be able to see clearly farther than about a yard, but this quickly improves.

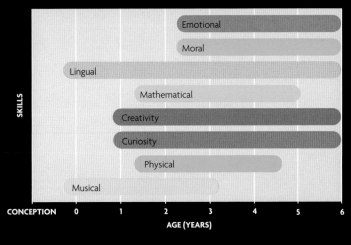

WINDOWS OF LEARNING

Human skills and faculties develop as the associated parts of the brain mature. The timetable is under genetic control, and no amount of teaching can instill in a child an ability that the brain is not ready to acquire. Until they are about three, for instance, infants cannot make moral judgments because their prefrontal cortex, where such decisions are made, is not fully "online." When the area is maturing, however, a child will learn the skill associated with it easily and rapidly, given the right stimuli. If a window of learning is missed, the child will have difficulty acquiring the skill later.

READY FOR BIRTH
This colored MRI scan shows a fetus during the 36th week of pregnancy. By this time, the fetus has usually shifted position so that its head faces the mother's cervix, ready to be born. Amazingly, babies are born with 100 billion neurons—the same number as an adult.

THE ADULT BRAIN

THE BRAIN DOES NOT STOP GROWING WHEN IT REACHES MATURITY. MORE THAN ANY OTHER ORGAN, IT CONTINUES TO REFORM ITSELF LONG INTO ADULTHOOD. NEW BRAIN CELLS CONTINUE TO BE CREATED, AND THE ARCHITECTURE OF THE BRAIN IS CHANGED CONSTANTLY IN RESPONSE TO LIFE EXPERIENCES.

REACHING MATURITY

Human brains are slow to reach full maturity. The prefrontal cortex is the last part to become fully active, and full myelinization, the sheathing of neuronal connections that allows information to flow freely along them, does not occur until a person is in their late twenties or early thirties. Once the prefrontal cortex is fully online, it becomes more active in situations that have emotional content. Whereas a teenager or child might be overwhelmed by emotion, the prefrontal cortex inhibits emotion when necessary, allowing a more thoughtful, deliberated response.

Sensory and motor cortices

Weak connection

Strong connection

Prefrontal cortex

Limbic area

Cerebellum

Basal ganglia
mediate movement

Prefrontal cortex
not fully developed

Corpus callosum
thickens

Amygdala
processes emotional information

CHANGING CONNECTIONS
Scientists have devised a typical growth chart of the human brain, formed by taking more than 200 fMRI scans of individuals with an age range of 7–10 years. They found that fibers connecting peripheral brain areas decreased, while increases occurred in those connecting the limbic areas with the frontal cortex as the brain matured.

KEY
INCREASED CONNECTION
DECREASED CONNECTION

TEENAGE YEARS
The prefrontal cortex is still developing, which is thought to be one reason for impulsiveness and rash decision-making. It is closely connected to the basal ganglia, which play an important role in motor skills. The fiber tract that links the hemispheres, the corpus callosum, is thickening, allowing for increased information-processing skills.

NEUROGENESIS

It used to be thought that the number of brain cells in the adult brain was fixed early in life and that laying down new memories and learning new things was achieved entirely by changes to existing neurons and their connections with one another. While this sort of rewiring is important for learning, it is now known that adults also benefit from the creation of new brain cells. Neurogenesis occurs mainly in the dentate gyrus of the hippocampus, the brain region that is centrally important for learning and memory. About one-third of the neurons in the adult hippocampus are replaced in a person's lifetime.

Dentate gyrus

Hippocampus

SECTION OF HIPPOCAMPUS

LOCATION OF HIPPOCAMPUS

MEMORY MAKER
The hippocampus is a vital part of the brain, essential for laying down and recalling memories. Neurogenesis helps it encode new information.

SITE FOR NEW CELLS
This light micrograph of sectioned hippocampal tissue shows nerve cells in the dentate gyrus, where new neurons are made.

MEASURING NEUROGENESIS

Neurogenesis is measured in animals by injecting their brains with a radioactive marker that attaches to dividing cells. Counting the marked cells when the animals die shows how many have multiplied. In humans, cell division is measured using tissue from cancer patients taking radioactive drugs. Scientists also discovered how to count new brain cells by carbon-dating tissue from donors who reached adulthood before the nuclear tests of the 1950s. The tests left radioactive molecules in the air that were absorbed into new cells, distinguishing them from older cells.

Corpus callosum fully developed to allow information flow between hemispheres

Basal ganglia

Prefrontal cortex processes information

Amygdala less involved in emotional processing

Hippocampus continues to produce new brain cells

STRENGTHENING CONNECTIONS

Learning new things helps make and keep the connections between neurons sheathed with myelin. When a neuron fires, it triggers activity in neighboring oligodendrocytes, a type of structural or glial cell (see p.69), which then wraps myelin around the axons of active cells. The myelin acts like insulation, allowing electrical impulses to flow swiftly along the axons. The white matter formed by myelin tends to shrivel with age if the connections are not kept in good repair, so keeping it intact by learning new things is an important way of preventing brain aging.

Myelin insulates axon

Cell body of oligodendrocyte

Myelin sheath wrapped around axon

Axon projects from neuron

MYELIN MAKER
Oligodendrocytes are found only in the brain, where they coat the axons of neurons with a fatty sheath called myelin.

AT 30 YEARS OLD
The prefrontal cortex is now fully developed, allowing for improved executive functions. This also means that the brain is less reliant on the amygdala to process emotional information. The other areas of the brain that were still developing in adolescence have now reached maturity.

NEW MEMORIES FOR OLD

The creation of new brain cells allows new information to be stored, but their arrival disrupts existing memories because they change the wiring pattern. Most memories form in the hippocampus and are transferred to long-term storage in other brain areas. For a while, the memory resides both in the hippocampus and elsewhere. After a few years, the memory is cleared from the hippocampus. Until the memory is fully transferred, the arrival of new cells in the hippocampus may weaken the connections encoding memories stored there. This may be why we rarely retain memories from when we were very young.

Cortex mirrors activity

Memory transferred

MEMORY TRANSFER
Memories are first formed as patterns of neural activity in the hippocampus, which are then echoed in areas of the cortex (see pp.160–61).

Hippocampus

PARENTHOOD

Having a child is a major event in most adult lives and usually brings about profound changes in behavior. These are accompanied by changes in the brains of both mothers and fathers. In both parents, raised levels of hormones, particularly prolactin and oxytocin, sensitize areas of the brain concerned with alarm (such as the amygdala) and action (the substantia nigra), making them more sensitive to their babies' cues, such as cries and expressions. Men's testosterone level falls and prolactin level rises, making their brains temporarily more like that of a female.

RIGHT HEMISPHERE

LEFT HEMISPHERE

BRAIN CHANGE
Research shows that becoming a parent produces a flurry of neurogenesis. MRI studies reveal an increase in cortical thickness in new mothers' brains, shown red in the scans above.

THE AGING BRAIN

THE TRADITIONAL VIEW OF AGING IS THAT THE BRAIN AND THE BODY START TO DEGENERATE. THIS IS TRUE IN THAT NEURONS ARE LOST AND, FOR THOSE THAT REMAIN, IMPULSES ARE TRANSMITTED MORE SLOWLY. THIS CAN LEAD TO SLOWING THOUGHT PROCESSES, MEMORY PROBLEMS, AND DETERIORATING REFLEXES, WHICH CAN CAUSE PROBLEMS WITH BALANCE AND MOVEMENT.

NATURAL DEGENERATION

In the past, it was rare for people to live to the age of 50 and beyond, so we have not evolved to use the brain in such advanced years. This makes the aging brain a relatively new phenomenon in human history and evolution. The natural degeneration of the brain and nervous system is not caused by disease, so it should not be confused with the pathology of dementia, which is associated with a pattern of specific brain changes. Recent research shows that most neurons actually remain healthy until you die, but brain volume and size decrease 5–10 percent from the age of 20–90. There are also changes in topography, with the grooves widening and tangles and plaques (small, disk-shaped growths) forming. However, the role of these deficits is not absolutely clear. They can occur in the brains of both healthy people and sufferers of Alzheimer's disease.

myelin -sheathed axons

decayed myelin sheath

MYELIN DECAY
The myelin sheath that insulates the axons of neurons is vital for effective cell-to-cell communication. This protein-based structure decays with age, leaving brain circuits less efficient, leading to balance and memory problems. The decayed myelin sheaths traveling from the cortex to spine are shown as blue and purple on this image, while the healthy ones are shown in green.

AGE AND EXCITEMENT LEVELS

Dopamine is a neurotransmitter that triggers excitement and rapid decision-making. Brain-imaging studies suggest that, as people age, activity in their dopamine circuits decreases. This might be reflected in behavioral changes, because dopamine is linked with thrill-seeking and risk-taking. Perhaps older people prefer a quieter life than younger people because dopamine is less abundant.

THE THRILL OF CHRISTMAS
Opening presents is highly exciting for children, but much less so for older people because dopamine, which is triggered by "rewards" (in this case, gifts), has less impact as you age.

Basal ganglia
These clusters of nerve cells appear normal in the young brain

Basal ganglia
The brighter areas are the product of iron accumulation

Subarachnoid space
The size of this area as shown here is normal in a 27-year-old

Subarachnoid space
As the brain becomes smaller due to lifelong loss of brain cells, this space enlarges

27-YEAR-OLD

87-YEAR-OLD

27-YEAR-OLD

87-YEAR-OLD

BASAL GANGLIA
This series of MRI scans shows the differences between crucial areas of the brain of a young adult compared to an elderly adult. The scans above show the basal ganglia, which plays a vital role in coordinating movement.

SUBARACHNOID SPACE
The subarachnoid space is the area around the outside edge of the brain, and is known as a potential site for brain hemorrhage (see p.221). It becomes notably larger as the brain ages, reflecting a general reduction in brain volume.

POSITIVE AGING

The brain can compensate for the effects of aging, and mental function can even improve with age. Myelin increases in the temporal and frontal lobes in the 45–50 age group may enable people to manage their knowledge better. Also, comprehension studies have shown that high-functioning older adults use either both hemispheres together, or a different hemisphere than either young adults or lower-functioning older adults.

This may be the brain's way of making up for declining functions, to keep thought and memory processes stronger.

**YOUNG ADULT
(LEFT HEMISPHERE)**   **YOUNG ADULT
(RIGHT HEMISPHERE)**

**ELDERLY ADULT
(LEFT HEMISPHERE)**   **ELDERLY ADULT
(RIGHT HEMISPHERE)**

BRAIN ACTIVATION CONTRASTS
One study compared fMRI scans of brain activity in young adults (top row) and older adults (bottom row) during sentence comprehension. The results suggest that older people with good comprehension compensate for the deficits in language areas of the brain by recruiting other areas.

PROTEIN ACCUMULATION

A recent study examined the brains of five people in their eighties, who had performed very well in memory tests, and compared them to the brains of "normal," nondemented elderly people of a similar age. The ones who performed well in the memory tests had fewer tangles consisting of a protein called tau in their brains than the other group. These tangles grow inside brain cells and are thought to eventually kill them.

FIBERLIKE TANGLES
Microscopic tangles (shown as dark masses) are often found in large numbers in the brains of Alzheimer's patients.

KEEPING THE BRAIN YOUNG

New research into brain aging indicates that the rate of decline may be slowed by lifestyle factors, such as regular exercise. Research has also found that reducing food intake, resulting in lower blood glucose levels, may slow the pace of change because blood glucose can cause damage to proteins. Certainly, people with elevated blood glucose levels, such as those with type 1 diabetes, show more signs of brain aging than nondiabetic individuals.

EXERCISE   **REST**

A HEALTHY DIET   **MENTAL FITNESS**

BENEFITS OF A HEALTHY LIFESTYLE
A number of lifestyle factors may help stimulate the growth of neural tissue. Gentle aerobic exercise, such as rapid walking, regular sleep, a good diet, and mental exercises help delay age-related mental decline and protect against age-related problems, such as memory loss.

Ventricles
These hollow spaces filled with cerebrospinal fluid are a normal size in the younger brain

Ventricles
These hollow spaces are much larger in the elderly brain

White-matter tract
This communication channel for the brain's information-processing gray matter is in good condition

White-matter tract
This changes in appearance during aging for as yet unknown reasons

27-YEAR-OLD   **87-YEAR-OLD**   **27-YEAR-OLD**   **87-YEAR-OLD**

VENTRICLES
The ventricles contain cerebrospinal fluid, which performs several functions, including protecting the brain from injury and transporting hormones. These areas become larger as the brain ages, as a result of the general loss of gray matter.

WHITE-MATTER TRACTS
The white matter contains mainly supporting (glial) cells, which are needed to support neurons. Because there are less supporting cells as the brain gets older, neurons function less efficiently.

THE BRAIN OF THE FUTURE

AS WE DISCOVER HOW THE BRAIN WORKS, THE PROSPECT OF CHANGING IT, ENHANCING IT, AND DEVELOPING ARTIFICIAL BRAINS IS FAST BECOMING FACT RATHER THAN FICTION. TECHNOLOGIES FOR MIND-READING, THOUGHT CONTROL, AND ARTIFICIAL INTELLIGENCE ARE ALREADY WITH US, AND ARE BECOMING MORE SOPHISTICATED EVERY DAY.

BRAIN–MACHINE INTERFACES

When a person is thinking, the brain produces electrical signals. Scientists have discovered ways in which the electrical signals can be picked up by sensors and sent wirelessly to other electrical devices, making it possible for a person to move or alter objects by thought alone. Most research in this field is directed toward developing devices to help people with nervous-system injuries regain the use of paralyzed limbs. The technology has also been picked up by some computer-game manufacturers, who have produced games that can be played using thought power.

HOPE FOR THE PARALYZED

A spinal cord injury left this man paralyzed from the neck down. Mind-control technology has enabled him to use a computer and other electrical devices remotely. His thoughts—in the form of electrical signals—are transmitted along a cable that connects to his brain via a microchip, which contains 100 electrodes.

THOUGHT-CONTROLLED GAMING
This device picks up electrical signals from a user's brain and uses them to control a virtual character in a computer game.

FICTION BECOMING FACT?
This still is taken from the science-fiction film *I, Robot*, which explores the idea of a robot experiencing emotions—a concept that may one day become fact.

MIND READING

The "picture" of neural activity created by fMRI scanning can be translated into a precise description of what a person is seeing and, to some extent, thinking. To achieve this, the output of a person's fMRI scan, captured while he or she is looking at a particular image, is processed by sophisticated computer software that translates the pattern of activity into a visual "read-out." Such "mind-reading" is made possible because neurons in the visual cortex are specialized for specific stimuli–horizontal or vertical lines, for example–so their firing patterns are indicative of the type of visual stimuli the neurons are registering.

SIGNATURE PATTERNS
In this experiment, the word "neuron" (shown in the top line) was shown to a volunteer. As each letter produces a distinct pattern of neural activity, through analyzing these patterns it is possible to reproduce the letters that the volunteer is seeing (shown in the bottom eight lines).

LIE DETECTION

Mind-reading is not limited to revealing what it is that a person is looking at. Brain-scanning studies have shown that, when a person is lying, the brain generates a different pattern of neural activity from when they telling the truth. This has been used to develop a "lie detector" that analyzes brain activity captured by fMRI. Although still in development, the technology is claimed to have an accuracy rate of over 90 percent–significantly greater than the accuracy rate of polygraph tests.

Medial frontal gyrus

Inferior frontal gyrus

LEFT HEMISPHERE

Medial frontal gyrus

REVEALING THE TRUTH
Different areas of the brain are activated according to when someone is telling the truth or lying. Here, the red areas show the telltale activity of a lie, while the blue areas are associated with telling the truth.

RIGHT HEMISPHERE

ARTIFICIAL INTELLIGENCE

Scientists have been working for decades on producing intelligent nonbiological systems, and have been very successful in developing computer programs that can equal, or sometimes outperform, the human brain. Chess programs, for instance, can now compete on even terms with the best players in the world. However, it has proved difficult to develop systems that are as flexible as the human brain, and thus able to operate in the constantly changing environments that constitute "real" life. To overcome this, the emphasis of artificial intelligence research has recently shifted from developing more advanced computers to creating "emotional" machines that are able to make crude but quick "holistic" or "intuitive" judgments that do not depend on enormous calculating capacity.

CHESS COMPUTER
Grandmaster chess player Garry Kasparov, regarded by many as the greatest chess player of all time, was unable to beat a computer program called X3D Fritz in 2003. Their game resulted in a tie.

AVATARS
An avatar is a digital representation of a person that is able to exhibit humanlike behavior. Although still primitive, there are concerns about how they could potentially manipulate human emotions.

CUTTING EDGE
ASIMO is a cutting-edge robot that can recognize faces and gestures, and distinguish sounds.

THE STATE OF TECHNOLOGY

Recent advances in biotechnology have made it possible to replace damaged limbs with artificial ones that can be controlled by thought, operating in much the same way as the original. Another advance involves altering brain function by inserting electrical pacemakers. Artificial sense organs, such as the bionic eye, are already on trial, and artificial brain parts such as memory add-ons and hippocampus replacements are not far behind.

Electrode

BRAIN PROBE
This X-ray shows an electrode inserted into the brain during a technique called deep-brain stimulation.

THE BIONIC EYE

People who have become blind as a consequence of eye conditions (as opposed to damage to areas of the brain associated with vision) may soon be able to see again thanks to the development of artificial eyes. A "bionic" eye prototype has been created, comprising a computer chip that sits in the back of the individual's own eye socket, which is linked up to a tiny video camera built into a pair of glasses. Images captured by the camera are beamed to the chip, which translates them into electrical impulses and sends them on to the visual cortex via the optic nerve.

With some eye conditions, light still enters iris, but photo-receptors that process light start to die

Retinal implant
Inserted into wall of retina

Camera
Mounted on frame of glasses; captures an image and sends it to microprocessor behind ear

Thalamus

Optic nerve

Iris

Retina cross section

Retinal implant
Receives signals from microprocessor and emits pulses, which travel via optic nerve to visual cortex in brain

Photoreceptors destroyed by disease

ETHICS AND TECHNOLOGY

As biotechnology advances, it generates ethical and moral dilemmas. Brain technologies are particularly sensitive because most of us consider the products of our brain—thoughts, feeling, desires—as the central part of our "selves." Stem cells—immature body cells that have the potential to turn into many different types of cells—might one day be used to restore damaged neurons. Their use in other areas of medicine has already generated huge debate, because initially they had to be harvested from human fetuses, but they can now be obtained another way.

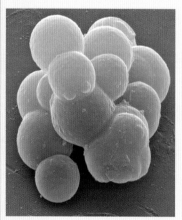

STEM CELLS
Stem cells like these can now be taken from blood flowing through the umbilical cord. Initially they came from fetuses, which caused much ethical debate.

NANOROBOTS
Microscopic robots could one day reengineer our bodies to be stronger, more intelligent, and resistant to disease, presenting complicated life choices.

BRAIN AND BODY ENHANCEMENTS
Practically every part of the body, including the sense organs, may soon have artificial counterparts. Some of these are already in development, although of those shown above only the vagus nerve stimulator is in widespread clinical use.

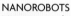

Memory chip

Artificial hippocampus
Two sets of electrodes send and
receive neural activity signals via
a memory chip

Optic radiation

Visual cortex
Signals from retinal implant
travel along optic nerve to
visual cortex (via thalamus and
optic radiation), where they are
processed into sight

Microprocessor
Converts data from camera into
an electronic signal and sends it
to retinal implant

Vagus nerve

Pacemaker
Tiny generator sends regular,
rhythmic pulses along tiny cable

Electrodes
These wrap around vagus
nerve and carry signal
generated from
pacemaker in
chest to brain

Computer
Processes impulses
and instructs arm
to make certain
movements

Plastic harness
Electrodes fitted to
this harness detect
electrical impulses
from rerouted sensory
nerves in the chest

Sensory nerves that
would normally travel
from spinal cord to
arm are rerouted to
muscles in chest

Prosthetic arm
With early versions of bionic
arms, patients were only able to
either bend their elbow or
open their hand, but the latest
versions allow both movements
simultaneously

VAGUS-NERVE STIMULATION

The vagus nerve is a cranial nerve, traveling from
the brainstem to various internal organs, that
has an important role in mediating brain
arousal. A number of different types of
brain disorders, such as chronic epilepsy
and severe depression, benefit from the
effects of stimulating this nerve. A small
disk with a tiny generator fueled by a
lithium battery is surgically implanted in
the chest, which sends regular, rhythmic
pulses along a wire that is tethered
to the left vagus nerve (the right vagus
nerve runs directly to the heart). The
frequency and intensity of the electrical
pulses can be altered according to the
severity of the condition.

THE BIONIC ARM

A bionic arm that is operated by the power of thought
alone is already in use, and future models, which are
currently being developed, are likely to be more lifelike
and increasingly dextrous. The current versions work
by rerouting motor nerves from the brain that
originally ran to the hand, and terminating them
instead in electrodes, which communicate with
computer-driven motors in the arm itself. Sensors
feed a limited degree of sensory information back
to the brain, so the user can determine both
temperature and pressure.

THE FUTURE

The rampant progress of biotechnology raises profound questions
about what it is to be human. This is particularly true with technology
that affects the human brain, because of all organs this is the one we
identify with the most closely. Some of the most common questions
raised include:

QUESTION	ANSWER
What changes in the way our brains function might we see if technology advances at its present rate?	"Thought" devices enabling us to control the world by mind power alone; synthetic brain "modules" to replace failing ones; conscious mood control by direct stimulation of the relevant brain areas.
Won't these things change what it means to be human? Will they even be acceptable?	Many of them, in crude form, are with us already and proving to be quite acceptable. We have "bionic" limbs, brain pacemakers, and even a prototype replacement hippocampus (see p.161).
What are the main technical problems still to be overcome?	The main problem is to do with mapping—despite the advances of the last ten years, the complex interconnections between different brain areas are still largely unknown.
Will machines ever be conscious?	There seems no reason why not. The ultimate challenge may not be technical at all, but rather the ethical implications of human consciousness being embodied in a nonhuman form.

THE PERCEPTION OF BRAIN DISORDERS AND THEIR CAUSES
HAS CHANGED PROFOUNDLY OVER THE COURSE OF HUMAN
HISTORY. EVEN TODAY, DIFFERENT CULTURES HOLD
MARKEDLY DIFFERENT VIEWS ABOUT THE DIVIDING LINE
BETWEEN NORMAL AND DISORDERED STATES OF MIND.
BUT, JUST AS OUR KNOWLEDGE OF HOW THE BRAIN
WORKS IS CURRENTLY UNDERGOING A REVOLUTION,

DISEASES AND DISORDERS

THE DISORDERED BRAIN

EVERY MENTAL STATE HAS A CORRESPONDING BRAIN STATE, CONSISTING OF A PARTICULAR PATTERN AND SEQUENCE OF NEURAL PROCESSES. UNTIL RECENTLY, MOST OF THESE PROCESSES WERE UNDETECTABLE, BUT THE ADVENT OF HIGH-TECH IMAGING HAS MADE THEM VISIBLE, WITH THE RESULT THAT MENTAL DISORDERS ARE INCREASINGLY BEING RECOGNIZED AS NEUROLOGICAL BRAIN DISORDERS.

EXORCISM
Exorcism is a ritual designed to expel bad spirits from the living. It was widespread in the Middle Ages, when demonic possession was often thought to be the cause of mental illness.

HISTORICAL THEORIES OF MENTAL ILLNESS

FOUR HUMORS
Hippocrates developed the idea that illness was the result of a lack of balance among four humors—blood, phlegm, and black and yellow bile.

Mental illness has commonly been regarded as disease of the spirit. In the Middle Ages it was assumed that devils (foul spirits) entered people and made them depressed (poor-spirited) or insane. Physical theories of mental illness include an imbalance of the "four humors," which were thought to determine a person's general mood and health, and fluctuations or blockages of various types of "forces." The 19th-century physician Franz Mesmer, for example, thought he had discovered "animal magnetism," which could cause ill health, including madness, if it was blocked. His treatment to control the magnetic flow was, effectively, hypnotism. Sigmund Freud (see p.189) popularized the concept of the unconscious, and believed that suppressed desires caused neurosis. He developed psychoanalysis, based on the idea of bringing hidden conflicts to consciousness.

HEALING ENERGY
"Mesmerists" healed anxious minds by hypnotism, although at the time they thought they were using animal magnetism (energy flow).

WHAT IS MENTAL DISORDER?

Mental illness is generally diagnosed when a person reports that they are experiencing the world in a way that is radically different from others or when their behaviour makes it difficult for them to function in society. The shifting nature of mental illness makes diagnosis notoriously difficult. Yet standard diagnosis is important because the presence or absence of mental illness may decide whether a person is criminally responsible, suitable for particular types of employment, or eligible for state aid. Medical practice also makes diagnosis essential before treatment can be given. The most commonly consulted guide to mental disorders is the US Diagnostic and Statistical Manual (DSM) published by the American Psychiatric Association (see panel below).

MODERN DIAGNOSTIC TOOLS
Some mental illnesses may be diagnosed by brain imaging—CT and MRI scans are good at showing tumors and areas of damage. Functional brain imaging may be used to explore abnormal brain patterns, such as those found in epilepsy.

DIAGNOSING MENTAL DISORDERS

The first edition of the DSM was published in 1952 following research by the US military during the Second World War. The current edition, DSM-5, was published in 2013 after 14 years of research. DSM-5 includes new diagnostic and classification criteria for some conditions—for example, Asperger's is now part of the autistic spectrum rather than a condition in its own right. But controversy has arisen over whether the manual has changed sufficiently to reflect advances in brain research. Diagnosis is still based firmly on behavioral tests not brain imaging or biological markers. The failure of DSM-5 to take a neuroscientific approach to mental illness has led the largest US center for psychiatric research, the National Institutes of Health, to reject the manual.

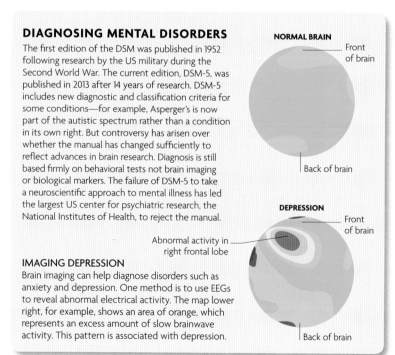

NORMAL BRAIN
Front of brain

Back of brain

DEPRESSION
Front of brain

Abnormal activity in right frontal lobe

Back of brain

IMAGING DEPRESSION
Brain imaging can help diagnose disorders such as anxiety and depression. One method is to use EEGs to reveal abnormal electrical activity. The map lower right, for example, shows an area of orange, which represents an excess amount of slow brainwave activity. This pattern is associated with depression.

PHYSICAL DISORDERS

All mental illness is physiological in that the behavior and experience associated with it is created by a pattern of neuronal activity, but only conditions that are clearly linked to damage are considered to be physical.

DEVELOPMENTAL Growing brains are very sensitive to environmental assault, such as oxygen deprivation. A problem before or during birth may cause permanent damage.

TRAUMATIC Brain trauma may arise from external events such as accidents that cause head injuries, and also from "cerebral" accidents, such as strokes and aneurysms.

DEGENERATIVE Brains, like all the organs, degenerate, and this can result in mental conditions such as memory loss, cognitive impairment, and, in severe cases, dementia.

ROOTS OF DISORDER

Some disorders are caused by physical damage, such as a head injury, or degeneration that disrupts normal brain function. Others are caused by "faulty" genes, or developmental problems—things that go wrong during gestation or infancy. In many cases, the root causes of mental illness cannot be traced and simply manifest as "functional" problems. Functional disorders may be marked by abnormalities in brain function, but it is often unclear if these are the cause or effect of the condition.

MANY CAUSES

Most mental illness is due to a combination of causes, as shown in this Venn diagram. The placements of the conditions are open to revision because in very few cases is the precise contribution of any one factor certain. As more is learned about the brain, the apparent causes may change.

DEGENERATION

I ALZHEIMER'S DISEASE

PARKINSON'S DISEASE I
MOTOR NEURONE DISEASE I

INJURY, TRAUMA, INFECTION

I EPILEPSY
I MENINGITIS
I ENCEPHALITIS
I HEMORRHAGE
I HYDROCEPHALUS
I CREUTZFELD–JACOB DISEASE

I MULTI-INFARCT DEMENTIA
I STROKE
I TUMORS

I MULTIPLE SCLEROSIS

NARCOLEPSY I
DOWN SYNDROME I
HUNTINGTON'S DISEASE I
NEURAL-TUBE DEFECTS I

DEVELOPMENTAL/GENETIC

I ABSCESS
I COMA
I PARALYSIS
I CEREBRAL PALSY

I DELUSIONAL DISORDERS
I DEPRESSION

I AUTISTIC SPECTRUM
I DEVELOPMENTAL DELAY
I ADDICTIONS

TOURETTE SYNDROME I
PERSONALITY DISORDERS I
ANXIETY DISORDERS I
EATING DISORDERS I
SEASONAL AFFECTIVE DISORDER I
OBSESSIVE–COMPULSIVE DISORDER I
SCHIZOPHRENIA I
SOMATIZATION DISORDER I

I CHRONIC FATIGUE SYNDROME
I BIPOLAR DISORDER
I POST-TRAUMATIC STRESS DISORDER

MULTIPLE SCLEROSIS

This MRI scan shows a demyelinated lesion (pink) in a person with MS (see p.235) It is the result of degeneration, which in turn may be due to genetic vulnerability or injury.

FUNCTIONAL

I ATTENTION-DEFICIT HYPERACTIVITY DISORDER
I MUNCHAUSEN'S SYNDROME
I PHOBIAS
I CONDUCT DISORDER
I BODY DYSMORPHIC DISORDER
I HYPOCHONDRIA

CONSTELLATIONS AND SPECTRUMS

Many disorders that have conventionally been seen as discrete conditions are now being recognized as related. People with autism, for example, have a core problem with understanding other people's mental processes. Around this core lies a constellation of symptoms grouped into three overlapping "suites" of behavior. These suites are conventionally seen as different types of problem, but their common relationship to the core deficit suggests that they share a genetic underpinning. Psychosis has a core that is characterized by over-interpretation of other minds. It too can be seen as the core of symptoms from overlapping suites.

Psychotic spectrum core
Hypermentalistic cognition and behavior; overly sensitive (to the point of delusion) about other minds

BIPOLAR DEPRESSION

UNIPOLAR DEPRESSION

SCHIZOPHRENIA

PSYCHOTIC SPECTRUM

RESTRICTED INTERESTS, REPETITIVE BEHAVIOR

AUTISTIC SPECTRUM   BALANCED   PSYCHOTIC SPECTRUM

KEY
MECHANISTIC COGNITION
MENTALISTIC COGNITION

COGNITIVE TASK PERFORMANCE

AUTISTIC-PSYCHOTIC CONTINUUM

OPPOSITE PROBLEMS?

Although they appear entirely different, autistic constellation disorders and psychotic spectrum conditions may actually be related. The two clusters of symptoms may be envisaged as existing on a single spectrum (above) with normal behavior in the middle.

Autistic spectrum core
Hypomentalistic—problems with understanding other people's mental processes or reflecting on one's own

PROBLEMS WITH SOCIAL RECIPROCITY

LANGUAGE, COMMUNICATION DIFFICULTIES

AUTISTIC SPECTRUM

SUITES OF BEHAVIOR

Psychotic and autistic spectrum disorders are shown here as separate suites of behavior, with the common symptoms forming the core of each spectrum.

HEADACHE AND MIGRAINE

Headache is a common symptom but the mechanism underlying it is not known for certain. The brain itself has no pain-sensitive nerve receptors. In many cases, it is thought that tension in the meninges or in blood vessels or muscles of the head and/or neck stimulates pain receptors, which send impulses to the sensory cortex of the brain, resulting in a headache. However, in some types of headache, such as migraine, the pain is thought to be due to overactivity of neurons that affects the brain's sensory cortex.

TENSION HEADACHE

ALSO KNOWN AS STRESS HEADACHES, TENSION HEADACHES ARE PROBABLY THE MOST COMMON TYPE OF HEADACHE.

The pain tends to be constant, although it may throb, and it may occur in the forehead or more generally over the head. The pain may be accompanied by tightening of the neck muscles and a feeling of pressure behind the eyes and/or tightness around the head. Tension headaches are typically brought on by stress, which causes tension in the muscles of the neck and scalp. This, in turn, is thought to stimulate pain receptors in these areas, which send "pain impulses" to the sensory cortex.

Tension in scalp muscles

Tension in neck muscles

MUSCULAR TENSION
Pain receptors in the muscles of the scalp and neck are stimulated by muscular tension, leading to the pain of a tension headache.

CLUSTER HEADACHE

THESE HEADACHES OCCUR IN CLUSTERS OF RELATIVELY SHORT ATTACKS OF SEVERE, OFTEN EXCRUCIATING, PAIN.

During cluster headaches there are several attacks (typically one to four) a day, followed by an attack-free remission period. The cluster period usually lasts from a few weeks to a couple of months. A remission period may last for months or even years, although some people experience no significant remissions. The cause of cluster headaches is not known, although there is some evidence that abnormal nerve cell activity in the hypothalamus may be involved.

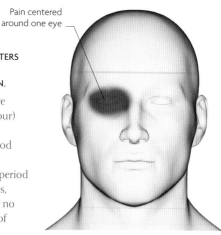

Pain centered around one eye

AREA OF PAIN
A cluster headache typically affects one side of the head and is centered around the eye, which may also water and become inflamed.

MIGRAINE

A MIGRAINE IS AN INTENSE, OFTEN THROBBING HEADACHE, MADE WORSE BY MOVEMENT AND OFTEN ACCOMPANIED BY SENSORY DISTURBANCES AND NAUSEA.

A migraine headache usually occurs at the front or one side of the head, although the area of pain can move during an attack.

Migraine is classified into two types: classical migraine and common migraine. In classical migraine, the headache is preceded by aura, a group of warning symptoms that includes: visual disturbances, such as flashing lights and other distortions; stiffness, tingling, or numbness; difficulty speaking; and poor coordination. In common migraine there is no aura. In both types there may be an early stage, known as prodrome, with features such as difficulty concentrating, mood changes, and fatigue or excessive energy. In common migraine, the prodrome is followed by the headache; in classical migraine, the prodrome is followed by aura, which is then succeeded by the headache. The headache gets worse with movement, and it is accompanied by symptoms including nausea and/or vomiting, and increased sensitivity to sound, light, and sometimes smells. It is often followed by a postdrome stage, in which there may be fatigue, difficulty focusing, poor concentration, and persistence of increased sensitivity.

Causes and triggers

The underlying cause of migraine is not known, but recent research suggests that it may be due to a surge of neuronal activity that sweeps through parts of the brain, eventually stimulating the sensory cortex, which results in the sensation of pain. However, many external factors that trigger migraine attacks have been identified: dietary factors, such as irregular meals, specific foods, and dehydration; physical factors, such as fatigue and hormonal changes; emotional factors, such as stress or shock; and environmental conditions, including changes in the weather or a stuffy atmosphere.

Sensory region of cortex

Cerebral cortex

Thalamus

Brainstem

MECHANISM OF MIGRAINE
The neurological pathways that cause migraine are unknown, but may involve intense neuronal activity in the brainstem, thalamus, and sensory cortex.

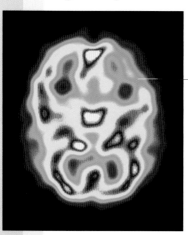

Area of low brain activity

DURING AN ATTACK
This SPECT scan shows different levels of brain activity during a migraine: red and yellow indicate high activity; areas of low activity are shown in green and blue.

Aura
Typically lasts about an hour

Headache
May last for hours or days

Prodrome
May last for hours or days

Postdrome
May last for hours or days

INTENSITY

TIME

COURSE OF MIGRAINE ATTACK
A classical migraine attack typically comprises four stages, which can vary in intensity and duration. Prodrome is followed by aura, with warning signs such as visual disturbances, abnormal sensations, poor coordination, and difficulty speaking. After the aura stage comes the headache, which is in turn followed by the postdrome stage.

CHRONIC FATIGUE SYNDROME

ALSO KNOWN AS MYALGIC ENCEPHALOMYELITIS (ME), CHRONIC FATIGUE SYNDROME IS A COMPLEX CONDITION THAT CAUSES EXTREME FATIGUE THAT LASTS FOR A PROLONGED PERIOD OF TIME.

The cause of chronic fatigue syndrome is not known. It can develop after a viral infection or a period of emotional stress, but in many cases there is no specific preceding factor. The principle symptom is persistent, overwhelming fatigue that lasts for at least several months.

Other symptoms vary, but commonly include poor concentration, impaired short-term memory, muscle and joint pain, and feeling ill and/or extremely tired after even mild exertion. The disorder is also often associated with depression or anxiety, but it is unclear whether these are a cause or a result of the condition.

Chronic fatigue syndrome is usually diagnosed from the symptoms, although various tests and psychological assessments can be carried out to exclude other possible conditions. It is a long-term disorder, although there may be periods of remission and sometimes the disorder clears up spontaneously.

Muscle pain
Muscles may be sore, without any swelling

Painful joints

Neurological problems
Persistent fatigue, poor concentration, short-term memory problems, headaches, and poor sleep

Sore throat

Tender lymph nodes

COMMON SYMPTOMS
The main indication of chronic fatigue syndrome is persistent, overwhelming fatigue. Other symptoms vary from person to person, but common symptoms are shown here.

HEAD INJURIES

HEAD INJURIES RANGE FROM MINOR BUMPS WITH NO LONG-TERM EFFECTS TO BRAIN DAMAGE THAT CAN BE FATAL.

Injuries to the head are often classified as closed, in which the skull is not broken, or open, in which the skull is fractured, leaving the brain exposed. Closed head injuries may cause indirect damage to the brain. For example, a hard blow to the head that does not fracture the skull may cause brain injury at the site of impact as the inside of the skull hits the brain. Such a trauma may also cause brain injury at the opposite side of the head (a contrecoup injury). Open head injuries are caused by a strong impact from a sharp object that fractures the skull and may penetrate the brain, for example, a stab wound.

Effects

Head injuries can rupture blood vessels, causing a brain hemorrhage (see p.229). Minor head injuries typically produce only mild, short-lived symptoms, such as a bruise on the head. In some cases, a temporary disturbance of brain function (concussion) may follow even relatively minor injuries, particularly if the injury has caused unconsciousness, and this may cause confusion, dizziness, and blurred vision, which may last for several days. Postconcussive amnesia can also occur. Repeated concussions eventually cause detectable brain damage, which may result in punchdrunk syndrome, symptoms of which may include impaired cognitive abilities, progressive dementia, parkinsonism (see p.234), tremors, and epilepsy.

Severe head injury may produce unconsciousness or coma, and usually brain damage, which in very severe cases may be fatal. In nonfatal cases, the effects of brain damage vary widely according to the severity and location of damage. The effects may include weakness, paralysis, problems with memory and/or concentration, intellectual impairment, and even personality changes. Such effects can be long-term or permanent.

FRACTURED SKULL
This three-dimensional CT scan of the skull reveals multiple fractures, including two large depressed fractures in which the skull has been pushed inward and fragmented. Such injuries are usually the result of a powerful blow from a blunt object and, in severe cases, may cause brain damage or even death.

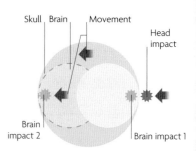

HEMATOMA
This color-enhanced CT scan shows a large extradural hematoma (orange)—a mass of clotted blood caused by a hemorrhage that occurred due to a head injury. If not treated, it may press on the brain, causing brain damage or death.

MOVING PERSON

Skull | Brain | Movement

1 In a person who is moving rapidly—for example, when traveling in a car—the skull and brain enclosed within it are moving at the same speed.

Skull | Brain | Movement
Head impact
Brain impact 2
Brain impact 1

2 If movement is suddenly stopped due to an impact, the brain hits the front of the skull, and a coutrecoup injury occurs when it rebounds and hits the back of the skull.

STATIONARY PERSON

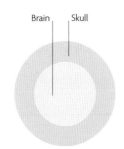

Brain | Skull

1 In a situation in which a person is stationary, both the skull and the brain within it are motionless at the time that they are struck.

Skull | Brain | Movement
Head impact
Brain impact 2
Brain impact 1

2 If the head is struck suddenly, the front of the skull is pushed against the brain, and the brain then rebounds and hits the back of the skull, causing a coutrecoup injury.

EPILEPSY

EPILEPSY IS A BRAIN FUNCTION DISORDER IN WHICH THERE ARE RECURRENT SEIZURES OR PERIODS OF ALTERED CONSCIOUSNESS.

Normally, neuronal activity in the brain occurs in a regulated way. However, during an epileptic seizure neurons start firing in an abnormal way, disrupting normal brain function. Although seizures are a defining symptom of epilepsy, they can occur without epilepsy being the cause.

The mechanism underlying epileptic seizures is not known for certain, but it is thought to involve a chemical imbalance in the brain. Normally, the neurotransmitter gamma-aminobutyric acid (GABA) helps regulate brain activity by inhibiting neurons in the brain. When the level of GABA falls too low–which itself may be due to abnormal amounts of enzymes that regulate GABA levels–neurons are not inhibited and they send a flood of impulses through the brain, resulting in a seizure. Epilepsy can have a number of causes, although in many cases the cause is unclear.

SEIZURE
This color-enhanced brain scan of a person with epilepsy reveals that the focus of seizure activity is in the right frontal lobe, as shown by the large orange cluster at the top right of the image.

A genetic factor may be involved in some cases. Other causes include head injury; birth trauma; an infection such as meningitis or encephalitis; a stroke; a brain tumor; and abuse of drugs or alcohol.

Many people find that specific factors can trigger a seizure. These triggers include stress; lack of sleep; fever; flashing lights; and drugs such as cocaine, amphetamines, Ecstasy, and opiates. Some women who suffer from epilepsy are more likely to have a seizure before the start of a menstrual period. Broadly, epileptic seizures fall into two main types:

generalized seizures and partial seizures (see table below). Seizures often start in one area of the brain, which might contain scar tissue or some structural abnormality, and then spread throughout the rest of the brain.

Some people experience a warning sign (called an aura) before an epileptic seizure. These warning signs may include a strange smell or taste; a feeling of foreboding; déjà vu; and a sense of unreality. In most cases, seizures stop by themselves. Sometimes a seizure can persist or seizures follow on from each other without the person recovering in between. This is known as status epilepticus and is a medical emergency.

PARTIAL EPILEPTIC SEIZURES
In a partial seizure, the seizure starts in and affects only part of the brain (above left). Sometimes, a seizure may start as a partial seizure and then become generalized and spread (above right).

GENERALIZED EPILEPTIC SEIZURE
In generalized seizures, most or all of the brain is affected by abnormal neuron activity.

STATUS EPILEPTICUS

Status epilepticus is the term used to refer to a potentially life-threatening condition in which there is a prolonged epileptic seizure or a series of repeated seizures that occur one after the other without recovery of consciousness between attacks. Precise definitions of status epilepticus vary, but generally it is defined as a single seizure that lasts for longer than 30 minutes, or a series of repeated seizures that lasts for longer than this time. In people who are known to have epilepsy, the most common cause of status epilepticus is failure to take antiepileptic medication. In other cases, the causes include a brain tumor, brain abscess, brain injury, cerebrovascular disease (such as a stroke), metabolic disorders, and drug abuse. Status epilepticus is a serious condition that may result in long-term disability or even death without prompt treatment with intravenous medications to control the seizures.

TYPES OF SEIZURES

Epileptic seizures can be categorized into two broad types, partial seizures and generalized seizures, depending on how much of the brain is affected by the abnormal neuron activity.

Partial seizures
In these types of seizures, abnormal neuron activity is restricted to a relatively small region of the brain. There are two main subtypes: simple partial seizures and complex partial seizures.

Simple partial seizures During these seizures there may be twitching on one side of the body; numbness or tingling; stiffness of the muscles in the arms, legs, and face; hallucinations of vision, taste, or smell; and sudden intense emotions. The person remains conscious throughout.

Complex partial seizures In these seizures the person is confused and unresponsive; may make peculiar, repetitive, apparently purposeless movements; and may scream or cry out, although there is no pain. The person remains conscious but usually has no memory of the seizure.

Generalized seizures
In these types of seizures, abnormal neuron activity affects most or all of the brain. There are six main subtypes, described below.

Tonic seizures In these seizures the muscles suddenly become stiff, which often causes the person to lose balance and fall over, usually backward. Tonic seizures tend to happen without warning, are usually short-lived, and the person recovers quickly.

Clonic seizures These seizures are very similar to myoclonic ones, causing jerking or twitching of the limbs or body, although they last longer, typically up to about two minutes. In addition, a person suffering a clonic seizure may lose consciousness.

Myoclonic seizures These generally happen shortly after waking up. During such seizures the arms, legs, or body twitch or jerk. A seizure usually lasts only a fraction of a second, but sometimes several seizures may occur in quick succession. Myoclonic seizures may occur on their own, but usually happen in association with other types, such as tonic–clonic seizures.

Atonic seizures These seizures are also sometimes called drop attacks. During the seizures the muscles suddenly relax and the person becomes floppy, which often causes them to lose balance and fall over, usually forward. Like tonic seizures, atonic seizures happen without warning, are short-lived, and the person recovers quickly after the seizure.

Tonic–clonic seizures Also sometimes known as grand mal, this type of seizure first causes the body to become rigid, this is followed by uncontrollable jerking or twitching. The person becomes unconscious and often loses bladder control. Typically, the seizure ends spontaneously after a few minutes, and afterward the person may be drowsy and confused.

Absence seizures Sometimes also known as petit mal, this type of epileptic seizure mainly affects children. During an absence seizure, the person loses awareness of his or her surroundings and appears to be staring vacantly into space. A seizure typically lasts for less than about 30 seconds, and in some cases seizures occur several times a day.

MENINGITIS

MENINGITIS IS INFLAMMATION OF THE MENINGES, THE MEMBRANES COVERING THE BRAIN AND SPINAL CORD, OFTEN AS A RESULT OF A VIRAL OR BACTERIAL INFECTION.

Typically, the infection reaches the meninges through the bloodstream from elsewhere in the body, although it may occasionally result from direct infection of the meninges after an open head injury. It may occur as a complication of various other diseases, including Lyme disease, encephalitis, tuberculosis, and leptospirosis. Viral meningitis may be caused by viruses such as herpes simplex or chickenpox virus. It tends to be relatively mild and causes symptoms similar to those of flu.

MENINGITIS BACTERIA
The five bacterial cells in the micrograph (right) are *Neisseria meningitidis* (also known as meningococcus), which is one of the most common causes of bacterial meningitis.

Rarely, it may cause serious symptoms, such as weakness or paralysis, speech problems, visual impairment, seizures, and coma.

Bacterial meningitis is less common than the viral form, but is more serious and can be fatal. It may be caused by various bacteria but is usually due to infection with meningococcal or pneumococcal bacteria. Symptoms may develop rapidly, over only a few hours, and include fever, stiff neck, severe headache, nausea, vomiting, abnormal sensitivity to light, confusion, and drowsiness, and sometimes seizures and loss of consciousness. In meningo-coccal meningitis, the bacteria may multiply in the blood, leading to a reddish purple rash that does not fade when pressed. If left untreated, bacterial meningitis can enter the cerebrospinal fluid, triggering an immune response that causes increased intracranial pressure, which in turn can cause brain damage.

ABSCESS DUE TO MENINGITIS
This color-enhanced MRI scan of a baby's brain shows a large abscess (pale orange at the upper left of the image) between the dura mater and arachnoid that has formed as a result of infection of the meninges.

Skull

Dura mater

Arachnoid

Pia mater

Brain tissue
The brain is not directly affected by meningitis, but it may become infected if meningitis bacteria spread to the bloodstream

Meninges
The meninges comprise the outer dura mater, the middle arachnoid, and the inner pia mater

SITES OF INFECTION
Usually the meninges become infected by the spread of bacteria or viruses (or rarely fungi) from elsewhere in the body. In some cases, infective bacteria may cause septicemia, which may affect the brain and other organs and may be fatal.

LUMBAR PUNCTURE

A lumbar puncture is a procedure in which a hollow needle is inserted into the subarachnoid space in the lower back to obtain a sample of cerebrospinal fluid or sometimes to inject drugs or other substances, such as dyes for specialized scans. The extracted fluid is examined to look for evidence of meningitis or other nervous system disorders, such as multiple sclerosis. The procedure is carried out under local anesthesia and takes about 15 minutes. There are usually no after-effects except occasionally a headache.

THE PROCEDURE
A hollow needle is inserted between vertebrae in the lower spine into the subarachnoid space and a sample of cerebrospinal fluid is withdrawn.

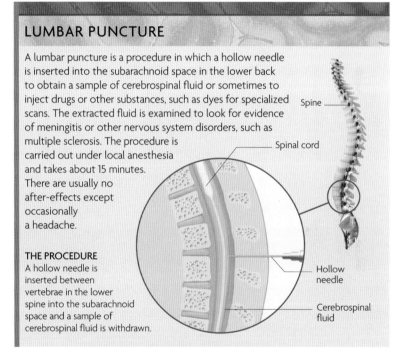

Spine

Spinal cord

Hollow needle

Cerebrospinal fluid

ENCEPHALITIS

ENCEPHALITIS IS INFLAMMATION OF THE BRAIN. IT IS USUALLY DUE TO INFECTION BY A VIRUS OR MAY OCCUR AS A RESULT OF AN AUTOIMMUNE REACTION.

A rare condition, encephalitis varies in severity from a mild, barely noticeable illness to one that can be life-threatening.

Only certain viruses are able to gain access to the central nervous system and affect nerves, and therefore potentially cause encephalitis. These viruses include the herpes simplex virus (which also causes cold sores), chickenpox virus, and measles virus. Occasionally, the infection may also affect the meninges, causing meningitis. In most cases, the immune system deals with the viral infection before it can affect the brain. However,

if the immune system is compromised, there is a greater risk of developing encephalitis. When encephalitis develops, the infection causes swelling, and parts of the brain may be damaged when it is compressed against the skull. Rarely, encephalitis is due to an autoimmune reaction, in which the immune system attacks the brain, leading to inflammation and brain damage.

Mild encephalitis usually causes only a slight fever and headache. In more severe cases, there may also be nausea and vomiting; weakness, loss of coordination, or paralysis; abnormal sensitivity to light; loss or impairment of speech; memory loss; uncharacteristic behavior; stiff neck and back; drowsiness; confusion; seizures; and coma. In very severe cases, encephalitis can cause permanent brain damage and may even be fatal.

VIRAL ENCEPHALITIS
This color-enhanced MRI scan of a brain reveals a large area of abnormal tissue in the temporal lobe (the pale orange area) that is due to infection with the herpes simplex virus, one of the most common causes of viral encephalitis.

BRAIN ABSCESS

AN ABSCESS IS A COLLECTION OF PUS, SURROUNDED BY INFLAMED TISSUE, THAT CAN FORM IN THE BRAIN OR ON ITS SURFACES. THERE MAY BE SEVERAL AT ONCE.

A brain abscess can result from a bacterial or, more rarely, a fungal or parasitic infection. Fungal and parasitic infections are usually restricted to people whose immune systems have been impaired–for example, those with HIV/AIDS, people undergoing chemotherapy, or those taking immunosuppressants.

A brain abscess can occur as a result of a penetrating head injury or an infection spreading from elsewhere in the body, such as from a dental abscess, middle-ear infection, sinusitis, or pneumonia. It can also result from injecting drugs using a nonsterile needle.

Symptoms and effects

Once an abscess has formed, the tissue around it becomes inflamed, which may cause brain swelling and increased pressure in the skull. Symptoms may develop over a few days or weeks and depend on the area of the brain affected. Common general symptoms include: headache; fever; nausea and vomiting; stiff neck; drowsiness; confusion; and seizures. A person

may also experience speech difficulties, vision problems, and weakness of the limbs.

A brain abscess can be diagnosed by a scan and tests to identify the infecting organisms. Without treatment, an abscess can cause unconsciousness, and a coma (see p.238) may develop. It may also lead to permanent damage, and in some cases can be fatal. Drug treatment can eliminate the infection and reduce the swelling in the brain, but a craniotomy (a procedure to make a small opening in the skull) may be needed to drain pus from a large abscess.

INFECTIOUS BACTERIA
A brain abscess may be caused by a wide variety of bacteria, including *Pseudomonas* (above left) and *Streptococcus* (above right), the most common cause.

ABSCESS IN BRAIN TISSUE
This color-enhanced CT scan shows a large abscess in the brain (orange area) of a person with AIDS. People who are immunocompromised, such as those with HIV/AIDS, are particularly vulnerable to abscesses.

TRANSIENT ISCHEMIC ATTACK

THIS IS AN EPISODE OF TEMPORARY LOSS OF BRAIN FUNCTION DUE TO AN INTERRUPTION OF THE BLOOD SUPPLY TO PART OF THE BRAIN.

Also called a "mini-stroke," a transient ischemic attack (TIA) is most commonly caused by a blood clot that temporarily blocks an artery supplying blood to the brain. It can also occur due to excessive narrowing of an artery as a result of atherosclerosis (buildup of fatty deposits on the artery wall). There are numerous risk

NARROWED CAROTID ARTERY
This X-ray shows an area of narrowing (circled) in the carotid artery in the neck. If an embolus temporarily lodges here, it may cause a TIA.

factors that contribute to the likelihood of a TIA, such as diabetes mellitus, previous heart attacks, high blood-fat levels, high blood pressure, and smoking.

Symptoms usually develop suddenly and vary according to the part of the brain affected by the restricted blood flow, but they include visual disturbances or loss of vision in one eye, problems speaking or understanding speech, confusion, numbness, weakness or paralysis on one side of the body, loss of coordination, dizziness, and possibly brief unconsciousness. If symptoms last for more than 24 hours, the attack is classed as a stroke. Having had a TIA indicates increased risk of stroke.

Treatment for TIA is aimed at preventing a stroke and includes endarterectomy (a procedure to remove the lining of an artery affected by atherosclerosis), anticoagulant drugs, or aspirin. It is also important to treat any risk factors, and stopping smoking is essential.

1 TEMPORARY BLOCKAGE
An artery supplying the brain, such as the carotid artery, may become temporarily obstructed by an embolus (a blood clot that originates elsewhere in the body) or by a thrombus (a clot that develops in the artery itself). The temporary arterial obstruction deprives the brain of oxygen and nutrients, producing the symptoms of a TIA.

Blockage (embolus or thrombus)

2 DISPERSAL OF BLOCKAGE
As blood flow breaks up the obstruction, blood supply to the brain resumes and the symptoms disappear as oxygen and nutrients once again reach the brain. Transient ischemic attacks tend to recur, and the occurrence of one or more attacks indicates an increased risk of a stroke.

Dispersed particles

Blocked blood flow

Blood flow resumes

Temporal artery

Maxillary artery

Facial artery

Common carotid artery

BLOOD SUPPLY TO HEAD AND NECK
The common carotid artery is the main blood vessel supplying oxygenated blood to the head and neck. A temporary blockage of the carotid artery can result in a TIA.

STROKE

DAMAGE TO PARTS OF THE BRAIN CAN OCCUR WHEN BLOOD SUPPLY TO THE BRAIN IS INTERRUPTED.

Interruption to the blood supply to the brain can occur as a result of a blockage of an artery in the brain (ischemic stroke), bleeding into the brain from a ruptured artery (hemorrhagic stroke), bleeding from a blood vessel in the brain (possibly from a ruptured aneurysm), or a subarachnoid hemorrhage (see below

right). Risk factors include age, high blood pressure, atherosclerosis, smoking, diabetes mellitus, heart-valve damage, previous or recent heart attack, high blood-fat levels, certain heart-rhythm disorders, and sickle cell disease.

Symptoms and effects

Symptoms develop suddenly and vary depending on the brain areas affected, but can include sudden headache, numbness, weakness or paralysis, visual disturbances, problems speaking or understanding speech, confusion, loss of coordination, and dizziness. If severe, a stroke can cause loss of consciousness, coma, and death.

Treatment depends on the cause– strokes due to a clot require drugs and hemorrhagic strokes may require surgery. Nonfatal strokes can cause long-term disability or impairment of function, for which rehabilitative therapies (such as physical therapy and speech therapy) may be required.

Blood vessel   Hemorrhage

HEMORRHAGIC STROKE
A hemorrhagic stroke is caused by bleeding into the brain from a ruptured blood vessel. High blood pressure is a significant risk factor because the increased pressure makes the vessels more likely to rupture.

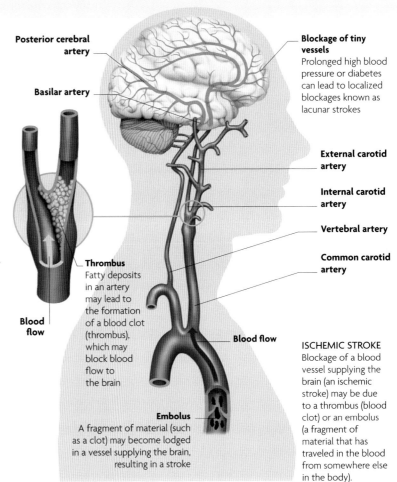

Posterior cerebral artery

Basilar artery

Blockage of tiny vessels
Prolonged high blood pressure or diabetes can lead to localized blockages known as lacunar strokes

External carotid artery

Internal carotid artery

Vertebral artery

Common carotid artery

Thrombus
Fatty deposits in an artery may lead to the formation of a blood clot (thrombus), which may block blood flow to the brain

Blood flow

Blood flow

Embolus
A fragment of material (such as a clot) may become lodged in a vessel supplying the brain, resulting in a stroke

ISCHEMIC STROKE
Blockage of a blood vessel supplying the brain (an ischemic stroke) may be due to a thrombus (blood clot) or an embolus (a fragment of material that has traveled in the blood from somewhere else in the body).

SUBDURAL HEMORRHAGE

A RUPTURED BLOOD VESSEL CAN CAUSE BLEEDING BETWEEN THE TWO OUTER MENINGES THAT SURROUND THE BRAIN.

The most common cause of a subdural hemorrhage is a head injury–it can occur from minor injuries, especially in the elderly.

After the injury, bleeding may occur rapidly (within minutes) in the case of an acute subdural hemorrhage, or slowly over days or weeks for a chronic subdural hemorrhage. The trapped blood forms a clot in the skull that compresses brain tissue and causes symptoms. These are variable and may fluctuate depending on the area of the brain affected. They may include headache, one-sided paralysis, confusion, drowsiness,

and seizures. In severe cases, there may be unconsciousness and coma. The long-term outcome depends on the size and location of the hemorrhage. A severe subdural hemorrhage may be fatal.

A subdural hemorrhage is usually diagnosed with a brain scan (CT or MRI). An X-ray may be taken if skull fracture is suspected. A small hemorrhage may not need treatment and can clear up on its own, but usually surgery is needed.

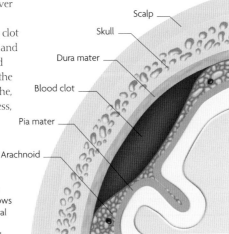

Scalp

Skull

Dura mater

Blood clot

Pia mater

Arachnoid

SUBDURAL HEMATOMA
A CT scan shows a large subdural hematoma (orange), which occurs when blood from a subdural hemorrhage forms a solid mass.

SITE OF SUBDURAL HEMORRHAGE
A subdural hemorrhage is bleeding into the space between the dura mater (outermost of the three meninges) and the arachnoid (the middle meninx).

SUBARACHNOID HEMORRHAGE

A SUBARACHNOID HEMORRHAGE IS CAUSED BY BLEEDING INTO THE SPACE BETWEEN THE TWO INNER MEMBRANES SURROUNDING THE BRAIN.

This type of hemorrhage is most commonly caused by rupture of a berry aneurysm or, rarely, is due to the rupture of an arteriovenous malformation. High blood pressure is a significant risk factor. Symptoms occur suddenly, without warning, and often develop rapidly (over minutes). Some people recover completely, some are left with residual disability, and some die. Arteries in the brain may constrict to reduce blood loss, which can reduce blood supply to part of the brain and cause a stroke.

Blood vessel

Neck of aneurysm

BERRY ANEURYSM
A berry aneurysm is a swelling that develops at a weak point in a blood vessel. It is usually present from birth.

Capillaries

NORMAL

ABNORMAL

ARTERIOVENOUS MALFORMATION
An abnormal knot of blood vessels on the brain's surface that is present from birth, an arteriovenous malformation is susceptible to rupture, causing a subarachnoid hemorrhage.

BRAIN TUMORS

BENIGN OR MALIGNANT GROWTHS CAN FORM IN THE BRAIN OR IN THE MEMBRANES AROUND THE BRAIN AND SPINAL CORD.

Primary brain tumors first develop in the brain itself and can be malignant or benign. They can arise in various types of brain cells and in any part of the brain, but primary tumors in adults are most common in the front two-thirds of the cerebral hemispheres.

Secondary tumors result from the spread of malignant cancer (metastasis) from elsewhere in the body, most commonly the lungs, skin, kidney, breast, or colon. Several secondary tumors can develop simultaneously and the cause of most tumors is not known. Rarely, some tumors may be associated with certain genetic conditions.

A tumor compresses the surrounding brain tissue and raises pressure inside the skull. Symptoms therefore depend on the size and location of the tumor, but may include severe, persistent headaches; blurred vision or other sensory disturbances; speech problems; dizziness; muscle weakness; poor coordination; impaired mental functioning; behavioral or personality changes; and seizures. If left untreated, a brain tumor may be fatal.

Brain tumors are diagnosed through brain scans and neurological tests. Treatment may involve a surgical removal (if possible), radiation therapy, and/or chemotherapy. Drugs to reduce the brain swelling may also sometimes be given.

MENINGIOMA
This micrograph shows a section through a meningioma, a type of benign tumor that develops in the meninges, the membranes that cover the brain and spinal cord.

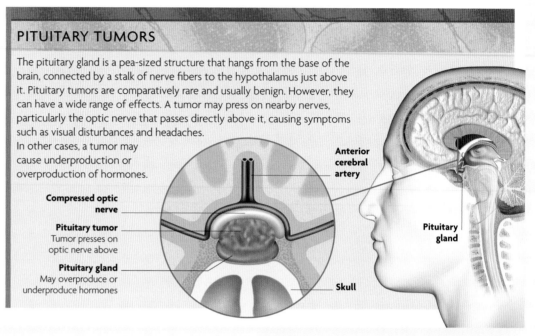

PITUITARY TUMORS

The pituitary gland is a pea-sized structure that hangs from the base of the brain, connected by a stalk of nerve fibers to the hypothalamus just above it. Pituitary tumors are comparatively rare and usually benign. However, they can have a wide range of effects. A tumor may press on nearby nerves, particularly the optic nerve that passes directly above it, causing symptoms such as visual disturbances and headaches. In other cases, a tumor may cause underproduction or overproduction of hormones.

Anterior cerebral artery

Compressed optic nerve

Pituitary tumor
Tumor presses on optic nerve above

Pituitary gland
May overproduce or underproduce hormones

Pituitary gland

Skull

DEMENTIA

THIS DISORDER IS CHARACTERIZED BY A GENERALIZED DECLINE IN BRAIN FUNCTION, PRODUCING MEMORY PROBLEMS, CONFUSION, AND BEHAVIORAL CHANGES.

Dementia is caused by microscopic damage to brain tissue that leads to atrophy. It can be caused by various disorders, some covered on the following pages. Most commonly, it is due to Alzheimer's disease (see opposite page). Another common cause is vascular dementia, in which reduced or blocked blood supply causes death of brain cells. This can occur suddenly due to a stroke or gradually through a series of small strokes. Other causes include frontotemporal degeneration; Lewy body dementia, in which small, round structures appear in brain cells, leading to the degeneration of affected brain tissue; and neurological deterioration associated with conditions such as AIDS, Wernicke–Korsakoff syndrome, Creutzfeldt–Jakob disease (see opposite page), Parkinson's disease (see p.234), Huntington's disease (see p.234), head injury, brain tumors (see above), and encephalitis (see p.227). In rare cases, it may occur due to vitamin or hormone deficiency, or as a side effect of certain medications. Rarely, dementia may be caused by inherited genetic mutations.

Symptoms and effects
Dementia is characterized by progressive memory loss, confusion, and disorientation. It can also give rise to atypical or embarrassing behavior, personality changes, paranoia, depression, delusions, unusual irritability, and anxiety. The affected person may make up explanations to account for memory gaps or strange behavior. As the condition progresses, a person with dementia may become indifferent toward other people and external events, as well as his or her own personal hygiene.

In rare cases, dementia may be due to a treatable cause, such as a side effect of medication or a vitamin deficiency, but usually there is no cure. Most forms are progressive, and a person may need total nursing care. Treatment with drugs may slow the deterioration of mental function and improve behavioral symptoms.

BRAIN ACTIVITY IN DEMENTIA
These two PET scans show the level of metabolic activity in a normal brain (left) and in the brain of a person with dementia (right), with yellow and red indicating areas of high activity, blue and purple areas of low activity, and black indicating minimal or no activity.

Blood vessel

Area of dead tissue

Clot blocking blood vessel

MULTI-INFARCT DEMENTIA
Vascular dementia can occur due to a series of blockages of blood vessels that supply the brain, usually due to clots. Each clot prevents oxygenated blood from reaching a small area of the brain, causing tissue death (infarct) in the affected area.

ALZHEIMER'S DISEASE

THE MOST COMMON CAUSE OF DEMENTIA, THIS IS A PROGRESSIVE DEGENERATIVE CONDITION IN WHICH PLAQUES CAUSE DAMAGE TO THE BRAIN.

Alzheimer's disease is rare before the age of 60, but increasingly common thereafter. Most cases occur without an identifiable cause. Mutations in several genes are associated with this disorder, however, and the genetic component is especially strong in the relatively rare cases of early onset disease (symptoms occurring before 60). In late-onset Alzheimer's disease, mutations in genes responsible for the production of a blood protein called apoliprotein E are implicated. These genes result in a protein (beta amyloid) being deposited in the brain as plaques, which leads to the death of neurons. Alzheimer's disease is also associated with reduced levels in the brain of the neurotransmitter acetylcholine. Additionally, it is thought that the disruption of the mechanism that controls the inflow of calcium ions into neurons may be involved, leading to excessive calcium in the neurons, which prevents them from receiving impulses from other brain neurons.

Symptoms may vary from one person to another, but typically Alzheimer's progresses through three stages (see panel, left). Alzheimer's disease is usually diagnosed from the symptoms, although brain scans, blood tests, and neuropsychological tests are also carried out.

Treatment

Treatment for this disorder is aimed at slowing down the degeneration, but it does not completely halt decline, and eventually complete nursing care is needed. Acetylcholinesterase inhibitors may slow progress of Alzheimer's disease in the early and middle stages, and memantine in the later stages.

ALZHEIMER'S HEALTHY BRAIN

ANATOMICAL CHANGES
These two vertical sections through the brain show the loss of brain tissue and increased surface folding in Alzheimer's disease (left) compared to a healthy brain (right).

PROTEIN FILAMENTS
Alzheimer's disease is often associated with the formation of tangled masses of protein filaments (shown in purified form in this micrograph), which may develop to form plaques.

STAGES OF ALZHEIMER'S DISEASE

The symptoms and progression of Alzheimer's disease vary from person to person. However, the symptoms become increasingly severe as the disease progresses and larger areas of the brain are damaged, although in some cases there may be periods in which the person seems to improve. Generally, there are three broad stages in the development of Alzheimer's disease.

STAGE	SYMPTOMS
Stage 1	The person becomes increasingly forgetful, and these memory problems may cause anxiety and depression. However, memory deterioration is a normal feature of aging and is not in itself evidence of Alzheimer's.
Stage 2	Severe memory loss, particularly for recent events, along with confusion about time and/or place; diminished concentration; aphasia (inability to find the right word); and anxiety, unstable moods, and personality changes.
Stage 3	In the third stage, confusion becomes very severe and there may be psychotic symptoms, such as delusions or hallucinations. There may also be abnormal reflexes and incontinence.

CREUTZFELDT–JAKOB DISEASE

DEMENTIA CAN BE CAUSED BY AN ABNORMAL PRION PROTEIN THAT ACCUMULATES IN THE BRAIN, CAUSING WIDESPREAD DESTRUCTION OF BRAIN TISSUE.

Prions are proteins that occur naturally in the brain, but their function is unknown. These proteins may become abnormally distorted, forming clusters in the brain and destroying brain tissue. This tissue destruction leaves holes in the brain, giving it a spongelike appearance, and results in various neurological dysfunctions, dementia, and finally death. There are four main types of Creutzfeldt–Jakob disease: sporadic CJD; familial CJD; iatrogenic CJD; and variant CJD, which is caused by infection with bovine spongiform encephalopathy (BSE).

Initial symptoms include memory lapses, mood changes, and apathy. These may be followed by clumsiness, confusion, unsteadiness, and speech problems. Toward the final stages there may be uncontrollable muscle spasms, stiffness of the limbs, impaired vision, incontinence, progressive dementia, seizures, and paralysis. Eventually, CJD is fatal.

TYPES OF CJD

There are four main types of Creutzfeldt–Jakob disease (CJD). They are differentiated principally by the cause of the disease, although there are also other differences between them, such as the typical age of onset and the general length of illness.

TYPE OF CJD	CHARACTERISTICS
Sporadic CJD	Also known as classic or spontaneous CJD, this is the most common form of the disease. It mainly affects people over 50, and usually progresses rapidly (over a period of months).
Familial CJD	This is an inherited form of CJD, caused by a genetic mutation. It first appears between the ages of 20 and 60 and typically has a long course, generally between 2 and 10 years.
Iatrogenic CJD	This rare form of CJD is due to contamination with blood, tissue, or other substances from an infected person as a result of a medical procedure, such as brain surgery or certain hormone treatments.
Variant CJD (vCJD)	This type of CJD is acquired by eating meat contaminated with BSE. Typically, the disease lasts about a year before causing death. This type is rare, as there are measures to prevent infected meat from entering the food supply.

VARIANT CJD AND BSE

Creutzfeldt–Jakob disease, previously an obscure illness, came to public prominence in the 1990s when a few people in the UK developed a form of the disease—known as variant CJD (vCJD)—after eating meat from cattle infected with bovine spongiform encephalopathy (BSE), commonly known as "mad cow disease." Initially it was thought that BSE was not transmissible to humans but this proved to be wrong, and stringent measures were introduced to prevent infected meat from entering the human food supply. As a result, the number of deaths in the UK from vCJD declined from a peak of 28 in 2000 to 1 in 2008.

BRAIN TISSUE IN CJD
This micrograph of brain cortex tissue from a person with variant CJD shows the characteristic spongelike appearance that is caused by the loss of neurons.

BRAIN SURGERY

SURGERY ON THE BRAIN IS A SPECIALIZED FIELD OF
NEUROSURGERY IN WHICH OPERATIONS ON THE BRAIN
OR MENINGES ARE CARRIED OUT THROUGH AN OPENING
MADE IN THE SKULL (A CRANIOTOMY) OR, MORE RARELY,
VIA THE NOSE AND NASAL CAVITY.

USES OF BRAIN SURGERY

Surgery may be used to treat various disorders. These include tumors
of the brain or the meninges; raised pressure inside the skull due to
a hemorrhage, hematoma, or hydrocephalus; traumatic brain injury,
for example due to a head wound; blood vessel abnormalities, such
as aneurysms; and brain abscesses. Less commonly, surgery may be
used to treat severe cases of epilepsy that have not responded to
medication, and to obtain biopsy samples. A highly experimental
form of brain surgery known
as deep-brain stimulation, which
involves placing electrodes inside
the brain, has been used to treat
a few patients with movement
disorders such as Parkinson's
disease (see p.234) and Tourette's
syndrome (see p.243).

STEREOTACTIC BRAIN SURGERY
A patient about to undergo deep-brain
stimulation first has a frame fixed to the
scalp. The frame helps the surgeon navigate
to the precise site in the brain where
electrodes are to be implanted.

TRANSNASAL SURGERY

A minimally invasive procedure, transnasal surgery involves inserting an endoscope
(viewing tube) through the nose to reach the base of the brain. The endoscope
enables the surgeon to view the operation site, and instruments can be passed
along it to perform surgical procedures. The main use of this type of brain surgery
is to remove tumors of the pituitary gland or of the meninges at the base of the
brain. It leaves no external scar, usually requires only a short hospital stay, and
tends to cause less pain afterward than traditional surgery.

REMOVING A BRAIN TUMOR
With the patient under anesthesia,
a flexible endoscope is passed
through the nasal cavity to the
base of the brain. The tumor
is then removed using
instruments passed along
the endoscope.

Tumor

Nasal cavity

Endoscope

DELICATE BRAIN SURGERY
In this operation, the surgeon is using an operating microscope while he removes a tumor. Having been under general anesthesia earlier in the operation, the patient is awake at this stage so that his responses can be assessed, thereby ensuring that brain damage is avoided.

PARKINSON'S DISEASE

THIS IS A PROGRESSIVE BRAIN DISORDER THAT CAUSES TREMORS, MUSCLE RIGIDITY, PROBLEMS WITH MOVEMENT, AND DIFFICULTY KEEPING BALANCE.

Parkinson's disease is caused by degeneration of cells in the substantia nigra nuclei of the midbrain. These cells produce dopamine, a neurotransmitter that helps control muscles and movement. Damage to the cells reduces dopamine production, leading to the characteristic motor symptoms of Parkinson's disease.

In most cases, the underlying cause is not known, although in a very few cases, specific genetic mutations have been linked to Parkinson's disease.

Symptoms usually develop gradually (over months or years), typically beginning with a tremor in a hand, arm, or leg that is worse when at rest. As the disease progresses, it becomes difficult to initiate voluntary movements; walking becomes a shuffling motion–it may be difficult to take the first step, and the normal arm swing when walking may be reduced or lost; muscles become rigid; handwriting becomes small and illegible; posture becomes stooped; and there may be loss of facial expression.

In the late stages, there may be problems speaking, swallowing may be difficult, and depression may occur. The intellect is usually unaffected, although dopamine depletion may cause symptoms of dementia.

Location of substantia nigra

DEEP IN THE BRAIN
This color-enhanced MRI scan of a horizontal section through the head shows the location of the substantia nigra, part of nuclei known as the basal ganglia, in the midbrain.

Substantia nigra | Cerebral aqueduct

HEALTHY BRAIN
This section of brain tissue shows the substantia nigra in a healthy brain, with the dark pigmented areas of the substantia nigra clearly visible.

Diminished substantia nigra | Cerebral aqueduct

DISEASED BRAIN
In this section of brain tissue of a person with Parkinson's disease, the pigmented neurons in the substantia nigra are significantly reduced.

PARKINSONISM

The term "parkinsonism" refers to any condition that causes the movement abnormalities that occur in Parkinson's disease resulting from the reduced production of dopamine (for example, tremors, muscle stiffness, and slow movements). Parkinson's disease is the most common cause of parkinsonism, but not everybody with parkinsonism has Parkinson's disease. Other causes include stroke, encephalitis, meningitis, head injury, prolonged exposure to herbicides and pesticides, other degenerative nerve diseases, and certain drugs, such as some antipsychotic drugs.

HUNTINGTON'S DISEASE

HUNTINGTON'S IS A RARE, INHERITED DISEASE IN WHICH NEURONS IN THE BRAIN DEGENERATE, LEADING TO JERKY, UNCONTROLLED MOVEMENTS AND DEMENTIA.

The underlying cause of Huntington's disease is a single abnormal gene that occurs when a group of DNA base pairs is repeated many times. The faulty gene generates an abnormal version of Huntingtin protein, which then builds up in nerve cells and leads to the degeneration of neurons in the basal ganglia and cerebral cortex.

Effects

Symptoms usually start to appear between the ages of 35 and 50, although they may sometimes start in childhood. Early symptoms include chorea (jerky, rapid, uncontrollable movements), clumsiness, and involuntary facial grimaces and twitches. Other symptoms then develop, including speech problems;

difficulty swallowing; depression; apathy; and dementia, which usually takes the form of lack of concentration, memory problems, and personality and mood changes (including aggressive or antisocial behavior). The disease usually progresses slowly, eventually causing death some 10–30 years after symptoms first appear.

A diagnosis of Huntington's disease is made from the symptoms, with brain scans, and also genetic (to test for the abnormal gene) and neuropsychological testing.

There is no cure for Huntington's disease, and drug treatment is aimed at reducing the symptoms. Keeping physically and mentally active is also advised.

Frontal lobe

AFFECTED AREAS
Huntington's disease causes degeneration of neurons in the basal ganglia (primarily in the caudate nuclei, putamen, and globus pallidus). It is also associated with degeneration in the frontal and temporal lobes.

Caudate nucleus

Putamen

External globus pallidus

Internal globus pallidus

Basal ganglia

Temporal lobe

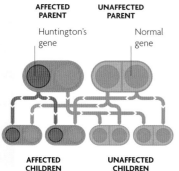

AFFECTED PARENT | UNAFFECTED PARENT

Huntington's gene | Normal gene

AFFECTED CHILDREN | UNAFFECTED CHILDREN

INHERITANCE PATTERN
Huntington's disease is inherited in an autosomal dominant fashion, which means that if one parent has a copy of the gene, each child has a 1 in 2 chance of inheriting the faulty gene and therefore of developing the disease in adulthood.

A C T G T T C A G C A G C A G

3 CAG REPEATS

GENETIC DEFECT
The genetic abnormality that causes Huntington's disease is a sequence of DNA on chromosome 4 in which a group of base pairs (CAG) is repeated numerous times. Whether or not a person develops the disease depends on the number of CAG repeats (see table, right).

HUNTINGTON'S DISEASE AND CAG REPEATS

NUMBER OF REPEATS	EFFECTS
0–15	No adverse effect; Huntingtin protein functions normally.
16–39	Huntington's disease may or may not develop.
40–59	Huntingtin abnormal; Huntington's disease will eventually develop.
60 or more	Huntingtin abnormal; Huntington's disease will develop early.

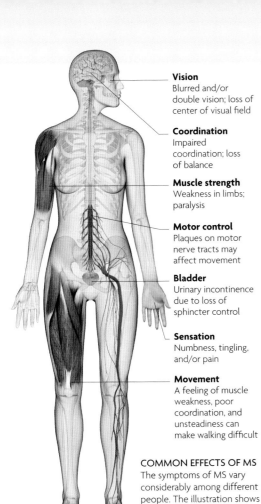

Vision
Blurred and/or double vision; loss of center of visual field

Coordination
Impaired coordination; loss of balance

Muscle strength
Weakness in limbs; paralysis

Motor control
Plaques on motor nerve tracts may affect movement

Bladder
Urinary incontinence due to loss of sphincter control

Sensation
Numbness, tingling, and/or pain

Movement
A feeling of muscle weakness, poor coordination, and unsteadiness can make walking difficult

COMMON EFFECTS OF MS
The symptoms of MS vary considerably among different people. The illustration shows some of the more common symptoms of the condition.

MULTIPLE SCLEROSIS

A PROGRESSIVE DISEASE, MULTIPLE SCLEROSIS CAUSES THE DESTRUCTION OF THE MYELIN SHEATHS THAT SURROUND NEURONS IN THE BRAIN AND SPINAL CORD.

Multiple sclerosis (MS) is thought to be an autoimmune disease in which the body's immune system destroys the cells that produce the myelin sheaths that surround and insulate neurons. Eventually hardened (sclerosed) plaques of scar tissue form over the demyelinated areas and the neurons themselves degenerate. The effect of these changes is to impair or block nerve impulses. The reason for this autoimmune reaction is not known, although there may be genetic, environmental, or infectious factors involved.

The course and symptoms of MS vary among individuals. In addition to common symptoms (see illustration, left), there may also be mental changes, such as poor memory, anxiety, and depression. The most common type is relapsing-remitting MS, in which attacks (relapses) of gradually worsening symptoms are followed by periods of remission. In progressive MS, symptoms worsen without remission. In most cases, relapsing-remitting MS may develop into progressive MS.

Macrophage

Myelin sheath   Nerve axon

Cell body

Demyelinated area

Damaged myelin sheath

EARLY STAGE
In the early stages of MS, the fatty myelin sheaths that surround the nerve axons are damaged. Macrophages, a type of white blood cell, remove the damaged areas, leading to demyelinated patches along the axons and impairing nerve conduction.

LATE STAGE
As the disorder progresses, there is an increasing amount of damage to the myelin sheaths and more nerves become affected, leading to a worsening of symptoms. Hardened (sclerosed) patches form over the demyelinated areas and eventually the nerve degenerates.

MOTOR NEURON DISEASE

IN THIS GROUP OF DISORDERS, PROGRESSIVE DEGENERATION OF MOTOR NEURONS LEADS TO INCREASING WEAKNESS AND WASTING OF MUSCLES.

In most cases, the cause of motor neuron disease (MND) is not known. However, genetic factors are thought to be important in affecting a person's susceptibility to the condition. Some rare types of MND are inherited. Motor neuron disease can affect the upper motor neurons (those originating in the motor cortex or brainstem) and/or the lower motor neurons (those in the spinal cord and brainstem that connect the central nervous system to the muscles). Damage to the upper motor neurons is indicated by spasticity, muscle weakness, and exaggerated reflexes. Damage to the lower motor neurons produces a weakening of muscles, paralysis, and atrophy of the skeletal muscles.

In addition to muscular symptoms, some people also experience personality changes and depression, but intellect, vision, and hearing remain unaffected.

There are many types of motor neuron disease, the most common of which are amyotrophic lateral sclerosis (ALS, or Lou Gehrig's disease) and progressive bulbar atrophy. Both these types affect both the upper and lower motor neurons.

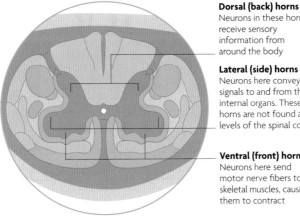

Spinal nerve   Spinal cord

Dorsal (back) horns
Neurons in these horns receive sensory information from around the body

Lateral (side) horns
Neurons here convey signals to and from the internal organs. These horns are not found at all levels of the spinal cord

Ventral (front) horns
Neurons here send motor nerve fibers to skeletal muscles, causing them to contract

NERVE TRACTS OF THE SPINAL CORD
Nerve fibers in the spinal cord are grouped into bundles, or tracts, depending on the type and direction of nerve impulses they convey. MND may affect the lower motor neurons, in the ventral horns of the spinal cord.

ASCENDING TRACTS
These nerve fibers convey sensory signals from the body to the brain.

DESCENDING TRACTS
These convey motor signals from the brain to the skeletal muscles of the torso and limbs.

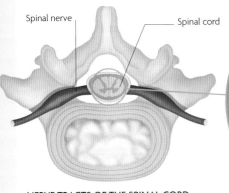

Mouth and throat
Difficulty swallowing, speaking, and chewing

Neck
Muscles in the neck become weak, causing the head to fall forwards

Chest and diaphragm
Difficulty breathing as muscles involved in breathing become weak

Leg and arm muscles
Weakness and stiffness in the legs, arms, and hands; muscles may occasionally cramp or spasm; eventually, inability to walk

AFFECTED AREAS
The effects of MND depend on the specific form of the disease, and there is also some variation among different individuals. In almost all cases, the disease is progressive and ultimately fatal. The principal effects of the main types of the condition are shown here.

PARALYSIS

PARTIAL OR COMPLETE LOSS OF CONTROLLED MOVEMENT DUE TO IMPAIRED MUSCLE FUNCTION MAY BE THE RESULT OF A NERVE OR MUSCLE DISORDER.

Paralysis can affect areas ranging from a single small muscle to most of the major muscles of the body. It is classified by the areas of body affected. Hemiplegia is paralysis of one half of the body. Paraplegia is the paralysis of both legs and sometimes part of the trunk. Quadriplegia is paralysis of all four limbs and the trunk. Paralysis may also be classified as "flaccid" (causing floppiness) or "spastic" (causing rigidity).

Paralysis can be caused by any injury or disorder that affects the motor cortex or the motor nerve pathways that run from the motor cortex via the spinal cord and peripheral nerves to the muscles. It may also result from a muscle disorder or myasthenia gravis (a disorder affecting the junction between nerves and muscles). The affected area sometimes feels numb.

Motor area affected

FRONT OF BRAIN

Opposite side of body paralyzed

Thoracic vertebra 1

Lumbar vertebra 1

Cervical vertebra 4

Cervical vertebra 7

HEMIPLEGIA
Paralysis of one half of the body may be caused by damage to the motor area of the brain on the opposite side.

PARAPLEGIA
Both legs and possibly part of the trunk may be paralyzed as a result of damage to the middle or lower spinal cord.

QUADRIPLEGIA
Damage to motor nerves in the lower neck causes quadriplegia. Damage higher in the neck is usually fatal.

DOWN SYNDROME

ALSO KNOWN AS TRISOMY 21, DOWN SYNDROME IS A CHROMOSOMAL ABNORMALITY THAT AFFECTS BOTH MENTAL AND PHYSICAL DEVELOPMENT.

One of the most common chromosomal abnormalities, Down syndrome is usually the result of an extra copy of chromosome 21; affected people therefore have 47 chromosomes in all of their body cells, rather than 46. It may also result when part of chromosome 21 breaks off and attaches to another chromosome, a process called translocation, so that cells have the normal number of chromosomes but chromosome 21 is abnormally sized. Very rarely, Down syndrome may be the result of mosaicism, in which some body cells have 47 chromosomes and some have 46. Exactly how these abnormalities produce the characteristic mental and physical features of Down is not known.

In most cases there is no identifiable reason for the chromosomal abnormality, although maternal age is a risk factor–after the early 30s, the risk of having a child with Down increases significantly. Paternal age can also be a risk factor, if the father is over 50. Parents who already have a child with Down or who have abnormalities of their own chromosome 21 have a higher risk of having a baby with Down syndrome.

Symptoms

There is considerable variation in the severity of symptoms, but typically they include slow motor and language development and learning difficulties. Physical symptoms may include a small face with upward-sloping eyes; a flattened back of the head; a short neck; a large tongue; small hands with a single horizontal crease on the palm; and short stature. There is also increased risk of various disorders, such as heart disease (often associated with congenital heart problems), hearing problems, underactivity of the thyroid gland, narrowing of the intestines, leukemia, and respiratory-tract and ear infections. Adults are at increased risk of eye problems such as cataracts. In older people there is a heightened risk of Alzheimer's disease. People with Down syndrome have lower than normal life expectancy, but some survive into old age.

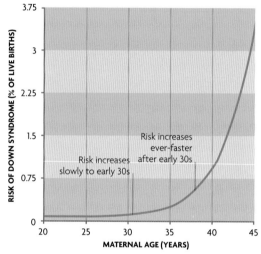

Risk increases ever-faster after early 30s

Risk increases slowly to early 30s

MATERNAL AGE AND DOWN SYNDROME
The risk of having a child with Down syndrome is related to the mother's age—increasing slowly up to the early 30s, and then at an ever-faster rate with increasing maternal age.

NORMAL CHROMOSOME COMPLEMENT
This karyotype (a photograph of the full set of chromosomes) shows the chromosome complement of a normal male, comprising a total of 46 chromosomes: 22 pairs of autosomes plus one pair of sex chromosomes (X and Y).

TRISOMY 21
This karyotype shows the chromosome complement of a male with Down syndrome. There are three chromosome 21s (hence the term "trisomy 21") instead of the normal two, resulting in the characteristic symptoms of Down syndrome.

14   21   14   21

Part of 21 breaks off

Part of 14 breaks off

Detached part of 14 reattaches to 21

Detached part of 21 reattaches to 14

BALANCED TRANSLOCATION
Down syndrome may be caused by a translocation, in which part of chromosome 21 breaks off and reattaches to another chromosome. A balanced translocation occurs when part of the other chromosome in turn moves to chromosome 21.

CEREBRAL PALSY

CEREBRAL PALSY REFERS TO A GROUP OF DISORDERS THAT AFFECT MOVEMENT AND POSTURE DUE TO BRAIN DAMAGE OR THE FAILURE OF THE BRAIN TO DEVELOP PROPERLY.

There are many possible causes of cerebral palsy, and often the cause is not identified. Usually, the brain damage occurs before or around birth. Possible causes include extreme prematurity; lack of oxygen to the fetus before or during birth (hypoxia); hydrocephalus (see below); infections transmitted from the mother to the fetus; or hemolytic disease, which is caused by a blood incompatibility between the mother and the fetus. After birth, infections such as encephalitis and meningitis, head injury, or a brain hemorrhage may cause cerebral palsy.

In addition to movement and posture abnormalities and the difficulties that these can cause (such as difficulty walking, talking, and eating), cerebral palsy may also give rise to various other problems, such as vision and hearing impairment and epilepsy. It may also sometimes cause learning difficulties. The severity of symptoms varies widely among different people, from slight clumsiness to severe disability.

There is no cure for cerebral palsy, but treatment includes physical therapy, occupational therapy, and speech therapy. Drugs may be used to control muscle spasms and increase joint mobility. Surgery may help correct any deformities that have developed as a result of abnormal muscle development. Cerebral palsy is not progressive.

BRAIN DAMAGE
This MRI scan shows the head of a child with cerebral palsy. The abnormal brain tissue (in the left side of the brain, but seen on the right of this image) has resulted in paralysis of the right side of the body.

TYPES OF CEREBRAL PALSY

Cerebral palsy can be classified into four main types, primarily on the basis of the type of movement abnormality, although there may also be other symptoms.

TYPE	CHARACTERISTICS
Spastic cerebral palsy	Exaggerated reflexes; stiff, difficult movement due to tight, stiff, and weak muscles.
Athetoid cerebral palsy	Involuntary writhing movements, especially in the face, arms, and trunk; difficulty maintaining posture.
Ataxic cerebral palsy	Problems maintaining balance; shaky movements of the hands and feet; and speech difficulties.
Mixed cerebral palsy	A combination of symptoms from the other types; often tight muscle tone and involuntary movements.

HYDROCEPHALUS

COMMONLY KNOWN AS WATER ON THE BRAIN, HYDROCEPHALUS IS AN EXCESSIVE BUILDUP OF CEREBROSPINAL FLUID WITHIN THE SKULL.

Hydrocephalus occurs either because excess cerebrospinal fluid is produced or because the fluid does not drain away normally. The fluid accumulates in the skull and compresses the brain, which may lead to brain damage.

This condition can be present at birth, often in association with other abnormalities, such as a neural-tube defect. The main symptom is an abnormally large head that continues to grow rapidly. Without treatment, severe brain damage may occur, which may lead to cerebral palsy or other physical or mental disabilities, or may even be fatal.

Hydrocephalus may occur later in life, as a result of a head injury, brain hemorrhage, infection, or a brain tumor. It usually clears up once the cause is treated.

ENLARGED VENTRICLES
In this MRI scan through the center of the head, the ventricles (black areas in the middle of the brain) are enlarged due to hydrocephalus. This abnormal accumulation of cerebrospinal fluid has compressed the brain.

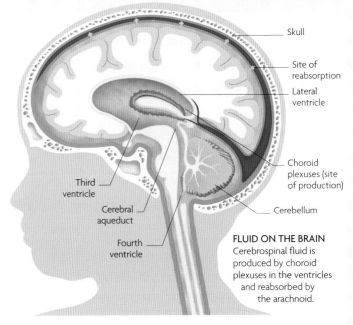

Skull

Site of reabsorption

Lateral ventricle

Third ventricle

Cerebral aqueduct

Fourth ventricle

Choroid plexuses (site of production)

Cerebellum

FLUID ON THE BRAIN
Cerebrospinal fluid is produced by choroid plexuses in the ventricles and reabsorbed by the arachnoid.

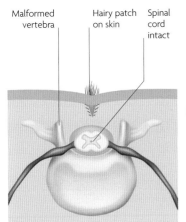

SPINA BIFIDA OCCULTA
In spina bifida occulta, the only defect is malformation of one or more vertebrae; the spinal cord is undamaged. There may be a hair tuft, dimpling, or a fatty lump at the base of the spine.

Malformed vertebra

Hairy patch on skin

Spinal cord intact

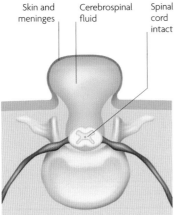

MENINGOCELE
In meningocele, the meninges protrude through the malformed vertebra, forming a sac filled with cerebrospinal fluid, which is called a meningocele. With this type of defect the spinal cord is not damaged.

Skin and meninges

Cerebrospinal fluid

Spinal cord intact

MYELOMENINGOCELE
This is the most severe form of spina bifida, in which the spinal cord is malformed and, contained within a sac of cerebrospinal fluid, protrudes through a defect in the skin.

Skin

Spinal cord malformed

NEURAL-TUBE DEFECTS

A NUMBER OF DEVELOPMENTAL ABNORMALITIES OF THE BRAIN OR SPINAL CORD CAN OCCUR WHEN THE NEURAL TUBE DOES NOT FORM PROPERLY.

The neural tube is the region along the back of an embryo that develops into the brain, spinal cord, and meninges. The cause of neural-tube defects is unknown, but they tend to run in families and have been associated with certain anticonvulsant drugs during pregnancy. A lack of folic acid during early pregnancy is also associated with the defects.

The most common types are anencephaly and spina bifida. In anencephaly there is a complete lack of a brain, which is always fatal. In spina bifida the vertebrae do not close completely around the spinal cord. In the most severe form of spina bifida, called myelomeningocele, the spinal cord is malformed and there may be paralysis of the legs and loss of bladder control.

NARCOLEPSY

THIS IS A NEUROLOGICAL DISORDER CHARACTERIZED BY CHRONIC DROWSINESS AND RECURRENT, SUDDEN EPISODES OF SLEEP THROUGHOUT THE DAYTIME.

This condition is thought to be due to abnormally low levels of proteins called hypocretins (also known as orexins) in the brain. Hypocretins are produced by cells in the hypothalamus and help regulate sleep and wakefulness. In people with narcolepsy, these cells are damaged. The underlying cause of the damage is not known, but it may be due to an autoimmune response, possibly triggered by an infection. A genetic factor may be involved, as the condition tends to run in families.

The main symptoms are overwhelming drowsiness and an uncontrollable urge to sleep–people with narcolepsy may fall asleep without warning at any time and place. Other common symptoms include a sudden loss of muscle tone (cataplexy) while awake and hallucinations at the start or end of sleep.

Hypocretin release

Hypothalamus

Locus coeruleus

Raphe nuclei

Hypocretin release

HYPOCRETIN SYSTEM
Produced by the hypothalamus, hypocretins affect many brain areas but particularly the locus coeruleus and raphe nuclei.

HYPOCRETIN RECEPTORS
This light micrograph of brain tissue shows a large number of neurons with hypocretin receptors (colored red).

COMA

A STATE OF UNCONSCIOUSNESS IN WHICH THERE IS A LACK OF RESPONSIVENESS TO INTERNAL AND EXTERNAL STIMULI IS CALLED A COMA.

Coma results from damage or disturbance to parts of the brain involved in maintaining consciousness or conscious activity, especially the limbic system and the brainstem. A wide range of problems can cause a coma, including head injury; lack of blood supply to the brain, as may occur after a heart attack or stroke; infections, such as encephalitis and meningitis; toxins, such as carbon monoxide or drug overdoses; and prolonged high or low blood-sugar levels, as can occur in diabetes mellitus.

Symptoms

There are varying degrees of coma. In less severe forms, the person may respond to certain stimuli and spontaneously make small movements. In the condition known as a persistent vegetative state there may be sleep–wake cycles, movements of the eyes and limbs,

and even speech, although the person does not appear to respond to any stimuli. In a deep coma, the person does not respond to any stimuli nor make any movements, although automatic responses such as blinking and breathing may be maintained. In severe cases, in which the lower brainstem is damaged, vital

functions such as breathing are impaired or lost and life support is necessary. Total and irreversible loss of brainstem function is classed as brain death.

Coma is diagnosed when a person remains persistently unconscious and unresponsive to stimuli. It is an emergency and requires immediate treatment.

1 Conscious Normal responses to stimuli such as sound, light, pain, and orientation (prompt response to questions about name, date, time, and/or location).

2 Confused The person is aware but bewildered and disoriented (does not respond promptly to questions about name, date, time, and/or location).

3 Delirious The person is disoriented, restless, or agitated, and shows a marked impairment of attention; there may be hallucinations or delusions.

4 Obtunded The person is sleepy, shows a marked lack of interest in the surroundings, and responds very slowly to stimuli.

5 Stuporous A sleeplike state with little or no spontaneous activity; typically, a person responds only to painful stimuli, by moving away or grimacing.

6 Comatose The person cannot be woken and does not respond to any stimuli, even painful ones; there is no gag reflex, and the pupils may not respond to light.

LEVELS OF CONSCIOUSNESS
There are various systems used to classify levels of consciousness, one of which is outlined here. The depth of a coma may also be assessed using a scale, most commonly the Glasgow Coma Scale.

BRAIN DEATH

Brain death is the irreversible cessation of functions of the brain and particularly the brainstem. The brainstem is responsible for maintaining vital functions such as breathing and heartbeat. If there is no activity in the brainstem and it is damaged so severely and irreversibly that these vital functions cannot be carried out independently without a life-support machine, a person may be diagnosed as brain dead. To confirm the diagnosis, a series of tests are carried out by two experienced physicians. These tests include checking responses to stimuli, checking functions controlled by the brainstem, and testing the ability to breathe without life support. Only if the two physicians are in agreement that brainstem and brain functions have been irreversibly lost is the diagnosis of brain death confirmed.

NORMAL EEG
Brain activity can be assessed by electroencephalography (EEG), in which electrodes are attached to the scalp and connected to a machine that records the levels of electrical activity in the brain.

NO ACTIVITY
Electroencephalography can be used to help diagnose brain death. If the EEG lines are flat, as in the recording above, it indicates that there is no activity in the brain, which is one of the criteria used to diagnose brain death.

DEPRESSION

DEPRESSION IS CHARACTERIZED BY PERSISTENT FEELINGS OF INTENSE SADNESS, HOPELESSNESS, AND LOSS OF INTEREST IN LIFE THAT INTERFERE WITH EVERYDAY LIFE.

In many cases, depression occurs without an obvious cause. A number of factors may trigger it, such as a physical illness; hormonal disorders or the hormonal changes during pregnancy (prenatal depression) or after childbirth (postpartum depression); or distressing life events, such as a bereavement. It may also occur as a side effect of certain drugs, such as oral contraceptives. Depression is more common in women, it tends to run in families, and various genetic mutations are associated with this disorder.

Various biological abnormalities have been found in the brains of depressed people, such as decreased levels of the neurotransmitter serotonin, raised levels of the enzyme monoamine oxidase, loss of cells from the hippocampus (an area of the brain involved in mood and memory), and abnormal patterns of neural activity in the amygdala and parts of the prefrontal cortex. However, the mechanisms by which such biological abnormalities may lead to depression are not known.

BEFORE TREATMENT   **AFTER TREATMENT**

DEEP BRAIN STIMULATION
In the PET scan on the left, a patient suffering from depression shows overactivity in the cingulate cortex (circled). After six months of deep brain stimulation, activity in this area (shown in the scan to the right) decreased and symptoms had improved.

SEASONAL AFFECTIVE DISORDER

Commonly known as SAD, seasonal affective disorder is a type of depression in which mood changes occur according to the season. The cause is not known, although it is thought that changes in daylight levels may cause alterations in brain chemistry that affect mood. Typically, the onset of winter brings depression, fatigue, lack of energy, cravings for sugary and starchy food, weight gain, anxiety and irritability, and avoidance of social activities. The symptoms then spontaneously clear up with the coming of spring. SAD can usually be treated with daily light therapy (sitting in front of a special light box that produces bright light similar to daylight) or antidepressants.

Symptoms and treatment

There is considerable variation among different people in the symptoms and in their severity. Most people experience several of the following: feeling unhappy most of the time; loss of interest and enjoyment in life; difficulty coping and making decisions; impaired concentration; persistent fatigue; agitation; changes in appetite and weight; disrupted sleeping patterns; loss of interest in sex; loss of self-confidence; irritability; and thoughts of, or attempts at, suicide. In some people, episodes of depression alternate with periods of extreme highs (manic episodes); this is known as bipolar disorder (see below).

Usually depression is treated with a talking therapy, antidepressant drugs, or both. Experimental treatment using deep brain stimulation (where implanted electrodes stimulate areas of the brain) is also being studied.

BRAIN AREAS
The biological basis of depression is not fully understood but several areas of the brain are thought to be involved, including the prefrontal cortex, hippocampus, and amygdala.

Prefrontal cortex
Amygdala
Hippocampus

BIPOLAR DISORDER

BIPOLAR DISORDER IS A MOOD DISORDER CHARACTERIZED BY MOOD SWINGS BETWEEN DEPRESSION AND MANIA.

The exact cause of bipolar disorder (sometimes called manic–depressive illness) is not known, although it is believed that it results from a combination of biochemical, genetic, and environmental factors. The levels of

BRAIN ACTIVITY IN BIPOLAR DISORDER
These PET scans show brain activity during normal periods (left) and increased levels of activity during a manic phase (right).

certain neurotransmitters in the brain, such as norepinephrine, serotonin, and dopamine, may play a role. Bipolar disorder tends to run in families and has a strong genetic component. However, environmental factors, such as a major life event, may act as triggers.

Symptoms

Typically, symptoms of depression and mania alternate, with each episode lasting for an unpredictable period. Between mood swings, a person's mood and behavior are often normal. Symptoms of a depressive episode may include feelings of hopelessness, disturbed sleep, changes in appetite and weight, fatigue, a loss of interest in life, and a loss of self-confidence; there may also be suicide attempts. Symptoms of a manic episode may include extreme optimism, increased energy levels, drive and activity, inflated self-esteem, racing thoughts, and risk-taking behavior.

CREATIVITY AND BIPOLAR DISORDER

Biographical studies suggest that bipolar disorder may be more common among accomplished artists than in the general population, and some artists seem to be able to utilize periods of mania as a spur to creativity. For example, the musical output of the German composer Robert Schumann (1810–56)—illustrated on the graph below—shows a link between his bouts of mania and the number of compositions he produced. He was most productive during manic phases and least productive when depressed. However, the quality of his work was not affected by his moods.

High number of compositions during manic phase
Decreased output when depressed

ANXIETY DISORDERS

THIS IS A GROUP OF DISORDERS IN WHICH FEELINGS OF ANXIETY AND/OR PANIC OCCUR FREQUENTLY ENOUGH TO CAUSE PROBLEMS IN COPING WITH EVERYDAY LIFE.

Temporary feelings of nervousness, apprehension, and even panic in stressful situations are normal and appropriate. However, when these anxiety reactions occur frequently in ordinary situations and disrupt normal activities, it is considered to be a disorder. In a few cases there may be an identifiable physical cause for persistent anxiety, such as a thyroid disorder or substance abuse, and sometimes generalized anxiety may develop after a stressful life event, such as a bereavement. In most cases the cause is not known, although a family history of an anxiety disorder increases the risk of developing one. The brain mechanisms underlying anxiety disorders are also unknown, although disruption of neurotransmitters in the frontal lobes or limbic system may be involved.

Whatever the underlying cause, the effect is to disrupt the body's normal control of its stress response –the "fight or flight" response. With anxiety disorders either the stress response fails to turn off or the stress response becomes activated at inappropriate times.

There are several forms of anxiety disorder. The most common is generalized anxiety disorder, which is characterized by excessive, inappropriate worrying that lasts for at least six months. Another form of anxiety disorder is panic disorder, in which there are sudden, unexpected attacks of intense anxiety or fear.

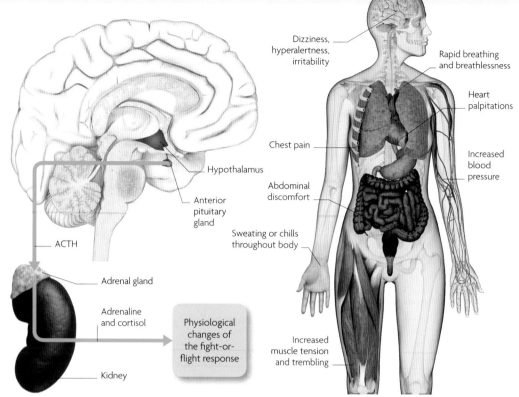

Hypothalamus

Anterior pituitary gland

ACTH

Adrenal gland

Adrenaline and cortisol

Physiological changes of the fight-or-flight response

Kidney

STRESS RESPONSE
In response to stress, the hypothalamus stimulates the pituitary gland to produce adrenocorticotropic hormone (ACTH). ACTH stimulates production of epinephrine and cortisol by the adrenal glands, and these hormones produce the fight-or-flight response.

Dizziness, hyperalertness, irritability

Rapid breathing and breathlessness

Heart palpitations

Chest pain

Increased blood pressure

Abdominal discomfort

Sweating or chills throughout body

Increased muscle tension and trembling

PHYSICAL EFFECTS OF ANXIETY
Activation of the body's flight-or-fight stress response produces widespread effects on the body. Normally, this response turns off when the stress disappears, but in anxiety disorders the stress response may be oversensitive or may fail to turn off.

FEAR OF SPIDERS
Arachnophobia is one of the most common phobias. Sufferers may experience anxiety about encountering a spider even when it is extremely unlikely.

AVIOPHOBIA
Fear of flying may occur by itself or as a manifestation of other phobias, such as acrophobia (fear of heights) or claustrophobia.

FEAR OF CROWDS
Enochlophobia may be associated with other fears, such as fear of catching a disease or being trampled.

ACROPHOBIA
Fear of heights is a generalized fear of being in a high place, even an enclosed space such as a high floor in a building.

PHOBIAS

A PHOBIA IS CONSIDERED TO BE A DISORDER WHEN PERSISTENT, IRRATIONAL FEARS OF PARTICULAR THINGS, ACTIVITIES, OR SITUATIONS DISRUPT EVERYDAY LIFE.

There are many different forms of phobia, but they can be categorized into two broad types: simple and complex. Simple phobias are fears of specific objects or situations, for example, spiders (arachnophobia) or enclosed spaces (claustrophobia). Complex phobias are more pervasive and involve several anxieties. For example, agoraphobia may involve fear of crowds and public places or of traveling in planes, buses, or other forms of public transportation; it also includes anxiety about being unable to escape to a safe place, usually home. Social phobia (also known as social anxiety disorder) is another complex phobia in which there is intense anxiety in social or performance situations (such as public speaking) because of fear of public embarrassment or humiliation.

Causes and effects

The causes of phobias are not known for certain, Some phobias tend to run in families, which may be a result of children learning a specific fear from their parents. In other cases, a phobia may develop in response to a traumatic event or situation.

The main symptom of a phobia is an intense, uncontrollable anxiety when confronted by the feared object or situation. Merely anticipating an encounter with the feared object or situation can cause anxiety. In severe cases there may be symptoms of a panic attack, such as sweating, palpitations, breathing difficulty, and trembling, when the object or situation is actually encountered. There is also usually a strong desire to avoid the feared object or situation, often to the extent of taking extreme measures. These effects can severely limit normal everyday activities and sometimes a person with a phobia may try using drugs or alcohol in an attempt to reduce the anxiety.

COMMON PHOBIAS	
NAME	**DESCRIPTION**
Astraphobia	Fear of thunder and lightning
Carcinophobia	Fear of cancer
Claustrophobia	Fear of enclosed spaces
Cynophobia	Fear of dogs
Mysophobia	Fear of contamination by germs
Necrophobia	Fear of death or dead things
Nosophobia	Fear of developing a specific disease
Nyctophobia	Fear of the dark
Ophidiophobia	Fear of snakes
Trypanophobia	Fear of injections or medical needles

POST-TRAUMATIC STRESS DISORDER

A SEVERE ANXIETY RESPONSE CAN DEVELOP AFTER A PERSON IS INVOLVED IN OR WITNESSES A DISTRESSING OR LIFE-THREATENING EVENT, SUCH AS A TERRORIST ATROCITY, NATURAL DISASTER, RAPE OR PHYSICAL VIOLENCE, SERIOUS PHYSICAL INJURY, OR MILITARY COMBAT.

The external cause of post-traumatic stress disorder (PTSD) is the experience of trauma. In the brain itself, various abnormalities in areas involved in memory, the stress response, and the processing of emotions have been identified. The amygdala (involved in memory and emotion processing) is overactivated in response to memories of traumatic events whereas the prefrontal cortex is under-responsive to fearful stimuli, which may result in its failure to inhibit the amygdala and thereby inhibit traumatic memories. The thalamus may also be involved; some people have a genetic constitution that is associated with an enlarged thalamus, which may in turn lead to an exaggerated response to fearful memories and an increased susceptibility to PTSD.

Symptoms and treatment

The symptoms of PTSD may develop immediately after a traumatic event or may not appear for months. They may include flashbacks or nightmares that trigger the same intense fear originally felt; emotional numbness; loss of enjoyment in usually pleasurable activities; memory problems; hypervigilance and an exaggerated startle response; sleeping problems; and irritability.

KEY
PTSD PATIENTS
CONTROLS

IMPAIRED MEMORY FUNCTION
Patients with PTSD and normal individuals (controls) were read a paragraph and asked to recall it immediately and after a delay. PTSD patients scored lower on both tests.

SHELL SHOCK

Stress reaction to the trauma of combat—shell shock—came to be widely recognized during World War I. Today, the term "shell shock" is categorized as "combat stress reaction" and refers to a collection of short-lived physical and mental symptoms, such as exhaustion and hypervigilance. If symptoms persist long-term, the condition is usually categorized as PTSD.

OBSESSIVE–COMPULSIVE DISORDER

COMMONLY KNOWN AS OCD, OBSESSIVE–COMPULSIVE DISORDER IS CHARACTERIZED BY RECURRENT THOUGHTS THAT CAUSE ANXIETY AND/OR OVERWHELMING URGES TO PERFORM REPETITIVE ACTS OR RITUALS IN AN ATTEMPT TO RELIEVE ANXIETY.

The exact cause of OCD is not known, but it is generally thought to be due to a combination of factors and may have different causes in different people. OCD tends to run in families, so there may be a genetic link in some cases. It has also been associated with childhood infection with Streptococcus bacteria. Brain imaging studies have found evidence of abnormal physiological connections in the communication loop between the orbitofrontal cortex, caudate nucleus, and thalamus involving the neurotransmitter serotonin. In addition, personality type may be a factor–perfectionists appear to be more susceptible to developing OCD.

Symptoms

Symptoms typically appear during the teenage or early adult years and may consist of obsessions, compulsions, or both. Obsessions are thoughts, feelings, or images that recur involuntary and provoke anxiety. For example, there may be an excessive fear of dirt that may be so powerful that the person fears leaving home in case he or she becomes contaminated. Compulsions are actions that a person feels compelled to carry out repeatedly in an effort to ward off anxiety, such as repeatedly checking things such as locks or doors. The person may recognize that the obsessions and/or compulsions are unreasonable but cannot control them.

Diagnosis and outlook

To be diagnosed with OCD, the symptoms must cause anxiety, must be present on most days for at least two weeks, and must interfere significantly with everyday life. With treatment most people recover, although symptoms may recur under stress. Deep brain stimulation, in which tiny electrodes are inserted into the brain to modulate the activity, is a promising new treatment for this condition.

COMPULSIVE BEHAVIOR
Compulsions, such as constant handwashing, are actions that a person feels compelled to carry out repeatedly.

Cingulate cortex
Caudate nucleus
Communication circuit between cortex and deeper brain structures
Orbital prefrontal cortex
Thalamus

BRAIN CIRCUIT IN OCD
This disorder may be associated with abnormalities in the communication circuit between the orbital prefrontal cortex and deeper brain structures.

BRAIN ACTIVITY IN OCD
These colored PET scans show patterns of brain activity associated with OCD. In the top pair, the colors show areas in which activity is increased when OCD symptoms get stronger. The bottom scans show areas of decreased activity when symptoms strengthen.

Frontal lobe
Parietal lobe
Frontal lobe
AREAS OF INCREASED ACTIVITY

Frontal lobe
Parietal lobe
Frontal lobe
AREAS OF DECREASED ACTIVITY

BODY DYSMORPHIC DISORDER

BODY DYSMORPHIC DISORDER (BDD) IS A MENTAL HEALTH PROBLEM IN WHICH A PERSON IS EXCESSIVELY CONCERNED ABOUT A PERCEIVED DEFECT IN HIS OR HER APPEARANCE AND THIS PREOCCUPATION WITH BODY IMAGE CAUSES SIGNIFICANT DISTRESS.

The cause of body dysmorphic disorder is unclear, although it is thought to be due to a combination of several factors, possibly including low levels of serotonin. It may occur in combination with other disorders, such as eating disorders, obsessive-compulsive disorder, and generalized anxiety disorder, although it is not clear whether there is a causative relationship with such disorders.

Many people are dissatisfied with some aspect of their appearance, but people with BDD are obsessed with one or more perceived flaws. Typical signs of BDD include refusing to be in photographs; trying to hide the "flaw" with clothing or makeup; constantly checking one's appearance in mirrors; frequently comparing one's appearance with that of others; often seeking reassurance about one's appearance; frequently touching the perceived flaw; and picking the skin to make it smooth. In addition, a person may feel anxious and self-conscious around other people because of the perceived flaw and may avoid social situations in which it might be noticed. In some cases, medical and surgical treatment may be sought to correct the perceived flaw.

Diagnosis

Body dysmorphic disorder is diagnosed by psychiatric evaluation. To be diagnosed with this disorder, preoccupations with appearance must cause considerable distress and interfere with everyday life.

Right hemisphere

Active area in left hemisphere

PROCESSING FACES IN BDD
Studies of BDD patients have revealed that they tend to use the left side of the brain, which normally processes complex detail, for processing pictures of faces. Normal people usually use their right hemisphere, unless they are examining a face closely.

AGE OF ONSET
Body dysmorphic disorder most commonly first appears during puberty or early adulthood. The peak age of onset is 11–15 years for both males and females, with about 40 percent of cases starting in this age group.

Bar chart: CASES (PERCENT) on y-axis (0 to 45), AGE (YEARS) on x-axis (0–5, 6–10, 11–15, 16–20, 21–25, 25+)

KEY
FEMALE
MALE

SOMATIZATION DISORDER

IN THIS CHRONIC PSYCHOLOGICAL PROBLEM, A PERSON COMPLAINS OF PHYSICAL SYMPTOMS FOR WHICH NO UNDERLYING PHYSICAL CAUSE IS FOUND.

A person with this disorder typically experiences several physical symptoms that persist for years. The symptoms are not generated intentionally and are often severe enough to interfere with everyday life, but no physical cause for them can be identified.

The symptoms may affect any part of the body, but complaints involving the digestive, nervous, and reproductive systems are the most common. If symptoms involve the voluntary central nervous system, such as paralysis, the condition is sometimes classed as conversion disorder (formerly known as hysteria).

The cause of somatization disorder is not known. In some cases it may be associated with other disorders such as anxiety and depression, but it is not clear whether these are causes or effects of the disorder.

LEFT HAND STIMULATED

RIGHT HAND STIMULATED

BRAIN ACTIVITY
Unusual patterns of brain activity may be detected in some cases of somatization disorder. These MRI scans show the brain of a person who experiences a loss of sensation in the left hand (the right side of the brain appears on the left in the images). The scans reveal an absence of brain activity (shown by the arrow) in the right somatosensory cortex when the left hand is stimulated. There is normal brain activity (circle) when the unaffected right hand is stimulated.

HYSTERIA

The term "hysteria" originates from the Greek word *hysterikos*, which referred to a medical disorder caused by disturbances of the uterus. The Austrian psychoanalyst Sigmund Freud (see p.189) suggested that hysteria was an attempt by the subconscious to protect the patient from stress. The term is no longer generally used in psychiatry, although it is still in everyday use to refer to a state of uncontrollable emotional excess.

DEMONSTRATION OF HYSTERIA
Hysteria was believed to be an inherited neurological disorder by the French neurologist Jean-Martin Charcot (1825–93), who used hypnosis to induce hysteria in patients and then studied the results.

HYPOCHONDRIA

THIS DISORDER IS CHARACTERIZED BY EXCESSIVE AND UNREALISTIC ANXIETY ABOUT HAVING A SERIOUS ILLNESS.

In hypochondria (also known as hypochondriases) trivial symptoms assume unrealistic significance. The symptoms are real, such as a cough or headache, but people with hypochondria are genuinely worried that they indicate a serious disease, such as lung cancer or a brain tumor. In mild forms, the person may simply worry constantly. In more severe cases, hypochondria can seriously disrupt everyday life, with the person making frequent visits to the doctor to have tests. Even when the test results prove negative, people may remain convinced that they have a serious illness and often seek other medical opinions. In addition, the person may believe they have a particular disease after hearing about it; for example, after hearing about Alzheimer's disease, an instance of momentary forgetfulness might lead the person to believe they have that disease. Many people with hypochondria also have other mental health disorders, such as depression, obsessive–compulsive disorder, phobia, or generalized anxiety disorder.

MUNCHAUSEN'S SYNDROME

SOMETIMES ALSO KNOWN AS HOSPITAL ADDICTION SYNDROME, MUNCHAUSEN'S SYNDROME IS A RARE PSYCHIATRIC CONDITION IN WHICH A PERSON REPEATEDLY SEEKS MEDICAL ATTENTION FOR FAKED OR SELF-INDUCED SYMPTOMS OF ILLNESS.

People with Munchausen's syndrome are aware that they are fabricating symptoms, unlike those with hypochondria, who truly believe they are ill. They do not fake illness in order to receive tangible benefits (such as financial gain). Instead, the motive seems to be to obtain investigation, treatment, and attention from medical personnel. People with the syndrome often have a good medical knowledge and create plausible symptoms and explanations for their faked illness, which makes diagnosis of Munchausen's syndrome very difficult. In addition to lying about symptoms, they may try to manipulate test results–for example, by adding blood to a urine sample–and may even inflict symptoms on themselves; they may injure themselves or ingest poisons, for instance. Typically, they attend many different hospitals, often repeatedly presenting the same symptoms.

In a related condition, known as Munchausen's by proxy or fabricated and induced illness (FII), people may invent or induce symptoms in somebody else. This usually involves parents faking or inducing symptoms in their child.

Diagnosis is difficult and involves carrying out various tests to exclude an underlying illness. If a genuine underlying cause is not found, a diagnosis is made from a psychiatric assessment.

FEIGNING DISEASE

Many people feign illness at some point in their lives, but in the majority of cases it is simply an occasional occurrence—to avoid going to work or school, for example. However, in some people fabricating illness is a pathological problem. This chart summarizes the ways in which feigning illness can be classified.

Nonpathological
This form of feigning typically involves using minor symptoms as a means of avoidance or of getting attention. The feigning tends to occur only sporadically and for no tangible gain.

Pathological
Pathological disease feigning, unlike the nonpathological form, tends to occur repeatedly and usually involves the feigner obtaining a significant tangible gain, such as a financial reward.

Malingering
This is the intentional use of false or exaggerated symptoms to obtain a significant gain, such as financial compensation or sympathy. It is not a disorder itself, but it may indicate a mental problem.

Factitious disorders
These involve intentional disease forgery to obtain emotional gain, such as sympathy, attention, and nurturing. Extreme forms of factitious disorders include Munchausen's syndrome.

TOURETTE'S SYNDROME

TOURETTE'S SYNDROME IS A NEUROLOGICAL DISORDER THAT IS CHARACTERIZED BY SUDDEN, REPETITIVE, INVOLUNTARY MOVEMENTS (CALLED MOTOR TICS) AND NOISES OR WORDS (CALLED VOCAL TICS).

In most cases, Tourette's syndrome runs in families and genetic factors may be involved, although the relevant genes and the mode of inheritance have not been identified. In some cases, known as sporadic Tourette's syndrome, there is no apparent inherited link. Various brain abnormalities have been implicated, including malfunctioning of the basal ganglia, thalamus, and frontal cortex, and abnormalities in the neurotransmitters serotonin, dopamine, and norepinephrine, although their causative relationship to Tourette's has not been established. Environmental factors may also play a role in the development of Tourette's syndrome.

Symptoms and effects
The characteristic symptoms of Tourette's syndrome are motor tics, such as blinking, facial twitches, shoulder shrugging, and head jerking, and vocal tics, such as grunting or repeating words. The involuntary utterances of swear words (coprolalia) is a well-known feature, but is comparatively rare. Other mental health problems, such as depression or anxiety disorders, may also develop. Typically, the symptoms first appear during childhood and get worse during the teenage years but then improve. However, in some cases the condition gets progressively worse and lasts throughout adulthood.

Diagnosis
For a positive diagnosis of Tourette's, both motor and vocal tics must be present and they must not be due to another medical condition, medications, or other substances. They must occur several times a day on most days or intermittently for more than a year.

TOURETTE'S MOTOR TICS
This long-exposure photograph illustrates the repetitive movements characteristic of Tourette's syndrome. A Tourette's sufferer, on the left, has had lights attached to his fingers to show his hand movements.

Basal ganglia
Responsible for implementing movement routines

Thalamus
Filters and relays nerve impulses to the cortex

Frontal cortex
Plays a key role in sequencing actions

IMPLICATED BRAIN AREAS
Brain studies of people with Tourette's have found abnormalities in certain areas of the brain, including the basal ganglia, thalamus, and frontal cortex, but it is not clear if these are a cause or effect of the disorder.

EXPERIMENTAL TREATMENT

Most people with Tourette's learn to live with it and do not require treatment. In severe cases, it is usually treated primarily with medication to help control the tics, although talking therapy may also be useful, particularly if there are other problems such as anxiety or obsessions. In a few, very severe, debilitating cases that have not responded to other treatments, deep-brain stimulation has been used. However, this procedure is still highly experimental and it is not yet clear whether the benefits outweigh the risks.

DEEP-BRAIN STIMULATION
This procedure involves surgically implanting a device known as a brain pacemaker into the brain (as shown here). The pacemaker sends electrical impulses to specific areas of the brain, thereby controlling their activity.

SCHIZOPHRENIA

A SERIOUS MENTAL HEALTH DISORDER, SCHIZOPHRENIA IS CHARACTERIZED BY DISTORTIONS IN THINKING, PERCEPTIONS OF REALITY, EXPRESSION OF EMOTIONS, SOCIAL RELATIONSHIPS, AND BEHAVIOR.

Contrary to popular belief, schizophrenia is not a "split personality," but rather a form of psychosis in which a person is not able to distinguish what is real from what is imagined.

The cause of schizophrenia is not known, although it is believed to result from a combination of genetic and environmental factors. Schizophrenia runs in families, and a person who has a close family member with the disorder is at increased risk of developing it. However,

it is believed that genetic susceptibility alone is insufficient to cause schizophrenia and environmental factors are also necessary. Among the environmental factors that may be involved are exposure to infection or malnutrition before birth, stressful life events, and the use of marijuana. Excess dopamine levels may also be involved since all antipsychotic drugs block dopamine, and drugs that release dopamine can trigger schizophrenia.

Various brain abnormalities have been identified in people with schizophrenia, including unusually low

Frontal lobe
Responsible for executive functions, such as attention, planning, motivation, and decision-making

Temporal lobe
Integrates and disseminates auditory information

Hippocampus
Involved in learning, memory, and linking emotion to memory

REDUCED GRAY MATTER
People with schizophrenia typically have reduced gray matter in the temporal lobes, hippocampus, and frontal lobes, but the significance of this finding is not clear.

HEARING VOICES
During auditory hallucinations, fMRI scans show activity mainly in right-hemisphere language areas, rather than in the left-hemisphere areas typically active in speech production. This may explain why the speech produced by the "voices" is simple and derogatory and why the patient mistakenly attributes them to an external source.

levels of glutamate receptors and a reduction of gray matter in certain brain regions, notably the hippocampus, frontal lobes, and temporal lobes. However, the significance of these abnormalities in schizophrenia has not been established.

Symptoms and treatment
Schizophrenia can take various forms (see panel, left). The symptoms typically develop during late adolescence or early adulthood in men, and some 4–5 years later in women. Different individuals may have different patterns of symptoms, and with varying degrees of severity. However, in general they may include delusions; hallucinations, especially auditory ones;

jumbled, incoherent speech (so-called "word salad"); lack of emotions or inappropriate emotions, such as amusement at bad news; disorganized thoughts; clumsiness; involuntary or repetitive movements; social isolation; neglect of personal health and hygiene; and unresponsive (catatonic) behavior.

Schizophrenia is diagnosed from the symptoms, but various tests are also usually performed to exclude other possible causes of abnormal behavior. Treatment is with medication, such as antipsychotic drugs, and talking therapy. About 1 in 5 people make a full recovery, but for the remainder schizophrenia is lifelong.

TYPES OF SCHIZOPHRENIA

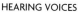

TYPE	DESCRIPTION
Paranoid schizophrenia	Delusions (particularly about being persecuted) and hallucinations are present, but thinking, speech, and emotions are often relatively normal.
Disorganized schizophrenia	Thinking and speech are confused and disordered, and emotions may be flat or inappropriate; behavior is disorganized and often disrupts everyday activities, such as cooking or washing.
Catatonic schizophrenia	Lack of responsiveness to the surroundings and immobility are typical features; in some cases, the person may exhibit strange postures or purposeless movements, or repeat overheard words.
Undifferentiated schizophrenia	Some of the symptoms of paranoid, disorganized, or catatonic schizophrenia are present, but the pattern of symptoms does not clearly fall into any of the types above.
Residual schizophrenia	Symptoms of schizophrenia are present, but these are now significantly less severe than when the schizophrenia was originally diagnosed.

LOSS OF TISSUE
These MRI scans of a pair of twins show that the ventricles (indicated by arrows) are enlarged—suggesting loss of brain tissue—in the twin on the right, who is schizophrenic. The twin on the left is not affected.

DELUSIONAL DISORDER

THIS DISORDER IS A TYPE OF PSYCHOSIS CHARACTERIZED BY THE PRESENCE OF PERSISTENT, IRRATIONAL BELIEFS THAT ARE NOT CAUSED BY ANOTHER MENTAL DISORDER.

In delusional disorder, the delusions are "non-bizarre" (involving things that are within the realms of possibility). Apart from the delusion and behavior related to it, someone with the disorder often functions normally, although preoccupation with the delusion can disrupt everyday life. The cause of delusional disorder is not known, but it is more common in

people with family members who have this disorder or schizophrenia. Socially isolated people tend to be more susceptible, and in some cases it may also be triggered by stress.

There are several types of delusional disorder: jealous (the delusion that their partner is unfaithful); persecutory (a belief that somebody is hounding or trying to harm them); erotomanic (somebody–often a celebrity–is in love with them); grandiose (an inflated sense of worth, power, talent, or knowledge); somatic (the delusion that they have a physical defect or medical problem); and mixed (two or more of the other delusional types).

DE CLERAMBAULT'S SYNDROME
Also called erotomania, de Clerambault's syndrome is a rare delusional disorder in which the sufferer believes that another person is in love with him or her. This disorder is a central theme in British novelist Ian McEwan's *Enduring Love*.

ADDICTIONS

AN ADDICTION IS A STATE OF BEING SO DEPENDENT ON SOMETHING THAT IT BECOMES DIFFICULT OR IMPOSSIBLE TO DO WITHOUT IT FOR ANY SIGNIFICANT PERIOD.

It is possible to become addicted to anything, but whatever the addiction is, the person cannot control it. An addiction may be to a substance or an activity.

It is believed that addictive substances or activities affect the brain so that it reacts in the same way that it responds to pleasurable experiences, by increasing the release of the neurotransmitter dopamine. It is not known why some people seem to be more likely to become addicted than others, although it is thought that genetic susceptibility and environmental factors probably play a role. For example, children who grow up in a family where there is drug or alcohol abuse are more likely to become addicted.

Although some symptoms are specific to the addictive substance or activity, there are several general symptoms that occur in all addictions. These include the development of tolerance–the need for increasing amounts to produce the desired effect; unpleasant physical and/or psychological withdrawal symptoms when the substance or activity is stopped; and continuing to use the substance or engage in the activity even though it may be detrimental to physical or mental health, or relationships.

ALLELE ONE
- Nicotine molecule binds loosely with protein
- Protein coded for by allele one

ALLELE TWO
- Nicotine molecule binds normally with protein
- Protein coded for by allele two

ALLELE THREE
- Nicotine molecule binds tightly with protein
- Protein coded for by allele three

GENES AND NICOTINE ADDICTION
Research indicates that there may be a genetic factor involved in some addictions. In people who carry one version (allele) of a particular gene, the allele may code for a protein that binds only loosely with nicotine. In people who carry other alleles, the proteins they code for may bind normally or tightly to nicotine. The tightness of binding alters the effects nicotine has on the body, which may, in turn, affect the susceptibility to nicotine addiction.

HEALTHY LIVER
A normal, healthy liver is dark red in color, has a smooth outer surface without lumps or scar tissue, and is free of areas of discoloration.

CIRRHOTIC LIVER
This liver shows advanced cirrhosis, with large areas of scar tissue, a lumpy surface, and general discoloration. Cirrhosis is one of the possible complications of alcohol addiction.

PERSONALITY DISORDERS

THIS IS A GROUP OF DISORDERS IN WHICH A PERSON'S HABITUAL BEHAVIOR AND THOUGHT PATTERNS CAUSE RECURRENT PROBLEMS IN EVERYDAY LIFE.

The cause of personality disorders is not known but they are thought to be due to a combination of genetic and environmental influences. Factors that may increase the risk of developing a personality disorder include a family history of such a disorder or another mental illness; abuse during childhood; a dysfunctional family life during childhood; and having conduct disorder (see p.248) in childhood.

There are many types of personality disorders (see panel, below), but in general they are all characterized by an inflexible way of thinking and behaving, irrespective of the situation. Symptoms tend to develop in adolescence or early adulthood and may vary in severity. Often a person with a personality disorder is not aware that the behavior and thought patterns are inappropriate, but may be aware of problems with personal, social, or work relationships, and these problems may cause distress. Specific symptoms depend on the type of personality disorder a person has.

TYPES OF PERSONALITY DISORDERS

Personality disorders are classified into three broad groups, known as clusters, according to the behavioral symptoms and types of thinking exhibited.

Cluster A The disorders that comprise this group are characterized by odd or eccentric behavior and/or thinking.

Paranoid People with paranoid personality disorder are suspicious and distrustful of others, may believe others are trying to harm them, and tend to be hostile and emotionally detached.

Schizoid Those with this disorder are uninterested in social relationships, introverted and solitary, and have a limited range of emotional expression; often they seem unable to recognize normal social cues.

Schizotypal People with this type are socially and emotionally detached and exhibit peculiarities of behavior and thinking, such as "magical" thinking (believing their thoughts can influence others).

Cluster B These are characterized by dramatic, erratic, or overemotional thinking and behavior.

Antisocial Previously called sociopaths, people with this personality disorder persistently disregard the feelings, rights, and safety of others; they may also persistently lie, steal, or behave aggressively.

Borderline Borderline types have problems with self-identity and fear being alone, yet often have volatile relationships; they engage in impulsive or risky behavior; and tend to have unstable moods.

Histrionic Histrionic types are highly emotional and constantly seek attention; they tend to be very sensitive to the opinions of others and overly concerned with their physical appearance.

Narcissistic Narcissistic types believe that they are superior to others, but still constantly seek approval; they tend to exaggerate their achievements and exhibit marked lack of empathy.

Cluster C The personality disorders that comprise this group are distinguished by habitual patterns of anxious, fearful, or inhibited thinking or behavior.

Avoidant People with avoidant personality disorder feel inadequate and are oversensitive to criticism or rejection; they are timid and extremely shy in social situations, which may lead to social isolation.

Dependent People with this type of personality disorder are extremely dependent on, and submissive toward, others; they feel unable to cope with everyday life alone and often feel an urgent need to be in a relationship.

Obsessive-compulsive Those with this personality disorder conform rigidly to rules and moral codes, are inflexible and often want to be in control; also tend to be perfectionists. This is not the same as OCD (see p.233), which is an anxiety disorder.

EATING DISORDERS

AN EATING DISORDER IS A CONDITION IN WHICH THERE ARE EXTREME PREOCCUPATIONS WITH FOOD AND/OR WEIGHT AND DISTURBANCES IN EATING BEHAVIOR.

The causes of eating disorders are not clear, although a combination of biological, genetic, psychological, and social factors are thought to be involved. The effects of social and peer pressure to be thin may be a contributory factor. Anxiety about body image, low self-esteem, and depression may also be involved.

Types of eating disorders

Eating disorders are most common in adolescent girls and young women, but also affect older women and men. The most common types are anorexia nervosa, bulimia nervosa, and binge-eating disorder.

Anorexia nervosa is characterized by self-starvation and excessive weight loss. Its main features are an intense fear of being fat or gaining weight; a resistance to maintaining normal weight; and the denial of the seriousness of low body weight. It can be fatal.

Bulimia nervosa is characterized by binge eating and then repeated compensatory actions to prevent weight gain, such as self-induced vomiting, laxative or diuretic use, excessive exercise, or fasting. It can result in life-threatening heart abnormalities due to an imbalance of electrolytes.

Binge-eating disorder is similar to bulimia nervosa but without the compensatory actions to counter the binges, which can lead to obesity.

BODY MASS INDEX
Body mass index (BMI) is a figure that indicates whether a person is within a healthy weight range. Adults with anorexia nervosa have a BMI of 17.5 or less.

KEY

UNDERWEIGHT BMI 18.4 OR LESS	OVERWEIGHT BMI 25–29.9
HEALTHY WEIGHT BMI 18.5–24.9	OBESE BMI 30–39.9
	VERY OBESE BMI 40 OR MORE

HEIGHT (METERS) — 1.5 to 2
WEIGHT (KILOGRAMS) — 40 50 60 70 80 90 100 110 120 130 140 150 160

WASTING AWAY
The extreme weight loss associated with anorexia nervosa leads to wasting of body tissues, as is evident in this photograph.

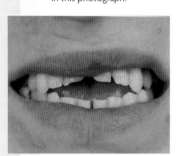

DENTAL EROSION
Repeated self-induced vomiting in bulimia nervosa can lead to erosion of tooth enamel by stomach acid, and this may lead to loss of teeth.

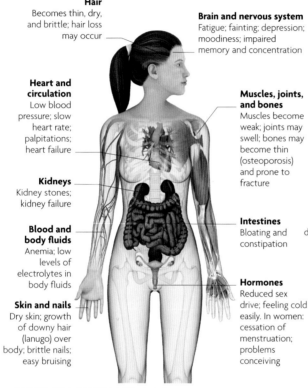

Hair
Becomes thin, dry, and brittle; hair loss may occur

Brain and nervous system
Fatigue; fainting; depression; moodiness; impaired memory and concentration

Heart and circulation
Low blood pressure; slow heart rate; palpitations; heart failure

Muscles, joints, and bones
Muscles become weak; joints may swell; bones may become thin (osteoporosis) and prone to fracture

Kidneys
Kidney stones; kidney failure

Intestines
Bloating and constipation

Blood and body fluids
Anemia; low levels of electrolytes in body fluids

Hormones
Reduced sex drive; feeling cold easily. In women: cessation of menstruation; problems conceiving

Skin and nails
Dry skin; growth of downy hair (lanugo) over body; brittle nails; easy bruising

EFFECTS OF ANOREXIA NERVOSA ON THE BODY
The most obvious effect of anorexia nervosa is extreme weight loss. However, it can also have a number of other effects on the body and may even be fatal.

Brain and nervous system
Dizziness; depression; low self-esteem; often a realization that eating behavior is abnormal

Mouth and teeth
Swollen, sore cheeks; gum disease; sensitive teeth; tooth erosion and decay; tooth loss

Heart and circulation
Low blood pressure; slow and/or irregular heart rate; heart-muscle disorders; heart failure

Throat and esophagus
Sore, irritated throat; inflammation of esophagus; esophageal rupture

Stomach
Pain; bloating; delayed emptying; ulceration; stomach rupture

Blood and body fluids
Anemia; low levels of electrolytes in body fluids; dehydration

Skin
Dry skin

Intestines
Irregular bowel movements; bloating; abdominal cramps; constipation; diarrhea

Muscles
Weakness

Hormones
Irregular or absent menstrual periods

EFFECTS OF BULIMIA NERVOSA ON THE BODY
Bulimia nervosa tends to have less obvious outward effects than anorexia nervosa as the person is often of normal weight. However, repeated bingeing and purging can have widespread physical effects.

ATTENTION DEFICIT HYPERACTIVITY DISORDER

COMMONLY KNOWN AS ADHD, ATTENTION DEFICIT HYPERACTIVITY DISORDER IS ONE OF THE MOST COMMON BEHAVIORAL DISORDERS OF CHILDHOOD.

ADHD is characterized by persistent difficulty paying attention and/or hyperactivity. It is most common in children, but it may persist into adulthood. ADHD tends to run in families and in most cases genetic inheritance, probably involving many genes, is thought to be the most probable underlying cause. However, this genetic predisposition interacts with various other factors, such as exposure to certain toxins (such as nicotine and alcohol) before birth, brain damage before birth or in the early years of life, and food allergies. There is no evidence that parenting problems cause ADHD, but they may influence its severity and a child's coping strategies. Some brain abnormalities have been found in children with ADHD, including low dopamine levels. Drugs that increase dopamine levels in the brain, such as Ritalin, may lessen symptoms. Symptoms usually appear during early childhood and may become worse when the child starts school. Due to the various ADHD-related problems, there may also be difficulty making friends, low self-esteem, anxiety, or depression.

TYPES OF ADHD
Attention deficit hyperactivity disorder can be categorized into three broad types, according to the predominant type of behavior exhibited.

Inattentive Symptoms include a short attention span; poor concentration; difficulty carrying out instructions; and changing activities often.

Hyperactive/impulsive Characterized by fidgeting; excessive activity; acting without thinking; excessive talking; and repeatedly interrupting a speaker.

Combined Symptoms include those of both other types, such as a short attention span, overactivity, and acting without thinking.

DEVELOPMENTAL DELAY

DEVELOPMENTAL DELAY IS A TERM USED WHEN A BABY OR YOUNG CHILD HAS NOT ACQUIRED THE SKILLS AND ABILITIES NORMALLY ACHIEVED BY A PARTICULAR AGE.

In the few first years of life there are important stages–developmental milestones–when a child is normally expected to have acquired certain basic physical, mental, social, and language skills. Child development is assessed in several areas, including physical and motor development; vision, hearing, speech, and mental development; and social development.

Generalized or specific delay

Delays can vary in severity and may affect one or more areas of development. Generalized delay affects most areas of development and may be due to various

WALKING UNAIDED
Being able to walk without help is one of the key developmental milestones. Typically, children manage this when between about 10 and 19 months old.

factors, such as severe visual or hearing impairment; brain damage; learning difficulties; Down syndrome; severe, prolonged disease, such as heart disease, muscle disease, or a nutritional disorder; or a lack of physical, emotional, or mental stimulation.

Developmental delay may also occur in specific areas only. Delay in movement and walking is quite common, and often a child catches up. However, there may be a serious underlying cause such as muscular dystrophy, cerebral palsy, or a neural-tube defect (see p.237). Delay in speech and language development may have various causes, including lack of stimulation, hearing problems, or more rarely, autism. Generalized difficulty with muscle control that affects speaking, which may be due to cerebral palsy, for example, can also cause delay in this area.

Diagnosis and treatment

Often delays are first noticed by parents, but a delay may also be detected during routine developmental checks. If a problem is suspected, a full developmental assessment is done, and the child may be referred to a specialist. Treatment depends on the severity and type of delay. It may include physical aids, such as glasses or hearing aids, therapies such as speech therapy, and possibly special educational help.

SCRIBBLING AND DRAWING
Normally, a child likes to scribble from about one year old, and by the age of about three most children are able to draw a reasonably straight line.

RIDING A TRICYCLE
The ability to pedal a tricycle is an indicator of motor-skill and physical development. Normally, this ability develops between about two and three years of age.

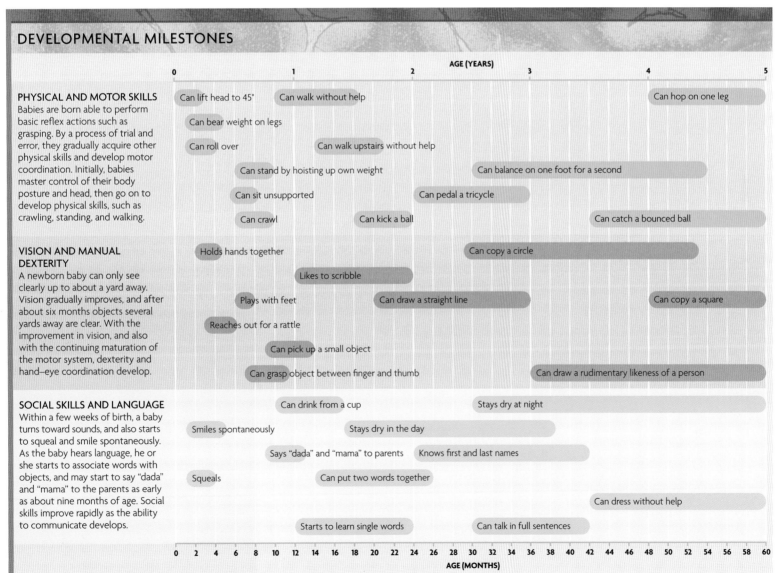

DEVELOPMENTAL MILESTONES

AGE (YEARS)

PHYSICAL AND MOTOR SKILLS
Babies are born able to perform basic reflex actions such as grasping. By a process of trial and error, they gradually acquire other physical skills and develop motor coordination. Initially, babies master control of their body posture and head, then go on to develop physical skills, such as crawling, standing, and walking.

- Can lift head to 45°
- Can walk without help
- Can hop on one leg
- Can bear weight on legs
- Can roll over
- Can walk upstairs without help
- Can stand by hoisting up own weight
- Can balance on one foot for a second
- Can sit unsupported
- Can pedal a tricycle
- Can crawl
- Can kick a ball
- Can catch a bounced ball

VISION AND MANUAL DEXTERITY
A newborn baby can only see clearly up to about a yard away. Vision gradually improves, and after about six months objects several yards away are clear. With the improvement in vision, and also with the continuing maturation of the motor system, dexterity and hand–eye coordination develop.

- Holds hands together
- Can copy a circle
- Likes to scribble
- Plays with feet
- Can draw a straight line
- Can copy a square
- Reaches out for a rattle
- Can pick up a small object
- Can grasp object between finger and thumb
- Can draw a rudimentary likeness of a person

SOCIAL SKILLS AND LANGUAGE
Within a few weeks of birth, a baby turns toward sounds, and also starts to squeal and smile spontaneously. As the baby hears language, he or she starts to associate words with objects, and may start to say "dada" and "mama" to the parents as early as about nine months of age. Social skills improve rapidly as the ability to communicate develops.

- Can drink from a cup
- Stays dry at night
- Smiles spontaneously
- Stays dry in the day
- Says "dada" and "mama" to parents
- Knows first and last names
- Squeals
- Can put two words together
- Can dress without help
- Starts to learn single words
- Can talk in full sentences

AGE (MONTHS)
0 2 4 6 8 10 12 14 16 18 20 22 24 26 28 30 32 34 36 38 40 42 44 46 48 50 52 54 56 58 60

LEARNING DISABILITY

LEARNING DISABILITY REFERS TO PROBLEMS IN UNDERSTANDING, REMEMBERING, USING, OR RESPONDING TO INFORMATION.

There are differences in opinion about what the term "learning disability" encompasses but, in general, it applies to conditions in which there is developmental delay. However, learning difficulty may also refer to a specific difficulty, for example, in reading or writing.

Types

Learning disabilities are commonly categorized as generalized or specific. Generalized learning disability affects all or almost all intellectual functions, leading to developmental delay. In addition to below-average intelligence, there may also be behavioral problems and, in severe cases, physical developmental problems as well, impairing motor skills and coordination.

DYSCALCULIA
Difficulty with mathematics—dyscalculia—is the numerical counterpart of dyslexia. It usually first becomes apparent in the early school years when a child has problems with learning number facts and calculations such as addition and subtraction.

FRAGILE X SYNDROME
This syndrome is a major cause of severe learning disability in boys. It is caused by a constriction near the end of an X chromosome (circled), making it prone to break.

Specific learning disabilities (see table, below) affect only one or a few areas of mental functioning and, in many cases, intelligence is not impared.

People with learning disability may also have various associated conditions, such as ADHD (see p.246), autistic disorder (see opposite page), or epilepsy (see p.226).

Causes

Learning disability can have a wide range of causes, including genetic abnormalities, such as Williams syndrome, or chromosomal abnormalities, such as

Down syndrome (see p.236) and fragile X syndrome (see below). Other factors include problems with brain development before or during birth, possibly due to exposure to toxins such as alcohol or drugs in the uterus, lack of oxygen, or premature or prolonged labor; and a head injury, malnutrition, or exposure to environmental toxins (such as lead) at a young age.

If a learning disability is suspected, a developmental assessment will be carried out. Hearing, vision, and other medical and genetic tests will also be done to check for underlying physical causes of the learning difficulties.

Left temporoparietal cortex

Left inferotemporal cortex — **NORMAL READERS**

Left inferior frontal gyrus — **DYSLEXIC READERS**

DYSLEXIC BRAIN
These two images show the areas of the brain that are active while reading in normal people (far left) and those with dyslexia (left). Only the left inferior frontal gyrus is active in those with dyslexia, whereas in normal readers other areas are also active.

COMMON SPECIFIC LEARNING DISABILITIES

TYPE	DESCRIPTION
Dyslexia	Impaired ability to learn to read and/or write. In addition to poor reading and spelling, there may also be difficulty with sequences, such as date order, and problems with organizing thoughts.
Dyscalculia	Difficulty performing mathematical calculations and trouble learning mathematical concepts, such as quantity and place value, and with organizing numbers.
Amusia	Commonly called tone deafness, the inability in a person with normal hearing to recognize musical notes, rhythms, or tunes or to reproduce them.
Dyspraxia	The inability to make skilled movements with accuracy. It can cause difficulty with establishing spatial relationships, such as positioning objects accurately.
Specific language impairment	Difficulties with understanding and/or expressing oral language in a child with no physical impediment to hearing or speaking and no generalized developmental delay.

CONDUCT DISORDER

CONDUCT DISORDER IS A BEHAVIORAL DISORDER IN WHICH A CHILD OR ADOLESCENT REPEATEDLY AND PERSISTENTLY BEHAVES IN A WAY THAT IS ANTISOCIAL.

Various factors put a child at increased risk of conduct disorder, including genetic factors, an unstable and/or violent family life, lack of supervision, abuse, and bullying. Learning disabilities (see above), attention deficit hyperactivity disorder (see p.246), and mental health problems such as depression also increase the risk. Children with conduct disorder also tend to have abnormal responses to reward and punishment.

Symptoms and effects

Symptoms vary from individual to individual, but they include aggressive behavior, physical cruelty, theft or persistent lying, deliberate destruction of property, and violations of rules, such as playing truant from school.

In some cases, a child may also engage in alcohol or drug abuse. Many children act in an antisocial or disruptive way from time to time, but in a child with conduct disorder the behavior occurs repeatedly over a period of several months or longer. As a result of such behavior, a child may find it difficult to make friends, have low self-esteem, and do poorly at school.

A diagnosis is usually based on a psychiatric assessment of the child's behavior patterns. Treatment of conduct disorder, through talking therapies such as cognitive-behavioral therapy, can be difficult, but early treatment is more likely to be effective. It is important that parents are involved in the treatment.

REDUCED BRAIN ACTIVITY
Children with conduct disorder tend to show reduced activity in the right orbitofrontal cortex (orange in this fMRI scan) when rewarded for a task. This supports the idea that this disorder arises from abnormal responses to the rewards and punishments that normally shape behavior.

AUTISM SPECTRUM DISORDERS

THIS IS A GROUP OF DEVELOPMENTAL DISORDERS
CHARACTERIZED BY PROBLEMS WITH COMMUNICATION,
SOCIAL RELATIONSHIPS, AND REPETITIVE BEHAVIOR.

There are several types of autism spectrum disorders, but the main ones are autistic disorder (sometimes referred to as "classic" autism) and Asperger's syndrome.

Autistic disorder usually appears in early childhood, before the age of about three years. It produces problems in three main developmental areas: impaired social skills, impaired communication, and restricted behavior. Typically, such children fail to respond to their name or to other speech directed at them; avoid eye contact; resist physical contact; start talking late and speak with an abnormal tone or rhythm; show abnormal response to social cues, such as faces and voices; perform repetitive movements, such as rocking; develop specific routines and become disturbed when they are changed; and may be unusually sensitive to sound, light, and touch, but sometimes ignore sensory signals. About half of all children with autistic disorder have learning difficulties and some children develop seizures. However, some children with autism have a high ability in one area, such as rote memory or precocious reading, and, rarely a child may have an

Basal ganglia
Involved in routine movements

Amygdala
Involved in emotional responses

Cerebellum
Refines balance and coordination

Hippocampus
Involved in memory formation

AFFECTED AREAS OF THE BRAIN
Autism has been associated with abnormalities in many brain regions (including those shown here), but their causal connection to autism is not yet clear.

Connective fiber

ORGANIZED CONNECTIONS
This diffusion tensor scan shows the clear, organized tracts of connective tissue in a healthy infant brain. These fibers are disorganized in a person that goes on to develop autism.

exceptional ability in a specific area (called savant syndrome), such as mathematics. Children with Asperger's syndrome tend to have similar symptoms, but in a less severe form. Many children are of average or above average intelligence and develop speech and language skills at the normal time. However, they have

very narrow interests, find it difficult to interact socially with their peers, and are usually inflexible in their behavior and routines.

There is no cure for autism spectrum disorders, and treatment is based on supportive education to help a child reach his or her potential.

RARE AUTISM SPECTRUM DISORDERS

TYPE	DESCRIPTION
Rett syndrome	This autism spectrum disorder affects females almost exclusively, and is caused by a mutation in a single gene. Typically, there is a period of normal development but then autism-like symptoms begin to appear, usually between about six and 18 months of age. The child's development then regresses: she shies away from social contact and no longer responds to her parents. The child stops talking, if she had been talking before, loses coordination of her feet, has repeated writhing movements of her hands, and has inappropriate outbursts of crying or laughter.
Childhood disintegrative disorder	This very rare form of autism spectrum disorder primarily affects males. As with Rett syndrome, there is a period of normal development followed by the onset of autism-like symptoms and regression. Symptoms typically appear between the ages of three and four years, although they may sometimes appear as early as two years. There are extensive and severe losses of previously acquired social, language, and motor skills, and there may also be loss of bladder and bowel control, repetitive, stereotyped behavior patterns, seizures, and severe intellectual impairment.

RESPONSE TO FACES
In these two MRI scans the yellow and red colors show areas of brain activity when looking at faces. In a normal person, there is activity in the fusiform gyrus of the temporal lobe (circled) but no corresponding activity in the brain of a person with autism.

NORMAL BRAIN
AUTISTIC BRAIN

RESPONSE TO VOICES
These two images show brain activity when normal people and those with autism listened to human voices. In the normal people, the superior temporal sulcus was active (the yellow and red area) whereas there was no activity in that area in those with autism.

NORMAL BRAIN
AUTISTIC BRAIN

TEMPLE GRANDIN

One of the best-known writers on autism, Temple Grandin is herself a high-functioning autist who has graphically described what it is like to have autism. Born in 1947 in the US, she was diagnosed with autism at the age of three. After a supportive early education, she attended ordinary schools, where she was often teased and picked on for being different. Nevertheless, she graduated from college and became a prominent researcher in animal science and welfare as well as an advocate for people with autism. In the field of animal welfare, she considers

her autism, hypersensitivity to stimuli, and unusual visual thought processes to be a positive advantage, giving her a unique insight into the stresses to which livestock are vulnerable. As a result of her early childhood experiences, Grandin is an advocate of early intervention and a supportive educational regime in autism, to help direct children with autism in productive directions. Even though autism affects every aspect of her life, Temple Grandin has said that she would not support a cure for all autism spectrum disorders.

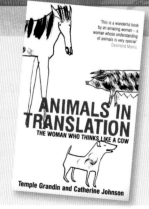

ANIMALS IN TRANSLATION
THE WOMAN WHO THINKS LIKE A COW
Temple Grandin and Catherine Johnson

ANIMALS IN TRANSLATION (2005)
In Temple Grandin's book, she uses her personal experience of both animal behavior and autism to put forward her often controversial theories about the mental processes of animals and how human and animal consciousness overlap.

GLOSSARY

A

acalculia The inability to perform numerical calculations due to neurological injury; see also *dyscalculia*.

acetylcholine A neurotransmitter that plays an important role not only in learning and memory but also in sending messages from the motor nerves to the visceral muscles.

action potential A brief pulse of electrical current that is generated by a neuron, and may be transmitted to neighboring cells.

adrenaline See *epinephrine and norepinephrine*.

afferent Traveling toward or entering; see also *efferent*.

agonist A molecule that binds to a receptor and stimulates the cell to fire; see also *antagonist*. An agonist is often a chemical that mimics the effect of a naturally occuring neurotransmitter.

agraphia The inability to write due to neurological injury.

alexia The inability to read due to neurological injury; also known as word blindness.

amnesia A general term for memory deficit.

amygdala A nucleus located in the limbic area of the temporal lobe that is crucial to emotion.

androgens The sex steroid hormones (including testosterone), which are responsible for male sexual maturation and associated with stereotypically masculine behavioral traits.

angular gyrus A ridge of the neocortex in the parietal lobe, next to the temporal and occipital lobe. It is concerned with the position of the body in space and linking sound and meaning.

anomia The inability to name objects.

anosmia The inability to smell.

anosognosia The failure, due to neurological injury, to be aware of a deficit in oneself, such as paralysis or blindness.

ANS See *autonomic nervous system*.

antagonist A molecule that blocks or prevents activation of a receptor.

anterior The front, or toward the front.

anterograde amnesia The loss of memory of things that occur after a brain injury, especially after concussion.

apraxia A partial or total inability to perform coordinated movements, including speech.

arachnoid membrane The middle of the three meninges (layers of tissue that cover the brain).

arcuate fasciculus The nerve-fiber tract that connects Broca's and Wernicke's areas.

ascending reticular formation A part of the reticular formation, responsible for the arousal and sleep–wake cycle.

association areas The regions of the brain that combine different types of information to produce a "whole" experience.

astrocyte A type of support cell that provides brain cells with nutrients and insulation.

ataxia A symptom of neurological disorder in which the sufferer experiences difficulty with balance and coordinated movement.

athetosis A condition in which muscles make slow, involuntary, writhing movements, seen in some forms of epilepsy.

attention deficit hyperactivity disorder (ADHD) A syndrome of learning and behavioral problems characterized by a short attention span and often by inappropriately energetic or frenzied activity. It usually occurs first in early childhood.

auditory cortex The region of the brain responsible for receiving and processing information relating to sound.

autonomic nervous system (ANS) A component of the peripheral nervous system, responsible for regulating the activity of internal organs. It includes both the sympathetic and parasympathetic nervous systems.

axon The fiberlike extension of a neuron that carries electrical signals to other cells. Most neurons have only one axon.

B

basal ganglia A bundle of nuclei in the base of the forebrain, including the striatum and globus pallidus. It is primarily concerned with selecting and mediating movements.

bilateral On both sides of the body; for example, both brain hemispheres.

bipolar disorder An illness that is characterized by dramatic mood swings.

blindsight The ability to respond to visual stimuli in spite of being blind due to damage to the visual cortex.

blood–brain barrier A network of tightly packed cells surrounding the brain, which prevents toxic molecules from entering.

bottom-up Usually refers to relatively "raw" information flowing from the primary sensory areas of the brain rather than from areas involved in thinking, imagining, or creating expectations.

brainstem The lower part of the brain that becomes the spinal cord.

brainwaves The regular oscillations (firings) of neurons. Different rates of firing indicates different mental states; see also *electroencephalograph (EEG)*.

Broca's area A frontal-lobe brain region, concerned with articulating speech.

Brodmann areas The microscopically distinct cortical areas that were mapped out by neurologist Korbinian Brodmann (1868–1918).

C

Capgras' delusion A rare syndrome in which people believe that a close friend or spouse has been replaced by a double. It is thought to be caused by damage to nerve pathways concerned with emotional recognition.

caudal Toward the tail end; see also *posterior*.

caudate nucleus A part of the striatum.

cell body The central structure of a neuron; also referred to as the soma.

central fissure Also called the central sulcus. A long, deep fissure that runs across the brain, dividing the parietal and frontal lobes.

central nervous system (CNS) The brain and spinal cord.

cerebellum The "small brain" behind the cerebrum that helps regulate posture, balance, and coordination.

cerebral cortex The outer, wrinkled "gray" part of the cerebral hemispheres.

cerebral hemispheres The two halves of the brain.

cerebrospinal fluid (CSF) The fluid found in the brain's ventricles, which brings nutrients to, and removes waste from, the brain.

cerebrum The major part of the brain, excluding the cerebellum and brainstem.

cerebellar penducles The short, stalklike extensions of the cerebellum, which connect it to the brainstem.

cholinergic system The nerve pathways that are activated by the neurotransmitter acetylcholine.

cingulate cortex The area of cortex that makes up the sides of the longitudinal fissure. It is closely connected to the underlying limbic system as well as to cortical areas of the brain, and is important in combining "top-down" and "bottom-up" information to guide actions.

circadian rhythm A cycle of behavior or physiological change lasting about 24 hours.

cochlea The spiral-shaped bony canal in the inner ear, containing the hair cells that transduce sound.

cognition Conscious and unconscious brain processes, such as perceiving, thinking, learning, and remembering information.

commisserectomy The surgical severing of the corpus callosum.

computed tomography (CT) A scanning technique that uses weak levels of X-ray to produce images of the brain and body.

concussion A brain trauma, usually caused by a blow to the head and resulting in temporary loss of consciousness.

cone A color-sensitive receptor cell in the retina, used primarily for daytime vision.

contralateral On the other side of the body or brain. Damage to the brain often leads to problems on the contralateral side of the body; see also *ipsilateral*.

coronal A vertical "slice" through the brain, running parallel to the shoulders.

corpus callosum The thick band of nerve tissue that connects the left and right hemispheres of the brain and carries information between them.

cortex See *cerebral cortex*.

Cotard syndrome A rare disorder in which patients assert that they are dead, often claiming to smell rotting flesh or feel worms crawling over their skin.

cranial fossa The various bowl-shaped cavities in the skull. The posterior cranial fossa houses the brainstem and cerebellum.

cranial nerves The 12 pairs of nerves that arise from the brainstem. These include the olfactory nerve, which conveys information about smell to the brain, and the optic nerve, which carries data about vision.

cranium The skull.

D

decussation The crossing of nerve fibers, as in the optic chiasm.

delusion A false belief that is not easily eradicated by exposure to evidence that reveals its falsity.

dementia A loss of brain function due to degeneration through age or cumulative damage to the brain.

dendrite A branch that extends from a neuron's cell body and receives signals from other neurons.

dentate gyrus The part of the hippocampus containing nerve cells that receive input from the entorhinal cortex.

depression A common illness characterized by intense and chronically low mood and energy levels.

diencephalon A part of the brain that includes the thalamus and the area that surrounds it.

dopamine A neurotransmitter that produces motivation and strong feelings of pleasurable anticipation.

dorsal At or toward the (upper) back.

dorsal horn The back part (in cross section) of the spinal cord, where nerve fibers, especially pain-carrying fibers, merge with the spinal cord to travel upward toward the brain.

dorsal route The pathway in the visual system that connects the visual cortex to the parietal lobe, also referred to as the "where" or "how" pathway; see also *ventral route*.

dorsolateral prefrontal cortex The area of the frontal lobe concerned with planning, organization, and various other executive functions of cognition.

dura mater The top of the three layers of tissue separating the brain from the skull; see also *meninges*.

dyscalculia A condition associated with difficulty in learning simple arithmetical operations in the absence of any other intellectual problems.

dyslexia A condition associated with difficulty in learning to read and write in the absence of any other intellectual problems.

E

EEG See *electroencephalograph*.

efferent Leading away from; see also *afferent*.

electroencephalograph (EEG) A graphic record of the electrical activity of the brain, made by attaching electrodes to the scalp that pick up the underlying brainwaves.

encephalin A type of endorphin.

encephalitis Inflammation of the brain.

endorphins A group of chemicals produced by the brain, which produce effects similar to those of opium.

entorhinal cortex The main route for information entering the hippocampus.

epilepsy An illness characterized by repeated seizures.

epinephrine and norepinephrine Hormones and neurotransmitters secreted by the adrenal gland; also referred to as adrenaline and noradrenaline.

event-related potential (ERP) The neural activity generated in response to a given stimulus recorded by EEG.

excitatory neurotransmitter A type of neurotransmitter that encourages neurons to fire; see also *inhibitory neurotransmitter*.

explicit memory The memories that can be consciously retrieved and reported.

F

fissure A deep cleft, or sulcus, on the surface of the brain.

fMRI See *functional magnetic resonance imaging*.

forebrain A major part of the brain, including the cerebrum, thalamus, and hypothalamus.

fornix An arching band of nerve tissue that carries signals around the limbic system from the hippocampus at one end, to the mammillary bodies at the other.

fovea The central part of the retina, composed of densely packed cones. It is the area of the retina that has the highest visual acuity.

frontal lobe The area at the front of the brain, responsible for thinking, making judgments, planning, decision-making, and conscious emotion.

functional imaging A range of techniques that allow neural activity to be measured and shown as visual images.

functional magnetic resonance imaging (fMRI) A brain-imaging technique in which magnetic resonance imaging is used to measure the changes in blood properties associated with neural activity; see also *magentic resonance imaging*.

fusiform gyrus A long cortical bulge on the underside of the temporal lobe, important for object and face recognition; see also *ventral route*.

G

gamma-aminobutyric acid (GABA) The major inhibitory neurotransmitter in the brain.

ganglion A cluster of interactive nuclei. The term also refers to light-sensitive cells in the retina.

Geschwind's territory A region of the brain concerned with language.

glial cells Also referred to as glia, the brain cells that support neurons by performing a variety of "housekeeping" functions in the brain. They may also mediate signals between neurons.

globus pallidus A part of the basal ganglia involved in movement control; see also *basal ganglia*.

glutamate The most common excitatory neurotransmitter in the brain.

grand mal See *seizure*.

gray matter The darker tissues of the brain, made up of densely packed cell bodies, as seen in the cortex.

gustatory cortex The area of the brain responsible for processing taste.

gyrus (*pl.* gyri) The bulges of tissue on the surface of the brain.

H

hallucination A false perception that occurs in the absence of any sensory stimuli.

hemiplegia A condition in which there is paralysis of one half of the body.

hemisphere One half of the brain.

hindbrain The back part of brain, adjoining the spine, which includes the cerebellum, pons, and medulla.

hippocampus A part of the limbic system lying on the inside of each temporal lobe. It is crucial for spatial navigation and encoding and retrieving long-term memories.

hormones The chemical messengers secreted by endocrine glands to regulate the activity of target cells. They play a role in sexual development, metabolism, growth, and many other physiological processes.

hypothalamus A cluster of nuclei that controls many body functions, including feeding, drinking, and the release of many hormones.

I

illusion A false perception or distortion of the senses often caused by unconscious brain processes.

implicit memory The memories that cannot be retrieved consciously, but are activated as part of particular skills or actions, or in the form of an emotion linked to an event that cannot be made conscious. Implicit memories underlie the learning of physical skills such as playing a ball game or tying a shoelace; see also *procedural memory*.

inferior Below or underneath.

inferior colliculi The principal midbrain nuclei of the auditory pathway.

inhibitory neurotransmitter A type of neurotransmitter that stops neurons from firing; see also *excitatory neurotransmitter*.

insula Also referred to as the insular cortex, the brain region that lies in a deep recess between the temporal and frontal lobes.

intelligence quotient (IQ) A score based on a range of tests that represents the relative intelligence of a person.

interneuron A "bridging" neuron connecting afferent and efferent neurons.

ipsilateral On the same side of the body as that in which a condition occurs; see also *contralateral*.

IQ See *intelligence quotient*.

K

Korsakoff syndrome A brain disease that is associated with chronic alcoholism. The symptoms include delirium, insomnia, hallucinations, and a lasting amnesia.

L

lateral On or to the side.

lateral geniculate nucleus (LGN) A nucleus in the thalamus that acts as a relay in the visual pathway.

lesion An area of injury or cell death.

limbic system A set of brain structures lying along the inner border of the cortex, crucial for emotion, memory, and mediating consciousness.

lobe One of four main areas of the brain that are delineated by function (occipital, temporal, parietal, and frontal).

longitudinal fissure Also called the longitudinal sulcus, the deep groove that marks the division of the two cerebral hemispheres.

long-term memory The final phase of memory, in which information storage may last anywhere from hours up to a lifetime.

long-term potentiation (LTP) A change in a neuron that increases the likelihood of it firing in unison with one that it has fired with before.

M

magnetic resonance imaging (MRI) A brain-imaging technique that provides high-resolution pictures of brain structures.

magnetoencephalography (MEG) A non-invasive functional brain-imaging technique that is sensitive to rapid changes in brain activity. Recording devices (SQUIDS) measure small magnetic fluctuations associated with neural activity in the cortex and present these in visual form.

magnocellular The pathways from large retinal ganglion cells to cortical visual areas. They are sensitive to movement.

mamillary bodies The small limbic-system nuclei that are concerned with emotion and memory.

medial In the middle.

medulla Also known as the medulla oblongata or myencephalon. A part of the brainstem situated between the pons and the spinal cord. It is responsible for maintaining vital body processes, such as breathing and heart rate.

melatonin A hormone that helps regulate the sleep–wake cycle. It is produced by the pineal gland.

meninges The three layers of protective tissue between the brain and the skull.

mesencephalon Also referred to as the "midbrain," the area of the brain between the forebrain and the brainstem, involved in eye movement, body movement, and hearing. It includes the basal ganglia.

midbrain See *mesencephalon*.

mind The thoughts, feelings, beliefs, intentions, and so on, that arise from the processes of the brain.

motor cortex The region of the brain containing neurons that send signals, directly or indirectly, to the muscles. It stretches around the brain like a horseshoe.

motor neuron A neuron that infiltrates muscle and causes it to contract or stretch.

MRI See *magnetic resonance imaging*.

myelencephalon See *medulla*.

myelin The fatty material that surrounds and insulates the axons of some neurons.

N

narcolepsy An illness characterized by uncontrolled bouts of sleeping.

near-infrared spectroscopy (NIRS) A functional imaging technique that shows varying levels of oxygen use in the brain (a marker of neural activity) by measuring the reflection of near-infrared light from cerebral tissues.

neocortex The wrinkled outer layer of the brain; also referred to as the cerebral cortex.

nervous system The nerve cells that connect to the brain and extend throughout the entire body. They are grouped into the central nervous system (CNS) and the peripheral nervous system (PNS).

neurogenesis The generation of new neurons in the brain.

neuron Also referred to as a nerve cell, a brain cell that signals to others by generating and passing on electrical signals.

neurotransmitter A chemical secreted by neurons that carries signals between them across synapses.

nociceptive Responding to painful or noxious stimuli.

norepinephrine An excitatory neurotransmitter, also known as noradrenaline; see also *epinephrine*.

nucleus A bound cluster or group of nerve cells with specialist functions.

nucleus accumbens A limbic-system nucleus that processes information related to motivation and reward.

O

occipital lobe The back part of the cerebrum, mainly dedicated to visual processing.

olfactory nerve/system The nerve/body system that responds to smell molecules.

opium A drug derived from poppy seeds that produces intense euphoria, pain relief, and relaxation.

optic chiasm The point of decussation (crossing) of the optic nerves from each eye; see also *decussation.*

optic nerve A bundle of nerve fibers carrying signals from retinal ganglion cells into the main part of the brain for processing.

oscillations The rhythmic firings of neurons.

oxytocin A neurotransmitter involved in social bonding.

P

parasympathetic nervous system A branch of the autonomic nervous system, concerned with the conservation of the body's energy. It inhibits the sympathetic nervous system.

parietal lobe The top-back subdivision of the cerebral cortex, mainly concerned with spatial computation, body orientation, and attention.

Parkinson's disease An illness characterized by tremors and slowness of action; it is thought to be caused by degeneration of dopamine-producing cells.

parvocellular The nerve pathways from small areas of the retina to cortical visual areas. They are sensitive to color and form.

peptides The chains of amino acids that can function as neurotransmitters or hormones.

peripheral nervous system (PNS) The part of the nervous system that includes all nerves and neurons outside the brain and spinal cord.

PET See *positron emission tomography*.

phantom limb An absent limb (usually amputated) that the person continues to experience as part of the body.

pia matter The innermost layer of the meninges; a thin, elastic tissue that covers the surface of the brain.

pineal gland A pea-sized gland located near the thalamus that produces melatonin, which regulates the sleep-wake cycle.

pituitary gland A hypothalamic nucleus that produces hormones, including oxytocin.

plasticity The capacity of the brain to change its structure and function.

pons A part of the hindbrain lying in front of the cerebellum.

positron emission tomography (PET) A functional imaging technique for measuring brain function in living subjects by detecting the location and concentration of small amounts of radioactive chemicals associated with specific neural activity.

posterior Toward the back or tail end. Also referred to as "caudal."

postsynaptic neuron A neuron that receives messages from another; see also *presynaptic neuron.*

prefrontal cortex The region of the brain in the forward-most part of the frontal cortex, involved in planning and other higher-level cognition.

premotor cortex A part of the frontal cortex concerned with planning movements.

presynaptic neuron A neuron that releases a neurotransmitter to carry signals across a synapse to another neuron; see also *postsynaptic neuron.*

primary cortex A region of the brain that first receives sensory information from organs, such as the primary visual cortex.

procedural memory A form of implicit memory relating to learned movements, for example, riding a bicycle.

proprioception Sensory information relating to balance and the position of the body in space.

prosopagnosia Inability to recognize faces.

psychasthenia A condition in which the sufferer experiences heightened sensitivity to negative stimuli, resulting in chronic anxiety.

psychedelic A drug that distorts perception, thought, and feeling.

psychoactive Changing brain function, usually referring to drugs.

psychosis A condition in which a person loses touch with reality.

psychotherapy The treatment of a mental disorder using psychological rather than medical methods.

putamen A part of the striatum, which itself is part of the basal ganglia, that is mainly concerned with regulating movement and procedural learning.

pyramidal neuron An excitatory neuron with a distinctive triangular body, found in the cortex, hippocampus, and amygdala.

Q

qualia The conscious, subjective sensations that arise from stimulation of sense organs, for example, pain, warmth, or seeing a color.

R

raphe nuclei The brainstem nuclei that mainly release serotonin and have wide-ranging effects on mental function.

rapid eye movement (REM) A phase of sleep characterized by rapid eye movements and vivid dreams.

reflex An involuntary movement, controlled by neurons in the spinal cord.

reticular formation A complex area in the brainstem containing various nuclei that affect arousal, sensation, motor function, and vegetative functions such as heartbeat and breathing.

retina The part of the eye containing light-sensitive cells, which send electrical signals to the visual area of the brain for processing into visual imagery.

reuptake The process by which excess neurotransmitters are removed from the synapse by being carried by transporter cells back into the axon terminals that first released them.

rhombencephalon See *hindbrain*.

rod A sensory neuron in the outer edge of the retina. It is sensitive to low-intensity light and is specialized for night vision.

rostral Toward or at the front side of the body; see also *anterior*.

S

sagittal A vertical plane passing through the brain from front to back. The midsagittal, or median, plane splits the brain into left and right hemispheres.

schizophrenia An illness characterized by intermittent psychosis.

seizure A disruption of normal neural activity. Grand mal seizures involve widespread synchronous neural firing, which produces unconsciousness.

serotonin A neurotransmitter that regulates many functions, including mood, appetite, and sensory perception.

short-term memory A phase of memory in which a limited amount of information may be held for several seconds to minutes; see also *working memory*.

single photon emission computed tomography (SPECT) An imaging process that measures the emission of single photons of a given energy from radioactive tracers in the brain, giving a measure of neural activity.

somatosensory cortex An area of the brain concerned with receiving and processing information about body sensations, such as pain and touch.

SPECT See *single photon emission computed tomography*.

SQUIDS See *magnetoencephalography*.

striate cortex An area of the visual cortex characterized (in cross section) by visually distinct strips of cells.

striatum A structure in the basal ganglia composed of the caudate and the putamen.

sulcus (*pl.* sulci) A valley or groove in the brain surface (the opposite of gyrus).

superior Toward or at the top.

superior colliculi Paired structures of nuclei of the midbrain that play a part in relaying visual information.

supplementary motor cortex An area in the front of the motor cortex involved in planning actions that are under internal control, such as actions done from memory rather than guided by current sensations.

survival value The benefit of a physical or behavioral characteristic to an individual's chances of surviving and reproducing.

sympathetic nervous system A part of the autonomic nervous system that speeds up heart rate, among other things, in response to stimulation; see also *parasympathetic nervous system*.

synesthesia The experience of having two or more senses "blended" in response to a stimulus–for example, a shape might be tasted as well as seen, or a sound may be seen as well as heard.

synapse A gap between two neurons that is bridged by neurotransmitters.

T

tegmentum The lower-back part of the midbrain.

telencephalon The largest part of the brain; see also *cerebrum* and *forebrain*.

temporal lobe A division of the cerebral cortex at the side of the head, concerned with hearing, language, and memory.

thalamus Large paired masses of gray matter lying between the brainstem and the cerebrum, the key relay station for sensory information flowing into the brain.

TMS see *transcranial magnetic stimulation*.

top-down A phrase used to distinguish "processed" information or knowledge that is used to interpret "raw" sensory data.

transcranial magnetic stimulation (TMS) A method by which electrical activity in the brain is influenced by a magnetic field, usually generated by a wand held on the scalp.

U

unilateral On one side of the body; see also *bilateral*.

V

V1 The primary visual cortex–other visual areas are often referred to as V2, V3, V4, and so on.

ventral Toward the lower, front surface (such as the abdomen of an animal).

ventral route The pathway in the visual system that connects the visual cortex to the temporal lobe, concerned with the recognition of objects and faces.

ventral tegmental area (VTA) A group of dopamine-containing neurons that make up a key part of the brain's reward system.

ventricle A cavity within the brain containing cerebrospinal fluid.

ventromedial prefrontal cortex A part of the prefrontal cortex, associated with emotions and judgment.

visual cortex The surface of the occipital lobe in which visual information is processed.

W

Wernicke's area The major language area, in the temporal lobe, concerned with comprehension. In most people, it is situated in the left hemisphere, near the junction with the parietal lobe.

white matter A type of brain tissue that is made up of densely packed axons that carry signals to other neurons. It is distinguished from cell bodies by the lighter color. White matter generally lies beneath the gray matter that forms the cortex.

working memory A process by which information is held "in mind" as active neural traffic until it is forgotten, or encoded in long-term memory.

INDEX

Page numbers in **bold** indicate extended treatments of a topic.

A

A-delta fibers, pain signals 107
abducent nerve 43
abscesses 227, **228**
absence seizures 226
acetylcholine 73
  Alzheimer's disease 231
  executing a movement 119
acrophobia 240
ACTH (adrenocorticotropic
  hormone) 61, 114, 240
action potentials 72
adaptive behaviors, emotions 129
addictions **245**
  cocaine 130
  oxytocin 137
  pleasure-seeking **130**
  to sugar **115**
adenosine, sleep-wake cycles 188
ADH (antidiuretic hormone) 61,
  114, 115
adipose tissue 102
adolescence
  emotions 39
adrenal glands 114, 240
adrenaline (epinephrine) 114
  and heat production 113
  stress response 240
  thrill-seeking 131
adrenocorticotropic hormone
  (ACTH) 61, 114, 240
aerobic exercise, effect on brain
  44
after-images 174
agency, self-consciousness **193**
aggression
  amygdala and 127
  body language 144
  personality markers 200
aging 44, **214–15**
agnosia, visual 85
agouti-related peptide (AgRP)
  115
alcohol
  addiction to 44, 245
  and brain shrinkage 44
  intoxication test 162
  and proprioception 104
alertness 186
alien beings 173
Alpha waves 181
  and creativity 170
alphabet, reading and writing
  152–53
altering consciousness **186–87**
alternating attention 182
altruism **141**
Alzheimer, Alois 9
Alzheimer's disease 230, **231**
  tangles and plaques 214, 215
ambiguous illusions **174**
American Psychiatric Association
  222
amino acids 73
amnesia, head injuries 225
amphibians, brains 48
amputation, phantom limbs **104**, 193
amusia 248
amygdala 53, 74, **127**, 209
  anticipation 130
  and body language 144
  and depression 239

amygdala cont.
  and dreams 189
  emotions 39, 126–29, 139, 212, 213
  functions 58
  gender differences 198
  and humor 171
  imaging **24**
  limbic system 64, 65
  memory 156, 160, 161
  morality 140
  and optimism 200
  pain signals 109
  phobias 127
  post-traumatic stress disorder
    241
  psychopaths 141
  recognizing faces 84
  self-awareness 139
  sense of smell and 97
  stria terminalis 126
amyotrophic lateral sclerosis 235
anesthesia, general **112**
analgesia, congenital 109
anarchic hand syndrome (AHS) 57
anatomy **50–73**
  brain cells **68–69**
  brain structures **52–55**
  brain zones and partitions **56–57**
  brainstem and cerebellum **62–63**
  cerebral cortex **66–67**
  early study of 8
  limbic system **64–65**
  nerve impulses **72–73**
  nuclei **58–59**
  scanning the brain 12
  thalamus, hypothalamus, and
    pituitary gland **60–61**
androstadienone 99
androstenone 99
anencephaly 237
aneurysm
  ruptured 229
  subarachnoid hemorrhage 229
anger
  adaptive behaviors 129
  facial expressions 136
angiotensin II 115
"animal magnetism" 222
animals
  evolution of brain **48–49**
  sense of smell 98
  social behavior 138
anorexia nervosa 246
ANS see autonomic nervous
  system
anterior cingulate cortex (ACC)
  creativity 170
  emotions 126, 128
  imaging **20**
  and optimism 200
  and pain 108, 109
  self-awareness 138, 139
anterior commissure, gender
  differences 198
anterior fissure, spinal cord 42
anterior intraparietal area (AIP) 83
anterior nucleus, hypothalamus
  113
anticipation 127, **130**
antidiuretic hormone (ADH) 61,
  114, 115
antisocial behavior, psychopaths
  141

antisocial personality disorder
  245
anxiety
  anxiety disorders **240–41**
  and decision-making 169
  eating disorders 246
  and experience of pain 109
  obsessive-compulsive disorder
    (OCD) **241**
  phobias **240**
  post-traumatic stress disorder
    (PTSD) **164**, **241**
  stria terminalis 126
aphasia 149, 151
apoliprotein E 231
apoptosis 209
appearance, body dysmorphic
  disorder **242**
appeasement 129
apperceptive agnosia 85
appetite control 115
arachnid
  arachnoid granulations 45
  skull 56
  spinal cord 42
arachnophobia 240
arbor vitae 63
archetypes, collective
  unconsciousness 193
arcuate fasciculus 148, 151
Aristotle 6, 8
arms
  bionic arms **219**
  executing a movement 118
  motor neuron disease 235
  phantom limbs **104**, 193
arteries 46–7
  arteriovenous malformation
    229
  carotid arteries 146
  Circle of Willis 45
  stroke **229**
  transient ischemic attacks 228
artificial intelligence **217**
artists, creativity 170
aspartate 73
aspartic acid 73
Asperger's syndrome 139, 172, **249**
association, accessing memories
  159
association areas
  emotions 129
  perceptions 39
associative agnosia 85
astraphobia 240
astrocytes 69, 70–71
asymmetry **57**
ataxic cerebral palsy 237
atherosclerosis 228
athetoid cerebral palsy 237
athletes 196
atonic seizures 226
ATP 106
atriopeptin 114
atrioventricular node 112
attachment **135**
attention
  and consciousness **182–83**
  laying down a memory 160
attention deficit hyperactivity
  disorder (ADHD) **246**
attraction, sexual 134
auditory canal, hearing 94

auditory cortex **91**
  and conversation 151
  hearing 94, 95
  laying down a memory 161
  music 93
  perception of sound 92
  reading 152
auditory frequency ranges **91**
auditory nerve 90
aura 172
  epileptic seizures 226
  migraine 224
auricular cartilage 90
autism **139**, 223
  autism spectrum disorders **249**
  autistic savants 164–65, 174, 249
  hyperlexia 153
  pattern-making 172
autoimmune diseases
  multiple sclerosis **235**
  narcolepsy **238**
automata 74
automatic movements 116
autonomic nervous system (ANS)
  40
  heart rate regulation **112**
  hypothalamus and 113
  phobias 127
  reticular formation 112
autopilot 185
avatars 217
aversion
  aversion behavior 129
  flavor-aversion learning 101
aviophobia 240
avoidant personality disorder 245
awareness 186
  agency and intention 193
  and consciousness 180
  types of 179
axons 68
  aging 214
  in brainstem 62
  cerebellum 63
  myelin sheaths 68, 69, 213
  nerve impulses 72, 73
  spinal cord 42
  synapses 69
  types of neurons 69

B

Baader–Meinhof Gang 205
babies
  attachment 135
  bonding with 135
  development of hearing **93**
  developmental delay **247**
  facial expressions 136
  maternal love 134
  number sense 169
  personality development 200
  sense of smell 99
backdating time **191**
bacteria
  brain abscesses 228
  meningitis 227
balance 118
  postural instability 119
  proprioception 104, 105
  vestibulocochlear nerve 43
ballism 119

auditory cortex **91** see above...
basal nuclei (ganglia) 53, **58**, 212, 213
  aging 214
  and brain "clocks" 190
  imaging **23**
  planning movement 117
  Tourette's syndrome 243
bases, DNA 196
basilar membrane 90
behavior and personality **194–205**
  adaptive behaviors 129
  autism spectrum disorders **249**
  aversion behavior 129
  conduct disorder **248**
  dementia **230**
  influencing the brain **198–99**
  morality **140–41**
  nature and nurture **196–97**
  obsessive-compulsive disorder
    (OCD) **241**
  personality **200–01**
  personality disorders **245**
  state-dependent memory 162
  strange brains **204–05**
belief systems **172–73**
belladonna 144
bereavement 239
Berger, Hans 9
berry aneurysm 229
beta amyloid 231
Beta waves, and consciousness 181
biceps muscle, proprioceptors 104
bilingualism **149**, 153
binge-eating disorder 246
binocular rivalry 87
biogenic amines 73
biometric sensors 129
bionic arms **219**
bionic eyes **218**
biotechnology **218–19**
bipolar disorder 223, **239**
bipolar neurons 69
birds, brains 49
bladder
  multiple sclerosis 235
  panic responses 127
bleeding see hemorrhage
"blind" smell 98
blind spot, retina 81
blindness 78
  bionic eyes **218**
  blindsight **79**
  inattention **183**
  seeing with sound **89**
Bliss, Timothy 9
blood clots
  stroke 229
  subdural hemorrhage **229**
  transient ischemic attacks 228
blood supply
  functional magnetic resonance
    imaging 13
  glucose 45
  oxygen in 45
blood vessels
  arteries 46–7
  arteriovenous malformation 229
  Circle of Willis 45
  hemorrhage 225
  panic responses 127
  stroke **229**
  and temperature control 113
  transient ischemic attacks **228**
  vascular dementia 230

body clock 63
body dysmorphic disorder (BDD) **242**
body language **144–45**
  and conversation 150
  tennis players 120
"body maps," self-consciousness 192, 193
body mass index (BMI) 246
body memories 157, 160
body weight, and brain weight 44
bonding
  love and 134
  oxytocin 135
bones
  in ear 90, 94
  skull 53, 54
borderline personality disorder 245
bottom-up processing **79**, **87**
bovine spongiform encephalopathy (BSE) 231
bowels, panic responses 127
bradykinesia 119
bradykinin 106
brain death **238**
"brain-in-a-vat" **180**
brain-machine interfaces **216**
brain waves
  and consciousness 181
  and creativity 170
  electroencephalographs 12
  in meditation 187
brainstem 52, **62–63**, 208, 209
  anatomy **62**
  brain death 238
  coma 238
  emotions 128, 129
  executing a movement 118
  functions 38, **63**
  hearing 94
  imaging **27**
  locked-in syndrome **63**
  reticular formation **112**
breastfeeding 135
breathing
  panic responses 127
  regulation of 112
Broca, Paul 9, **10**
Broca's aphasia 149
Broca's area 10, **148**
  conversation 151, 203
  imaging **25**
  and memory 157, 203
  reading 152
Brodmann, Korbinian 9, **67**
brown fat 113
BSE (bovine spongiform encephalopathy) 231
bulbous corpuscles 102
bulimia nervosa 246
bullies **141**

C

C-fibers, pain signals 107
calcium
  Alzheimer's disease 231
  executing a movement 119
  ion channels 65
camphor 96
cancer
  brain tumors 230
  fear of 240
carbohydrates 45
carbon dioxide, regulation of breathing 112
carcinophobia 240

carotid arteries
  stroke 229
  transient ischemic attacks 228
  Wada test 146
cars, driving 116
cartoons, humor 171
cataplexy 238
catatonia **190**
catatonic schizophrenia 244
cats
  brains 49
  expressions 136
caudate nucleus 52, 54, 58
  and memory 156, 157
  and obsessive-compulsive disorder 241
cells
  cell membrane 68
  cerebral cortex 67
  and consciousness 181
  retina 81
  stem cells 218
  support cells **69**, 70–71
  see also glial cells; neurons
central executive, memory 157
central nervous system (CNS) **40–41**
  evolution of 48
central sulcus, imaging **29**
cerebellar cortex 63, 117
cerebellar hemispheres see cerebellum
cerebellar peduncles 62
cerebellum 52, 53, 55, 56, 62, **63**, 208, 209, 212
  anatomy 63
  and conversation 151
  disorders 119
  functions 63
  imaging **32**
  internal structure 63
  and memory 156, 157
  planning movement 117
cerebral cortex 55, **66–67**
  and consciousness 180
  development 208
  evolution 49
  functional areas **67**
  functions 57
  hippocampus 65
  imaging **18**
  landmarks **66**
  limbic lobe 65
  memory 157
  pain signals 106, 108
  sense of taste 101
  structure **67**
cerebral hemispheres see hemispheres; left hemisphere; right hemisphere
cerebral palsy **237**
cerebrospinal fluid (CSF) 44, 57
  aging 215
  flow of **45**
  hydrocephalus **237**
  lumbar puncture 227
  protection of brain 45
  in spinal cord 42, 45
cerebrum 53, 208, 209
  see also hemispheres; left hemisphere; right hemisphere
cervical region, spinal nerves 42
cervical spinal cord 53
cervical vertebra 53
Charcot, Jean-Martin 242
chess 217
chest, motor neuron disease 235
chickenpox virus 227
childbirth 135
  postpartum depression 239

children
  attention deficit hyperactivity disorder (ADHD) 246
  autism spectrum disorders **249**
  childhood disintegrative disorder 249
  conduct disorder **248**
  developmental delay **247**
  dyslexia 153
  factors in intelligence 168
  maternal love 134
  personality development 200
  reading and writing 152
  see also babies
chimpanzees
  brains 49
  language areas 147
Chinese room, theory of consciousness **179**
chloride ions, nerve impulses 72
chloroform 112
cholinergic circuits 130
chorea 58, 119, 234
choroid, eye 81
choroid plexuses, cerebrospinal fluid 45
chromosomes 196
  Down syndrome **236**
chronic fatigue syndrome **225**
cilia, hair cells 94
cingulate cortex
  and aggression 200
  and depression 239
  emotions 126
  self-consciousness 192
  social cognition 184
  see also anterior cingulate cortex; posterior cingulate cortex
cingulate gyrus 64, 65
cingulate sulcus 65
circadian rhythm 63
Circle of Willis 45, 46
circuits
  emotion circuits 128
  forming memories 158
CJD (Creutzfeldt-Jakob disease) **231**
claustrophobia 240
"clocks" 190
clonic seizures 226
clots see blood clots
cluster headaches **224**
CNS see central nervous system
co-operation, personality markers 200
co-ordination, multiple sclerosis 235
cocaine addiction 130
coccyx 42
cochlea 90, 92, 94
cochlear duct 90
cochlear implants **91**, 94
cochlear nerve 90, 92, 94, 95
cochlear nucleus 95
cocktail-party effect 92
cognitive illusions **174–75**
cold, thermoreceptors 102, 113
collateral fissure 65
collective unconscious **193**
color
  color vision **83**
  illusions 87
  language and 147
  visual perception 87, 89
column of fornix 64
coma 225, **238**
commitment 134
communication **142–53**
  autism 223

communication cont.
  body language and gestures **144–45**
  conversation **150–51**
  expressions **136–37**
  gestures and body limbic system **144–45**
  limbic system areas 148–49
  origins of language **146–47**
  reading and writing **152–53**
  smell and **99**
complex partial seizures 226
complicated grief **130**
comprehension, and aging 215
compulsions 241
computed tomography (CT) scans 12, 222
computers
  artificial intelligence **217**
  brain-machine interfaces 216
  consciousness 219
concentration 179, 186, 187
concha, ear 94
concrete-mindedness 172
concussion 225
conduct disorder 245, **248**
conduction aphasia 149
cone cells, retina 81, 88
congenital analgesia 109
congruence 139
conjunctiva, eye 80
connective tissue, support cells 70–71, 249
connectivity 39
Connectome 9, 74
conscious awareness 179, 180
conscious movement 116, 117
conscious vision 84
consciousness 6, **174–91**
  altering **186–87**
  attention and **182–83**
  dissociation 186
  emotions 126, **128–29**
  investigating the brain 8
  and language 146
  levels of 192
  locating **180–81**
  in machines 219
  proprioception 104
  requirements of **181**
  self **192–93**
  sensory information **79**
  sleep and dreams **188–89**
  time **190–91**
  types and levels of **179**
  what is consciousness? **178–79**
constellations, mental disorders **223**
contrecoup injury 225
control see movement and control
conversation **150–51**
conversion disorder 242
coprolalia, Tourette's syndrome 243
cornea, eye 80
corpus callosum 52, 53, 56, 74, 204, 212, 213
  altered brain states 186
  and emotions 126
  gender differences 198
  split brain 204
corpus striatum 58
cortex see cerebral cortex and individual cortices
cortisol, stress response 240
Cottingley fairies 173
covert attention 182
cranial nerves 42, **43**, 53, 55, 208

cranial nerves cont.
  brainstem 62
  peripheral nervous system 40
  taste and smell 101
craniotomy 11, 232
creativity **170–79**
  and bipolar disorder 239
Creutzfeldt-Jakob disease (CJD) **231**
CSF see cerebrospinal fluid
CT (computed tomography) scans 12, 222
cuddling babies 135
cultural influences **199**
cynophobia 240
cytoplasm 68, 69

D

Dale, Henry H 9
Dali, Salvador 191
danger, thrill-seeking 131
Darwin, Charles 9
day length 190
daydreaming 186
De Clerambault's syndrome 244
deafness 78, 91
death **238**
decision-making 11, **169**
  and aging 214
  agency and intention 193
  morality 140
"declarative" memories 158, 160
deep brain stimulation 218
  for depression 239
  for movement disorders 232
  for Tourette's syndrome 243
default-mode network (DMN) 184
defenses, physical **45**
degenerative disorders 222, 223
déjà vu **163**
Delgado, José **10**
Delta waves, sleep 181
delusions
  delusional disorder **244**
  schizophrenia 244
dementia 203, 214, **230**
  Alzheimer's disease 230, **231**
  artificial hippocampus 161
  Creutzfeldt-Jakob disease **231**
  Huntington's disease **234**
demons, exorcism 222
dendrites 68, 69
  synapses 69
dendritic spines 69
dentate gyrus 65, 212
dentate nucleus, cerebellum 117
dependent personality disorder 245
depolarization, nerve impulses 72
depression 185, 222, 223, **239**
  and creativity 170
  grief and 129
  pacemakers and 219
depth, vision **83**, 89
dermatomes **42**
dermis 102
Descartes, René 6, 8, **178**
desire **130**
  and dreams 189
development and aging **206–19**
developmental delay **247**
  learning disability 248
developmental disorders 222, 223
devils, history of mental illness 222
diabetes, and aging 215
diagnosis, mental disorders **222**
Diagnostic and Statistical Manual (DSM) of Mental Disorders 222

diaphragm, motor neuron disease 235
diencephalon 53, 60
diet *see* food
diffusion tensor imaging 13
digestive system, panic responses 127
direction, attention to 183
disbelief 172
diseases and disorders **220–49**
  causes **223**
  constellations and spectrums **223**
  historical theories of **222**
  diagnosis **222**
  see also individual disorders
disgust 128
  adaptive behaviors 129
  bad odors 98
  facial expressions 136
dislocated self **193**
disorganized schizophrenia 244
dissociation **186**
dissociative identity (DID) **201**
distorting illusions **175**
distraction, and experience of pain 109
divided attention 182
DNA **196**
  Huntington's disease 234
  in neurons 68
dogs
  brains 49
  expressions 136
  sense of smell 97, 98
dolphins, brains 49
dopamine 73
  and addiction 130, 245
  and aging 214
  anticipation 130
  and attention deficit hyperactivity disorder 246
  bipolar disorder 239
  and brain "clocks" 190
  and desire 130
  and emotions 127, 128
  "falling in love" 134
  genetic influences 197
  and humor 171
  Parkinson's disease 234
  and pattern-making 173
  reward system 115, 130
  and schizophrenia 244
  substantia nigra 58
  thrill-seeking 131
dorsal horn, pain signals 106
dorsal pathway, vision **84–85**, 89
dorsal root, spinal nerves 42
dorsal striatum 58
dorsolateral prefrontal cortex
  and consciousness 180
  and morality 140
Down syndrome **236**, 248
drawings, autistic savants 164–65, 174
dreams **189**
  conscious perception 181
  lucid dreams **189**
driving, movements 116
drop attacks 226
drowsiness 188
  narcolepsy **238**
drugs
  addiction to 130
  altering consciousness 186
  opiates 107
  placebo effect 109
  and proprioception 104
  sleeping drugs 189
dualism 178
Duchenne, Guillaume 137
"Duchenne" smile 137

dura mater
  skull 56
  spinal cord 42
dyscalculia 248
dyslexia 149, **153**, 248
  limbic system differences 153
  left-handedness and 199
  treating 153
dysphasia 149
dyspraxia 248

E

eardrum 90, 91, 94
ears **90–95**
  anatomy **90**
  balance 105
  deafness 78, 91
  hearing **94–95**
  nerves 43
  sending information to thalamus 60
earthworms 48
East Asia, cultural influences 199
eating disorders 242, **246**
Ebbinghaus illusion 175
echolocation 91
ecstasy
  out-of-body experiences 193
  supernatural experiences 173
ECT *see* electroconvulsive therapy
EEG *see* electroencephalography
Egypt, ancient 6, 8
Einstein, Albert 204–05
electrical impulses 38
  brain-machine interfaces **216**
  executing a movement 119
  imaging techniques 9
  nerve impulses **72–3**
  scanning the brain 12, 13
electroconvulsive therapy (ECT) 202
electrodes 9
electroencephalography (EEG) 6, 12, 202
  brain death 238
elephants
  brains 49
  impossible drawing 175
embodied cognition 138
embolus
  stroke 229
  transient ischemic attacks 228
embryonic disc 208
emotions 39, **124–31**
  artificial intelligence 217
  avatars 217
  body language 144
  conflicting emotions 137
  conscious emotions **128–29**
  and consciousness 179
  and conversation 150
  and decision-making 160
  desire and reward **130–31**
  and dreams 189
  empathy and sympathy 140
  and experience of pain 109
  expressing **136**
  feeling **128**
  gender differences 198
  gestures 145
  laying down a memory 160, 161
  limbic system 126
  mirroring **123**
  morality 140
  post-traumatic stress disorder **164, 241**
  reading **137**
  and recognition 163
  recognition of faces 84

emotions *cont.*
  responding to 139
  robots 216
  schizophrenia 244
  and sense of smell 96, 99
  and the supernatural 173
  teenagers 203
  timing **129**
empathy **140**
  facial expressions and 139
  mirror neurons 11
encephalins 107
encephalitis **227**
endocrine system **114–15**
  pituitary gland 61
endoplasmic reticulum 68
endorphins 107
endoscopes, transnasal surgery 232
energy, sources of **45**
English language, dyslexia 153
enochlophobia 240
entorhinal cortex, memory 161
environment
  influence of 196
  and intelligence 168
  and schizophrenia 244
epidermis, skin 102
epigenetic alteration 196
epilepsy **226**
  pacemakers and 219
  seizures 181
  split brain 204
epinephrine (adrenaline) 114
  and heat production 113
  stress response 240
  thrill-seeking 131
episodic memory 157, 160
epithelium, olfactory **97**
erotomania 244
erythropoietin 114
Escher, M. C. **175**
ether 112
ethics, biotechnology **218**
ethmoid bone 54
euphoria 130, 134
eustachian tube 90
evolution **48–49**
  and aging 214
  of language **147**
  sense of smell 98
  sense of taste 100
excitatory neurotransmitters 73
  and personality 200
  and subjective time 190
excitement, and aging 214
exercise
  and aging 215
  effect on brain 38, 44
exorcism 222
expressions 127, **136–37**, 139
exterior globus pallidus 53, 54
extradural hematoma 225
extroversion, personality markers 200
eyes **80–89**
  attention 182, 183
  bionic eyes **218**
  blindness 78
  blindsight **79**
  bonding with babies 135
  brainstem functions 63
  communication **144**
  eye contact 144
  eye-tracking studies 86–87
  facial expressions 136–37
  iris 208
  macular degeneration 218
  nerves 43
  neurons 69
  panic responses 127

eyes *cont.*
  retina **81**, 208
  seeing **88–89**
  sending information to thalamus 60
  structure **80–81**
  visual pathways **80, 84–85**
  visual perception **86–87**

F

fabricated and induced illness (FII) 243
face
  autism spectrum disorders 249
  bones 54
  expressions 127, **136–37**, 139
  pain 107
  pattern-making 173
  recognition 83, 84, **85**, 139, 163
  sending information to thalamus 60
  sexual attraction 134
  smiling 129, **137**
  symmetry 134
facial nerve 43
facial nucleus 58
factitious disorders 243
factual recognition, faces 84
fairies 173
"falling in love" 134
false memory **164**
fasciculus cuneatus 62
fasciculus gracilis 62
fat tissues
  brown fat cells 113
  regulation of hunger 115
fatigue, chronic fatigue syndrome **225**
fatty acids 100
fatuous love 134
fear
  adaptive behaviors 129
  body language 144
  facial expressions 127, 136
  hemispheres and 128
  hypothalamus and 126
  and moods 129
  phobias 127, **240**
feedback mechanisms
  neuroendocrine system **114**
  proprioception 104
feelings *see* emotions
feigning disease **243**
femininity
  female brain 198
  and sexual attraction 134
fetus, development of hearing 93
field sobriety tests 104
"fight or flight" response 127, 129, 240
filum terminale 42
fish, brains 48
fissures
  cerebellum 63
  cerebral cortex 66
flashbacks, post-traumatic stress disorder 164, 241
flavor-aversion learning 101
flight response 127, 129, 240
flocculonodular lobe 63
fMRI (functional magnetic resonance imaging) 7, 12, 13
focused attention 182
folia, cerebellum 63
folic acid 237
"folk memory" 193
follicle-stimulating hormone (FSH) 61, 114

food
  and aging 215
  appetite control 115
  eating disorders **246**
  and intelligence 168
  taste **100–01**
foramen magnum 53, 62
foramina, facial bones 54
forebrain 53
  forgetting 156, **164**
  Alzheimer's disease 231
  blocking memory 164
form, visual perception 89
fornicate gyrus 65
fornix 53, 55, 65
fovea **81**
fractures, skull 225
fragile X syndrome 248
free will 11
Freeman, Walter 11
"freezing," motor disorders 119
Freud, Sigmund 9, 184, 222
  and dreams **189**
  on hysteria 242
friendship 134
frogs, brains 48
frontal bone 54, 66
frontal cortex
  bilingualism 149
  and consciousness 180
  emotions 126, 128, 129
  false memory 164
  functions 138
  and limbic system 64
  pain signals 108
  planning movement 117
  Tourette's syndrome 243
frontal lobe 66
  altered brain states 186
  attention 182
  and consciousness 180
  and creativity 171
  decision-making 169
  and dreams 189
  emotions 128
  imaging **17**
  intelligence 168
  meditation 187
  memory 156, 157, 160
  visual pathways 84, 85
  visual perception 88
frontal-polar cortex, imaging **16**
functional brain imaging 12
functional disorders 223
functional magnetic resonance imaging (fMRI) 7, 12, 13
fungi, brain abscesses 228
fusiform gyrus
  emotions 129
  face recognition 139
  imaging **31**
future prospects **216–17**

G

GABA *see* gamma-aminobutyric acid
Gage, Phineas 8, **10, 141**
Galen 8
Gall, Franz Joseph 9, **10**
Galvani, Luigi 8
games, brain-machine interfaces 216
gamma-aminobutyric acid (GABA) 73
  and emotions 127
  epilepsy 226
  and sleep 188
Gamma waves
  and creativity 170
  meditation 187

ganglia *see* nuclei
ganglions, sensory nerves 42
gender differences
  emotions 126, 127
  and facial symmetry 134
  influencing the brain 198
  stria terminalis 126
general anesthetics **112**
generalized anxiety disorder 240, 242
generalized seizures 226
genes and genetics **196–97**
  and addictions 245
  Alzheimer's disease 231
  attention deficit hyperactivity disorder 246
  autism spectrum disorders 249
  and individuality 38
  and intelligence 168
  and personality 200
  personality disorders 245
genetic diseases
  Huntington's disease **234**
  motor neuron disease (MND) **235**
  schizophrenia **244**
  Tourette's syndrome **243**
geniculate nuclei 53, 60
Geschwind's territory 148
gestures **145**
ghosts **173**
ghrelin 115
glands
  neuroendocrine system 114
  see also adrenal glands; pituitary gland
Glasgow Coma Scale 238
glial cells 44, **69**
  cerebellum 63
  cerebral cortex 67
global aphasia 149
globus pallidus **58**, 117
glossopharyngeal nerve 43, 101
glucagon 114
glucose **45**
  and aging 215
  PET scans 12
glutamate 73
glutamic acid 73
glycine 73
Golgi, Camille 9
Golgi cells 63
Golgi complex 68
"goose bumps" 113
gorillas
  brains 49
  language abilities 147
grammar 146
  of gestures 145
grand mal epilepsy 226
Grandin, Temple **249**
grandiose delusional disorder 244
granule cells, cerebellum 63
gray matter 44
  bilingualism 149
  cerebral cortex 67
  spinal cord 42
  in thalamus 60
greebles 83
Greece 8
grief 129
  complicated grief **130**
growth of brain 39
growth hormone (GH) 61, 114
gustatory areas 101
gymnasts 105
gyri (gyrus) 54, 209
  cerebral cortex 66

H
hair cells, in ear 90, 91, 94
hairs
  "goose bumps" 113
  touch receptors 102
hallucinations
  schizophrenia 193, 244
  supernatural experiences 173
halothane 112
hands
  anarchic hand syndrome (AHS) 57
  bionic arms **219**
  gestures **145**
  handedness 57, **199**
  manual dexterity 247
  phantom limbs 104
  touch receptors 103
happiness, facial expressions 137
"hard" problems, vision 88
hatred 128
head
  cranial nerves **43**
  injuries 6, **225**
  see also face; skull
headaches **224**
hearing **90–95**
  conversation **150**
  development of **93**
  hearing loss **91**
  perception of sound **92–93**
heart
  hormones 114
  panic responses 127
  regulation of heart rate **112**
heart attack, referred pain 107
heat, thermoreceptors 102, 113
Helmholtz, Hermann von 8
hematoma 225
  subdural 229
hemorrhage 225
  hemorrhagic stroke 229
  subarachnoid hemorrhage **229**
  subdural hemorrhage **229**
hemiplegia **236**
hemispheres
  and aging 215
  basal nuclei 58
  missing 205
  split brain **11**, **204**
  tumors 230
  see also left hemisphere; right hemisphere
Hensen's cells 90
herbivores, sense of taste 100
heroin
  addiction 130
  pain relief 107
Herpes simplex virus 227
heterosexuality 198
hierarchy of brain **53**
hindbrain 53, 62
hippocampus 53, **65**, 209
  artificial hippocampus **161**, 219
  cellular organization 59
  and consciousness 180
  and depression 239
  and dreams 189
  emotions 126, 127
  imaging **24**
  limbic system 64, 65
  memory 65, **156–63**, 164
  and novelty-seeking 200
  reading 152
  smell and 99
  spatial memory 162
Hippocrates 222
histamine 73, 106
history
  investigating the brain **8–9**
  neuroscience **10–11**

histrionic personality disorder 245
HM (Henry G. Molaison) **11**, 159
Holmes, Gordon Morgan 9
homeostasis 114
Homo erectus 49
Homo habilis 49
Homo neanderthalensis 49
homosexuality 198
hormones
  and day length 190
  and emotions 126, 127
  feedback mechanisms **114**
  neuroendocrine system **114–15**
  oxytocin **135**
  pituitary gland 61
  pituitary tumors 230
hospital addiction syndrome 243
human genome 196
humor **171**
"humors," history of mental illness 8, 222
hunger **115**
Huntington's disease **234**
hydra 48
hydrocephalus **237**
hydrogen atoms, magnetic resonance imaging 13
hypchondria, and creativity 170
hyperactive ADHD 246
hyperkinesia 119
hyperlexia **153**
hyperventilation 127
hypnosis **186**, 222
hypochondria **242**
hypocretins 238
hypodermis 102
hypoglossal nerve 43
hypokinesia 119
hypomania, and creativity 170
hypothalamus 53, 55, 56, **61**
  anticipation 130
  appetite control 115
  and dreams 189
  emotions 126, 127, 128
  functions **113**
  gender differences 198
  hormones 114
  limbic system 64
  narcolepsy 238
  neuroendocrine system 114
  oxytocin 135
  sleep–wake cycles **115**
  stress response 240
  thermoreceptors 113
hysteria **242**
  and creativity 170

I
"I," self-consciousness 192
"ice-pick" lobotomy 11
illness *see* diseases and disorders *and individual disorders*
illusions
  cognitive illusions **174–75**
  Mona Lisa illusion 85
  motion 85
  visual perception 87
imagination, and creativity 170
imaging techniques 6–7, **9**, **12–13**, 222
immune system
  autoimmune diseases 235, 238
  brain abscesses 228
  encephalitis 227
implants
  artificial hippocampus **161**, 219
  bionic eyes 218
  cochlear **91**, 94
  early experiments 10

implicit memory 157, 160
impulses *see* nerve impulses
impulsive ADHD 246
inattention blindness **183**
inattentive ADHD 246
incubi 189
incus 90
individuality 38, 198
infatuation 134
infections
  encephalitis **227**
  meningitis **227**
inferior colliculus 62, 95, 118
inferior temporal lobe, visual pathways 85
inflammation 106
  brain abscesses 228
  encephalitis **227**
  meningitis **227**
influencing the brain **198–99**
information
  creativity 170
  dreams 189
  illusions 174
  processing 38
  sensations 39
  signaling speed 39
infrared light, hearing **94**
inhibitory neurotransmitters 73, 190
injuries
  head injuries **225**
  and language problems 149
  pain 106–07
inkblot test 201
"inner ear" 157
"inner speech" 39
insomnia 188
instability, postural 119
instincts
  collective unconsciousness 193
  empathy and sympathy 140
  language 146
  morality 140–41
insula 66
  conflicting emotions 137
  and cooperative behavior 200
  and disbelief 172
  emotions 128, 129
  imaging **22**
  self-awareness 138, 139
  sense of taste 101
insular cortex 108
insulin 114, 115
insulin-like growth factor (IGF) 196
intelligence **168–69**
  artificial intelligence **217**
  decision-making **169**
  IQ ("intelligence quotient") 168, 170
  and size of brain 44, 168, 205
intention
  mirroring **123**
  self-consciousness **193**
interior globus pallidus 53, 54
intestines, hormones 114
intimacy 134, **135**
intoxication test 162
intracranial cavity 44
intraparietal sulcus 169
introspection 192
invertebrates, evolution of brain **48**
investigating the brain **8–9**
ion channels, in hippocampus 65
ions, nerve impulses 72, 73
IQ ("intelligence quotient") 168, 170

iris, eye 80
iron, in basal ganglia 214
ischemic stroke 229
Italian language, dyslexia 153
itching 102

J
jamais vu **163**
jaw bones 53
jealous delusional disorder 244
joints, proprioceptors 104
judgments, morality **140–41**
Jung, Carl 193

K
Kasparov, Garry 217
kidneys
  hormones 114
  thirst 115
kissing 135
knee, patellar spinal reflex 116
knowledge
  and aging 215
  self-consciousness 192
  taxi drivers 162
Koko (gorilla) 147

L
L-dopa 173
language 38
  autism 223
  bilingualism **149**, 153
  brain imaging 13
  Broca's area 10, **148**
  conversation **150–51**
  definition 146
  developmental milestones 247
  dyslexia **153**
  evolution of **147**
  gender differences 198
  and handedness 199
  language areas **148–49**
  language problems **149**
  and memory 157
  mother tongue 153
  origins of **146–47**
  and perception **147**
  reading and writing **152–53**
  specific language impairment 248
  and thinking 179
  Wernicke's area 10, **148**
larynx, and evolution of language 147
lateral corticospinal tract 118
lateral geniculate nucleus 80, 81
lateral hypothalamic area 113
lateral hypothalamic nucleus 115
lateral lobes, cerebellum 63
lateral sulcus 66
  asymmetry 57
  Einstein's brain 205
laughter 171
  and visual illusions 87
Leaning Tower of Pisa 175
learning **154–65**
  anticipation 130
  flavor-aversion learning 101
  intelligence 168
  long-term potentiation 197
  memory 156, 157
  reading and writing 152
learning disability **248**
  Down syndrome 236
  language problems 149
left-handedness 57, **199**

left hemisphere 53
  bilingualism 149
  and conversation 151
  functions **57**
  and language 146
  split brain 204
legs
  executing a movement 118
  motor neuron disease 235
  phantom limbs **104**, 193
lemurs 138
lens, eye 80
lentiform (lenticular) nucleus 58
Leonardo da Vinci 174
leptin 115
letters, reading and writing 152–53
Lewy body dementia 230
Libet, Benjamin 9, **11**, 191, 193
lie detection **216**
life, quality of 134
life-support machines 238
lifestyle, and aging 215
ligaments, proprioceptors 104
light
  after-images 174
  hearing light **94**
  seasonal affective disorder 239
  sleep-wake cycles 115
  vision 80, 82, 88
liking 130
limbic lobe 64, **65**, 66
limbic system **64–5**, 74
  and desire 130
  emotions 39, 126
  "falling in love" 134
  functions 57
  hypothalamus and 113
  and recognition 163
  smells and 64, 96, 98, 99
limbs
  executing a movement 118
  phantom **104**, 193
  prosthetic 104, **219**
lipids 44
listening
  Broca's area 148
  conversation **150**
literacy 152
literal-mindedness 172
liver, alcohol addiction 245
lobes, cerebral 66
  see also individual lobes
lobotomy **11**
location, attention to 183
locked-in syndrome **63**
Lomo, Terje 9
long-term memory **156**, 158, **160–61**
long-term potentiation 158, 197
longitudinal fissure 66
loss, emotions 128
Lou Gehrig's disease 235
love **134–35**
lucid dreams **189**
lumbar puncture **227**
lumbar region, spinal nerves 42
lumbar vertebrae 42
lungs
  panic responses 127
  regulation of breathing 112
luteinizing hormone (LH) 61, 114

M

macaques, language areas 147
McCain, John 199
McEwan, Ian 244
McGurk effect 78
machines
  artificial intelligence **217**
  brain-machine interfaces 216
  consciousness 219

macular degeneration, eyes 218
"mad cow disease" 231
madeleine effect, sense of smell **99**
madness, and creativity 170
magic mushrooms 187
magnetic encephalography (MEG) 7, 12, 13
magnetic resonance imaging (MRI) 7, 9, **13**, **14–35**, 74, 222
male brain 198
malingering 243
malleus 90
mamillary body 55
  and emotions 126
  functions 58, 64
  memory 156
mammals, brains **49**
manic-depressive illness **239**
manual dexterity, developmental milestones 247
mapping the brain **10**
maps
  "body maps" 192, 193
  spatial memory 162
marijuana, and schizophrenia 244
Mars, canals on 174
masculinity
  male brain 198
  and sexual attraction 134
massa intermedia 198
material universe, and consciousness 178
maternal love 134
mathematics 205
The Matrix (film) 180
maxilla 53
mazes, spatial memory 162
ME (myalgic encephalomyelitis) **225**
"meaningfulness" 186
measles virus 227
medial frontal cortex 184
medial frontal gyrus 140
medial preoptic nucleus 113, 198
median sulcus 62
medicine
  biotechnology **218–19**
  see also drugs
meditation **187**
medulla 53, 56, 62
  functions 57, 63
  pain signals 106
  sense of taste 101
MEG (magnetic encephalography) 7, 12, 13
Meinhof, Ulrike 205
Meissner's corpuscles 102
melanin 58
melanocortin 115
melanocyte-stimulating hormone (MSH) 61, 114
melatonin 114
  circadian rhythm 63
  sleep-wake cycles 115
membranes
  cell membrane 68
  see also meninges
memory 38, **156–65**
  accessing memories **159**
  Alzheimer's disease 231
  anticipation 130
  artificial hippocampus **161**, 219
  association 159
  autism 249
  blocking 164
  collective unconsciousness 193
  and conversation 150, 151
  déjà vu and jamais vu **163**
  dementia **230**
  distribution in brain **158**
  and emotions 126

memory cont.
  forming memories 158
  head injuries 225
  hippocampus and 65, **156–63**, 164
  HM (Henry G. Molaison) **11**, 159
  inability to store **159**
  laying down a memory **160–61**
  location of **161**
  long-term potentiation 158, 197
  movement memory 120
  multiple personalities 201
  oxytocin and 135
  and personality 200
  phobias 127
  post-traumatic stress disorder 164, 241
  principles of **156–57**
  reading 152
  recall and recognition 84, **162–63**
  short- and long-term memory **156**
  sleep and 188
  smell and **99**
  spatial memory **162**
  storage **158–59**
  suppressing 158
  types of **157**
  unusual memory **164–65**
men
  emotions 126, 127
  influences on the brain 198
  male brain 198
  and sexual attraction 134
meninges
  skull 45, 54
  spinal cord 42
meningitis **227**
meningocele 237
menstrual cycle 99
Merkel's disks 102
mesencephalon 53
mesenchephalon 53
Mesmer, Franz Anton 8, 222
metabolic rate, and heat production 113
metastases, brain tumors 230
microglia 69
microtubules 68
mid-frontal area, and numbers 169
midbrain 53, 55, 62
  disorders 119
  limbic system 64
migraine **224**
Milner, Brenda 9
mimicry
  mirror neurons 11
  personality development 200
mind
  consciousness **178–79**
  dualism 178
  mind-control technology 216
  mirror neurons 11
  theory of **139**
mind reading **216**
"mini-strokes" **228**
mirror illusion, phantom limbs 104
mirror neurons **11**, **122–23**, 139
mitochondria 68
mixed cerebral palsy 237
mixed delusional disorder 244
modiolus 90
modules 38
Molaison, Henry G. (HM) **11**, 159
molecules 41
  neurotransmitters 73
  smell 96, 97
Mona Lisa illusion 85
Monism 178
Moniz, Egas 9, 11

monkeys
  attachment 135
  and facial symmetry 134
  language areas 147
monoamine oxidase, and depression 239
monoamines 73
moods **129**
  bipolar disorder **239**
  and decision-making 169
  neurotransmitters and 197
morality **140–41**
morphine
  addiction 130
  pain relief 107
mosaicism 236
Moscow Brain Research Institute 205
mother tongue 153
motion see movement and control
motor control
  developmental milestones 247
  executing a movement 119
  multiple sclerosis 235
  nuclei 58
  paralysis 236
  Parkinson's disease 234
motor cortex
  and consciousness 180
  disorders 119
  executing a movement 118
  pain signals 108
  planning movement 117
  self-awareness 139, 192
  speech 151
motor nerves
  bionic arms 219
  disorders **119**
  executing a movement 119
  reflex actions 116
  spinal cord 42
motor neuron disease (MND) **235**
motor tics, Tourette's syndrome 243
mouth
  facial expressions 136–37
  motor neuron disease 235
  sending information to thalamus 60
  sense of taste 100, 101
  speech 151
movement and control **110–23**
  attention 183
  blindsight 79
  cerebral palsy **237**
  executing a movement **118–19**
  illusions 85
  mirroring **122**
  motor disorders **119**
  multiple sclerosis 235
  neuroendocrine system **114–15**
  nuclei 58
  parkinsonism 234
  planning **116–17**
  proprioception 104
  reflex actions **116**
  regulation **112–13**
  unconscious action **120–21**
  vision 85, 89
"Mozart effect," listening to music **93**
MRI (magnetic resonance imaging) 7, 9, **13**, **14–35**, 74, 222
multi-infarct dementia 230
multi-sensory perceptions 39
multi-tasking 182
multiple sclerosis (MS) 69, 223, **235**
multipolar neurons 69
Munchausen's by proxy 243
Munchausen's syndrome **243**

muscles
  cataplexy 238
  executing a movement **118–19**
  facial expressions 136–37
  motor disorders **119**
  motor neuron disease 235
  moving 117
  multiple sclerosis 235
  paralysis **236**
  proprioceptors 104, 105
  sleep paralysis 189
music 196
  amusia 248
  creativity 170
  hearing **93**
myalgic encephalomyelitis (ME) **225**
myasthenia gravis 236
myelin sheaths 68
  and aging 214, 215
  manufacture of 69
  multiple sclerosis 69, 235
myelinated axons, nerve impulses 72
myelomeningocele 237
Myers-Briggs personality test 201
myoclonic seizures 119, 226
mysophobia 240

N

nanorobots 218
narcissistic personality disorder 245
narcolepsy 188, **238**
nasal cavity 53
natural morality 141
nature and nurture **196–97**
navigation, spatial memory 162
Neanderthals 49
"Near Death Experiences" 193
neck, motor neuron disease 235
Necker cubes 87
necrophobia 240
neglect 85
Neisseria meningitidis 227
neocortex 74, 138
nerve fibers
  nuclei **58**
  pain fibers **107**
  spinal cord 42
  see also axons; dendrites
nerve impulses 42, **72–3**
nerve tracts, in brainstem 62
nerves
  cranial nerves **43**
  paralysis **236**
  spinal nerves **42**
nervous system **40–43**
  aging 214
  damage to 107
  evolution of 48
nervousness 129, 240
networks, neural 41
neural correlates of consciousness 181
neural crest 208
nueral groove 208
neural plate 208
neural tube 208
neural tube
  defects **237**
neurites 68
neurocranium 54, 66
neuroendocrine system **114–15**
neurofeedback 202
neurogenesis 69, 197, 212, 213, 215
neuroglia 70–71
neuromuscular junction 119
neuron progenitor cells 69, 197

neurons 41, **68–9**
  aging 44, 214–15
  Alzheimer's disease 231
  attention 183
  in cerebral cortex 67
  connectivity 39, 168
  epilepsy 226
  general anesthetics 112
  hippocampus 65, 212
  learning 156, 157
  memory 156, 158, 160, 161
  mind reading 216
  mirror neurons **11, 122–23,**
    139
  motor neuron disease
    235
  multiple sclerosis 235
  nerve impulses 42, 72
  neural networks 41
  neurogenesis 69, 197, 212, 213, 215
  nuclei **58–9**
  plasticity **197**
  regeneration 39, **69**
  signal transmission 38
  spinal cord 42
  spindle cells 126
  synapses **69**
  in thalamus 60
  and time 190
  types of **69**
neuropathic pain 107
neuropeptide (NPY) 115
neuroscience, history of **10–11**
neurostimulation 202–203
neurosurgery **232–33**
neurotransmitters 38, **73**
  and aging 214
  Alzheimer's disease 231
  anxiety disorders 240
  bipolar disorder 239
  and depression 239
  and desire 130
  and emotions 128
  executing a movement 119
  "falling in love" 134
  gene expression and 196
  and mood 197
  nerve impulses 72, 73
  Parkinson's disease 234
  and personality 200
  sleep–wake cycles 188
  and time 190
neurotubules 73
neurulation **208**
nicotine addiction 130, 245
nightmares, post-traumatic stress
    disorder 241
Nixon, Richard 136
nocebo effect 109
noise
  hearing **93**
  Tourette's syndrome 243
nonpathological disease feigning
    243
noradrenaline (norepinephrine) 73,
    239
noradrenergic receptors 130
nose
  facial expressions 136–37
  sense of smell **96–97**, 101
  transnasal surgery **232**
nosophobia 240
novelty-seeking, personality
    markers 200
nuclei 53, **58–9**
  in brainstem 62
  in hypothalamus 61, 113
  in thalamus 60
nucleus accumbens 115, 130
numbers **169**
  dyscalculia 248
  language and 147

nurture, and intelligence 168
nutrition see food
nyctophobia 240

O

Obama, Barack 199
objective time 190
objects, recognition **83**
obsessive-compulsive disorder
    (OCD) **241**, 242
obsessive-compulsive personality
    disorder 245
occipital bone 53, 54, 66
occipital cortex 121
occipital lobe 66
  imaging **33**
octanoic acid 96
octanol 96
oculomotor nerve 43
odors, sense of smell 96
oestrogen 114
olfaction see smell
olfactory bulb 64, 96, 101
olfactory cortex
  emotions 126
  functions 97, 101
  memory 162
olfactory epithelium **97**
olfactory nerve 43, 55, 101
olfactory receptors 96
olfactory tract 97
oligodendrocytes 68, 69, 213
olivary nuclei 53
olives 53
omnivores, sense of taste 100
ophidiophobia 240
opiate drugs 107, 130
opiate system
  pain relief 107, 130
  sugar addiction 115
optic chiasm 53, 80, 88
optic disk 80, 81
optic nerve 43, 80, 88, 208
optic radiation 80, 81, 88
optic tracts 80
optical illusions **174**
optimism, personality markers 200
orbital frontal gyri **19**
orbitofrontal cortex
  anticipation 130
  and body language 144
  conduct disorder 248
  conflicting emotions 137
  and consciousness 180
  decision-making 169
  emotions 128
  morality 140
  and obsessive-compulsive
    disorder 241
  sense of smell 97
orexins 238
organ of Corti 90, 91, 94, 95
organelles 68
orgasm 135
orthonasal smell 96, 97, 101
ossicles, ear 90, 94
otitis media 91
otosclerosis 91
out-of-body experiences (OBEs)
  parietal lobe and 186
  self-consciousness and 193
  and spiritual transcendence 172
  supernatural experiences 173
ovaries, hormones 114
overt attention 182
oxygen **45**
  regulation of breathing 112
oxytocin 61, **135**
  and fear 127
  functions 114, 213

P

pacemakers 218, **219**, 243
Pacinian corpuscles 102
pain **106–109**
  brain surgery 39, 109
  experiencing **108–9**
  headache and migraine **224**
  inability to feel 109
  morality 140
  pain relief **107**
  phantom limbs 104
  receptors 39, 102
  reflex actions 116
  social rejection 139
  types of **107**
pair bonding 134
pancreas, hormones 114
panic
  panic attacks 240
  phobias 127, 240
papillae, taste buds 100
paradox illusions **175**
parahippocampal gyrus 64, 65
paralysis **236**
  brain-machine interfaces 216
  motor cortex damage 119
  sleep paralysis 189
paranoia
  and creativity 170
  paranoid personality disorder 245
  paranoid schizophrenia 244
paraplegia 236
parasites, brain abscesses 228
parietal bones 54
parietal cortex 209
  attention 182
  disorders 119
  and dreams 189
  executing a movement 118
  false memory 164
  maths enhancement 203
  pain signals 108
  self-consciousness 192
  unconscious action 120
parietal lobe 66
  altered brain states 186
  emotions 128
  imaging **28**
  intelligence 168
  meditation 187
  memory 156
  morality 140
  out-of-body experiences 173,
    186
  unconscious movement 117
  visual pathways 84
parietal-temporal junction, and
    consciousness 180
parkinsonism **234**
Parkinson's disease **234**
  nuclei problems 58
  pacemakers and 219
  and time 190
partial seizures 226
partitions and zones **56–7**
passion 134
passivity, sadness 129
patellar spinal reflex 116
pathological disease feigning 243
pattern-making **172–73**
Pavlov, Ivan 205
Penfield, Wilder 9, **10**, 103
Penrose triangle 175
perception
  backdating time **191**
  and consciousness 179
  illusions 174–75
  language and **147**
  multisensory perceptions 39
  self-awareness 180
  visual perception 84, **86–7**

peripheral nervous system (PNS)
    40–41, 74
  evolution of 48
persecutory delusional disorder
    244
Persinger, Michael 173
persistent vegetative state 238
personality 38, **200–15**
  learning **200**
  multiple personalities **201**
  and obsessive-compulsive
    disorder 241
  personality assessment **201**
  personality disorders **245**
perspective illusions 175
PET (positron emission
    tomography) 7, 12, 13
petit mal epilepsy 226
pets, expressions 136
phantoms
  phantom limbs **104**, 193
  visual phantoms **181**
phenylethylamine, "falling in love"
    134
phenylthiocarbamide (PTC) 100
pheromones 99
philosophy, investigating the
    brain 8
phobias 127, **240**
phonological deficit hypothesis,
    dyslexia 153
photoreceptors 80, 81
phrenology **10**
physical skills
  developmental milestones 247
  disorders 222
pia mater
  skull 56
  spinal cord 42
pictures, visual perception **86–87**
piloelection 113
pineal gland 55, 62, 114
  sleep-wake cycles 115
pinna 90, 94
Piraha Indians 147
Pisa, Leaning Tower of 175
pituitary gland 53, 56, **61**
  emotions 126
  hormones 114
  hypothalamus and 113
  neuroendocrine system 114
  oxytocin 135
  pain relief 107
  stress response 240
  thirst 115
  tumors **230**, 232
placebo effect 109
plaques, aging brain 214, 215
plasticity 38, **197**
Plato 8
pleasure 127, **130–31**, 135
pons 53, 56, 62
pontine nucleus, cerebellum 117
position, proprioception 104
positron emission tomography
    (PET) 7, 12, 13
post-traumatic stress disorder
    (PTSD) **164**, **241**
posterior cingulate cortex
  imaging **34**
  morality 140
  pain signals 108
posterior cranial fossa 55
posterior nucleus, hypothalamus
    113
posterior parietal complex 108
posterior temporal sulcus
  morality 140
  self-awareness 139
postpartum depression 239
postural instability 119
potassium ions, nerve impulses 72

potentiation, forming memories
    158, 161, 197
precuneus, imaging **34**
prefrontal cortex 66, 74, 209, 212,
    213
  and brain "clocks" 190
  conscious movement 117
  and consciousness 138, 180,
    192
  decision-making 169
  and depression 203, 239
  and doing two things at once
    168
  and dreams 189
  emotions 128
  morality 140
  post-traumatic stress disorder
    241
  reward system 130
  social rejection 139
  thalamus and 60
pregnancy
  prenatal depression 239
premotor cortex
  conscious movement 117, 118
  decision-making 169
  thalamus and 60
prenatal depression 239
primary auditory cortex **30**,
    95
primary geniculate nucleus 95
primary motor cortex 117, 118
primary visual cortex
  and consciousness 180
  imaging **35**
  visual perception **88–89**
primates
  and language 146, 147
  sexual attraction 134
  social behavior 138
prions, Creutzfeldt-Jakob disease
    231
procedural memory 157, 160
"processing gap," and doing two
    things at once 168
production aphasia 149
progesterone 114
progressive bulbar atrophy 235
projective tests, personality 201
prolactin 61, 114, 213
proprioception 102, 104–05
propylthiouracil (PROP) 100
prosencephalon 53
prosopagnosia **85**
prostheses 104, **218–19**
proteins 197
  accumulation in brain 215
  Alzheimer's disease 231
  amino acids 73
  Creutzfeldt-Jakob disease 231
  narcolepsy 238
Proust, Marcel 99
Pseudomonas 228
psilocybin 187
psychastenia, and creativity
    170
psychoanalysis 222
  and dreams **189**
psychopaths **141**
psychosis 223
psychotic deviation, and
    creativity 170
punchdrunk syndrome 225
pupil, eye 80, 88, 144
Purkinje cells 63
pus, brain abscesses **228**
putamen 52, 54, 58
  body memory 120
  memory 156, 157
  planning movement 117
pyramid 53
pyramidal decussation 118

Q

quadriplegia 236
quality of life 134

R

Ramón y Cajal, Santiago 9
rapid eye movement (REM) sleep
    188, 189
Rasmussen, T. 9
rationality **141**
rats, investigating the brain 8
reaction pathways **120–21**
reading **152–53**
    dyslexia **153**, 248
    hyperlexia **153**
reality, and consciousness 178
recall and recognition **162–63**
receptor cells
    sense of smell **96–7**
    thermoreceptors 102, 113
    touch 102
recognition **163**
    faces 83, 84, **85**, 139, 163
    objects **83**
    oxytocin and 135
    visual perception 89
recollection, memory 156
red nucleus, cerebellum 117, 118
referred pain **107**
reflex actions **116**, 193
    and body language 144
regeneration, neurons 39, **69**
regulation, movement and
    control **112–13**
Reissner's membrane 90
rejection, social 139
relaxation 186
religion **172**
renin 115
repetitive behavior 223
repolarization, nerve impulses 72
reptiles, brains 48
"reptilian brain" 48
residual schizophrenia 244
resting-state networks 184
reticular activating system (RAS)
    112
reticular formation **112**
    altered brain states 186
    and consciousness 180
    and dreams 189
reticular laminar 90
reticulospinal tract 118
retina 80, **81**
    bionic eyes 218
    neurons 69
    optic nerve 43
    seeing 88
    sending information to
        thalamus 60
retronasal smell 96, 101
Rett syndrome 249
reward **130–31**
    and aging 214
    altruism 141
    emotions 127
    and humor 171
    sex, love and survival **134–35**
rhinal sulcus 65
rhombencephalon 53
ribosomes 68
right and wrong **140–41**
right-handedness 57, **199**
right hemisphere 53, **55**
    emotions **128**
    functions **57**
    and language 146, 151
    split brain 204
rigidity, motor disorders 119

Ritalin 246
rituals
    altering consciousness 186
    collective unconsciousness 193
Rizzolatti, Giacomo 9, **11**
robots 216–17
    and mirror neuron system 139
    nanorobots 218
rods, retina 81, 88
romantic love 134
root hair plexus 102
rootlets, spinal nerves 42
Rorschach inkblot test 201
rough endoplasmic reticulum 68
rubrospinal tract 118
Ruffini corpuscles 102

S

sacral region, spinal nerves 42
SAD (seasonal affective disorder)
    239
sadness 128, 129
    adaptive behaviors 129
    facial expressions 137
Salem witch trials 172
Sally-Ann test 139
salt, thirst 115
satisfaction 130
savants, autistic 164–65, 174, 249
scalp
    nerves 54
    skin 54
scanning the brain **12–13**, **14–35**
scepticism, and pattern-making
    173
schizoid personality disorder
    245
schizophrenia 185, 203, 223, **244**
    and agency 193
    catatonia 190
    and creativity 170
schizotypal personality disorder
    245
Schumann, Richard 239
Schwann cells 67, 69
sclera 80, 81
Searle, John 179
seasonal affective disorder (SAD)
    239
sebaceous glands 102
seeing **88–9**
seizures
    epilepsy 181, **226**
    status epilepticus **226**
selective attention 182
self
    agency and intention 193
    consciousness and 179, 180,
        192–93
    social behavior **138–39**
    split brain experiments 11
semantic memory 157, 160
semicircular canals, ear 90
sensations 39
    and consciousness 179
    laying down a memory 160
    multiple sclerosis 235
"sensed presence" 172
senses **76–109**
    attention 182–83
    dermatomes **42**
    ears **90–95**
    eyes **80–89**
    information sent to brain 38
    mixed senses 78
    pain **106–09**
    proprioception **104–05**
    sensory aphasia 149
    smell **96–9**, **101**
    spinal cord 42

senses cont.
    synesthesia **78**
    taste **100–01**
    touch **102–103**
sensory cortex
    emotions 127
    laying down a memory 160, 161
    phantom limbs 104
sensory nerves 208
    reflex actions 116
    spinal cord 42
serotonin 73
    bipolar disorder 239
    and body dysmorphic disorder
        242
    and depression 239
    genetics and 197
    and obsessive-compulsive
        disorder 241
sex **134–35**
sex hormones 114, 127
shell shock **241**
shivering 113
short-term memory **156**, 161
shrinking-body illusion 174
sign language, gorillas 147
signal transmission 38, 39
Silbo language 146
simple partial seizures 226
singing 151
sinoatrial node 112
sixth sense **104–05**
size of brain **44**
    and aging 214
    and evolution of brain 49
    and intelligence 44, 168, 205
skills, plasticity of brain 38
skin
    dermatomes **42**
    injuries 106
    itching 102
    proprioceptors 105
    scalp 54
    structure 102
    touch receptors **102**
skull 53, 54
    and cerebral cortex 66
    craniotomy 11, 232
    fractures 225
    head injuries 225
    phrenology **10**
    protection of brain 45
    and size of brain 44
    trepanation 8
sleep **188**
    and aging 215
    brain waves 181
    circadian rhythm 63
    consolidation of memories 161
    dreams **189**
    narcolepsy **238**
    sleep paralysis 189
    sleep-wake cycles **115**
    sleeping drugs 189
    sleepwalking **188**
smell, sense of **96–9**
    brain areas **101**
    chemistry of **96**
    and emotions 126
    limbic system 64
    perception of smell **98–9**
smiling 129, **137**
smoking, nicotine addiction 245
smooth endoplasmic reticulum
    68
sniffing, sense of smell 96
social brain **132–39**
    autism spectrum disorders 223,
        249
    developmental milestones
        247
    expressions **136–37**

social brain cont.
    personality markers 200
    the self and others **138–39**
    social awareness **138–39**, 184
social groups 134
    and size of neocortex 138
social phobia 240
soma, neurons 68, 69
somatic delusional disorder 244
somatic sensory system,
    proprioception **104–05**
somatization disorder **242**
somatosensory cortex **103**
    executing a movement 118
    pain 108
    phantom limbs 104
    self-consciousness 192
    sense of taste 101
sound
    attention 183
    dyslexia 153
    hearing 90, 91, **92–5**
    language 146
    localization 92
    seeing with (soundscapes) **89**
    Tourette's syndrome 243
spastic cerebral palsy 237
spasticity 119
spatial awareness 65
spatial memory **162**
spatial relationships, visual
    pathways 85
spatial skills 157
specific language impairment 149
spectrums, mental disorders **223**
speech
    conversation **150–51**
    development of 93
    dyslexia **153**
    hearing 93
    hyperlexia **153**
    language areas 148
    origins of language **146–47**
    problems **149**
    stuttering **149**
    Wernicke's area 92
Sperry, Roger 9, **11**
sphenoid bone 53, 54
spina bifida occulta 237
spinal accessory nerve 43
spinal cord **42**, 53, 208
    cerebrospinal fluid 45
    disorders 119
    executing a movement 118–19
    lumbar puncture 227
    motor neuron disease 235
    neural-tube defects **237**
    pain signals 106
    reflex actions 116
    spinal tracts 118–19
spinal nerves 40, **42**
    patellar spinal reflex 116
spindle cells 126
spiritual experiences 172, 173
split brain **11**, **204**
sports, and left-handedness 199
stammering **149**
stapes 90, 91, 94
state-dependent memory **162**
status epilepticus 226
stem cells 197, 218
stereocilia 90
stereograms 83
stereoscopic smell **98**
stereotactic brain surgery 232
stimulus and reward 130
stomach
    hormones 114, 115
    panic responses 127
storage, memory **158–59**
strange brains **204–05**

Streptococcus 228, 241
stress
    anxiety disorders 240
    post-traumatic stress disorder
        (PTSD) **164**, **241**
    shell shock **241**
    stress response 240
    stria terminalis 126
stress headaches 224
stria terminalis 126
striatum, and social behavior
    200
stroke 203, 228, **229**
    brain remodelling 197
    and language problems 149
    motor disorders 119
    neurostimulation 203
    speech problems 151
    vascular dementia 230
structures of the brain **52–5**
stuttering **149**, 199
subarachnoid hemorrhage **229**
subarachnoid space 56
    aging 214
    lumbar puncture 227
    spinal cord 42
subcutaneous tissue, pain signals
    107
subdural hematoma 229
subdural hemorrhage **229**
subfornical organ 115
subjective time 190
substantia nigra **58**
    and brain "clocks" 190
    Parkinson's disease 58, 234
    planning movement 117
subthalamic nuclei 53, 55, **58**
    planning movement 117
succubi 189
sugar addiction **115**
sulci (sulcus) 54
    cerebral cortex 66
Sumerians 8
"superhighway," intelligence **168**
superior colliculus 53, 62
    attention 182
    emotions 129
superior olive, hearing 95
superior sagittal sinus 56
superior temporal sulcus
    and body language 144
    conflicting emotions 137
    and numbers 169
supernatural **173**, 193
superstition **172–73**
"supertasters" 100
supplementary motor cortex
    conflicting emotions 137
    conscious movement 117, 118
    and consciousness 180
    disorders 119
    pain signals 108
support cells **69**, 70–71
suprachiasmatic nucleus (SCN) 113,
    115
surgery **109**, **232–33**
    deep brain stimulation 218
    general anesthetics **112**
    lobotomy **11**
    transnasal surgery **232**
surprise
    adaptive behaviors 129
    facial expressions 136
survival
    morality and 141
    sex, love and **134–35**
sustained attention 182
swearing, Tourette's syndrome
    243
sweat glands 99, 102
Swift, Jonathan 205
Sylvian fissure 57, 66

symbols
  collective unconsciousness 193
  communication 146
  dreams and 189
  reading 152
symmetry of brain, and language 146
symmetry of face, and sexual attraction 134
sympathy **140**
synesthesia **78**
synapses 68, **69**
  nerve impulses 72, **73**
  neural networks 41
synaptic cleft 69, 73, 119
synaptic vesicles 73

T

tangles, aging brain 214, 215
taste **100–01**
  laying down a memory 160
  taste associations **101**
tau 215
taxi drivers, spatial memory 162
technology **218–19**
tectorial membrane 90
teenagers
  emotions 39
telencephalon 53
temperature, thermoreceptors 102, **113**
temperoparietal junction, self-awareness 139
temporal bones 54
temporal lobe 66
  altered brain states 186
  and consciousness 180
  and conversation 151
  imaging **21**
  memory 156, 157
  morality 140
  olfactory cortex 101
  reading 152
  and the supernatural 173
  visual pathways 84
  weird experiences 172
tendons, proprioceptors 104, 105
tennis players 120–21
tension headaches **224**
testosterone 213
thalamic bodies 60
thalamus 53–6, **60**
  altered brain states 186
  and consciousness 180
  and dreams 189
  emotions 126, 127, 128
  functions 57, 58
  gender differences 198
  general anesthetics 112
  hearing 94, 95
  imaging **26**
  laying down a memory 160
  limbic system 64
  memory 156
  and obsessive-compulsive disorder 241
  pain relief 107
  pain signals 108
  planning movement 117
  post-traumatic stress disorder 241
  sense of taste 101
  Tourette's syndrome 243
  visual perception 88
theory of mind (ToM) **139**
  empathy and sympathy 140
thermoreceptors 102, **113**

thinking 39, **166–75**
  belief and superstition **172–73**
  brain-machine interfaces 216
  cognitive illusions **174–75**
  and consciousness 179
  controlling prostheses 218, 219
  creativity **170–71**
  decision-making **169**
  emotions 126
  humor **171**
  intelligence **168–69**
  language and 179
  number sense **169**
  self-consciousness **192–93**
thirst **115**
thoracic region, spinal nerves 42
thoracic spinal cord 53
thought see thinking
threat, emotions 128
three-dimensional brain imaging 12
three-dimensional vision **83**
  paradox illusions **175**
thrill-seeking 131, 200, 214
throat
  and evolution of language 147
  motor neuron disease 235
  speech 151
thrombus
  stroke 229
  transient ischemic attacks 228
thymus gland 114
thyroid gland 114
thyroid-stimulating hormone (TSH) 61, 114
tics 119
  Tourette's syndrome 243
timbre, music 93
time **190–91**
tiredness 115
  chronic fatigue syndrome **225**
tobacco, addiction 130
Tomatis, Alfred 93
tone deafness 248
tongue
  sense of taste **100**
  speech 151
tonic-clonic seizures 226
tonic seizures 226
top-down processing **79**, 87
touch, sense of **102–103**
  mirroring **122**
Tourette's syndrome **243**
trait tests, personality 201
trances 186
transcortical motor aphasia 149
transcortical sensory aphasia 149
transcranial direct current stimulation (tDCS) 203
transcranial magnetic stimulation (TMS) 171
transient ischemic attacks (TIA) **228**
translocation, chromosomes 236
transnasal surgery **232**
transsexuals, stria terminalis 126
trauma
  laying down a memory 160
  post-traumatic stress disorder (PTSD) **164**, **241**
  traumatic disorders 222, 223
  traumatic memory **164**
trepanation 8, 11
triangle, Penrose 175
tribar 175
trigeminal nerve 43, 53
  facial pain 107
  sense of taste 101
"trigger points," facial pain 107
trisomy 21 (Down syndrome) **236**
trochlear nerve 43

truth telling 216
tryanophobia 240
tumors **230**
  surgery 232, 233
tunnel of Corti 90
turtles, brains 48
twins
  genetics 197
  and intelligence 168
  left-handedness 199
  religion 172
"two minds" 82
tympanic canal 90
tympanum 90, 94

U

unconscious mind
  decision-making **11**
  emotions **127**
  memories 160
  proprioception 104
  psychoanalysis 222
  sensory information **79**
  unconscious action 116, 117, **120–21**
  unconscious vision 84
unconsciousness 192
  collective unconsciousness **193**
  coma **238**
  epileptic seizures 226
  general anesthetics 112
  head injuries 225
  sleep 188
understanding 179
undifferentiated schizophrenia 244
unipolar depression 223
unipolar neurons 69
United States of America, cultural influences 199

V

vacuoles 68
vagus nerve 43
  pacemakers **219**
values, morality 140
Van Gogh, Vincent 170–9
variant CJD **231**
vascular dementia 230
vassopressin 135
"vegetative" centers 57
veins, arteriovenous malformation 229
ventral pathway, vision **84–5**, 89
ventral pontine syndrome 63
ventral striatum 128
ventral tegmental area (VTA) 115, 130
ventricles 57
  aging 215
  cerebrospinal fluid 45, 57
  hydrocephalus 237
ventrolateral prefrontal cortex 169
ventrolateral preoptic nucleus 188
ventromedial nucleus, hypothalamus 113
ventromedial prefrontal cortex (VMPC)
  and belief 172
  morality 140
vermis 63
vertebrae 54
  spina bifida 237
  spinal nerves 42
vertebrates, evolution of brain **48**
Vesalius, Andreas 8

vestibular canal 90, 94
vestibulocochlear nerve 43, 90
vestibulospinal tract 118
vibrations
  hearing 90, 91, 94, 95
  touch receptors 102
violence, psychopaths 141
virtual reality
  "brain-in-a-vat" 180
  pain relief 109
  virtual body experiment 193
viruses
  encephalitis 227
  meningitis 227
visceral pain 107
vision **80–89**
  bionic eyes **218**
  developmental milestones 247
  multiple sclerosis 235
  reactions to visual stimuli 120–21
  seeing **88–9**
  split brain 204
  visual agnosia 85
  visual attention defects 85
  visual neurons 78
  visual pathways **84–5**
  visual perception **86–7**, **88–9**
  visual phantoms **181**
visual cortex 81, **82–83**
  and consciousness 180
  and dreams 189
  imaging **35**
  and memory 157, 158, 161
  mind reading 216
  reading 152
  and recognition 163
  thalamus and 60
  visual perception **88–9**
visual word-recognition area 152
vocal tics, Tourette's syndrome 243
voices, autism spectrum disorders 249
volume of brain **44**
vomeronasal region (VMO) 99

W

Wada test 146
wanting 130
water
  in brain 44
  thirst **115**
water on the brain (hydrocephalus) **237**
weight of brain **44**
Wernicke, Karl 9, **10**
Wernicke's aphasia 149
Wernicke's area 10, 92, **148**
  conversation 150
whistles, Silbo language 146
white blood cells 45, 106
white matter 44
  aging 215
  cerebellum 62, 63
  spinal cord 42
  in thalamus 60
Williams syndrome 248
Willis, Thomas 8
Wiltshire, Stephen 164–65
wine tasters 100
women
  emotions 126, 127
  female brain 198
  and sexual attraction 134
words 146
  "inner ear" 157
  Tourette's syndrome 243
  see also language
working memory 156, 157, 161

worms 48
worrying 240
  hypochondria **242**
writers, creativity 170
writing **152–53**
  dyslexia **153**, 248
  hyperlexia **153**

X, Y, Z

X-rays, computed tomography (CT) 12
Yakovlevian torque 57
yawning 138
zones and partitions **56–7**

ACKNOWLEDGMENTS

For the revised edition, Dorling Kindersley would like to thank: Roz Hitchcock and Gemma Casajuana at DK Digital Production, London; Manjari Rathi Hooda, Lakshmi Rao, Justin C. Murik, Nain Rawat, Abhay Pratap, Vinit Dubey, Vishal Gupta, Jay Pandey, and Hari Dutt of the DK Digital Media Division, Delhi; Ehtisham Sayed at Testronic Laboratories; Henry Fry, Nicholas Hayne, Jessica Cawthra, Susmita Dey, Himani Khatreja, and Vineetha Mokkil for editorial assistance; Amit Malhotra and Charlie Noon for design assistance; and Bimlesh Tiwari for DTP assistance.

The publisher would like to thank the following for their kind permission to reproduce their photographs:
(Key: a-above; b-below/bottom; c-center; f-far; l-left; r-right; t-top)

Edward H. Adelson: 87cr; **Alamy Images:** Alan Dawson Photography 146bl, allOver photography 45tr, Bubbles Photolibrary 186cr, Mary Evans Picture Library 174br, Everett Collection Historical 212br, Photo by M. Flynn / © Salvador Dali, Gala-Salvador Dali Foundation, DACS, London 2009 191t, Paul Hakimata 200tl, Barrie Harwood 202cr, Hipix 10bc, Kirsty McLaren 130c, Mira 44bc, 115cr, Robin Nelson 179c, Old Visuals 92cra, Photogenix 122tl, Pictorial Press 200-201, Picture Contact 217br, Print Collector 178bl, Simon Reddy 116t, Supapixx 153br, Tetra Images 123tl, vario images GmbH & Co. KG 190cr; **American Medical Association:** Archive of General Psychiatry Vol 62 No 7, July 2005 799-805, Niels Birbaumer et al, Deficient Fear Conditioning in Psychopathy, © 2005. Reprinted with permission of American Medical Association / Image: Ralf Veit 141bc; **Arionauro Cartuns:** 171cr; **Helen Barbas:** Scientific American Feb 2009 p70 (US edition); Claus C. Hilgetag & Helen Barbas, Exploring the folds of the Brain – And Their Links to Autism 66bl; **Dr Jason J.S. Barton:** 85cr; **George Bartzokis, M.D, UCLA Neuropsychiatric Hospital and Semel Institute:** 214cl; **Dr Theodore W Berger, University of Southern California:** 161tl; **Blackwell Publishing:** European Journal of Neuroscience Vol 25, Issue 3, pp863-871, Renate Wehrle et al, Functional microstates within human REM sleep: first evidence from fMRI of a thalamocortical network specific for phasic REM periods. © 2007 John Wiley & Sons / Image courtesy Renate Wehrle 189fcr; **Bloomsbury Publishing Plc:** Temple Grandin & Catherine Johnson, Animals in Translation: the woman who thinks like a cow, 2005 249br; © **EPFL / Blue Brain Project:** 74cb, 75c, Thierry Parel 75cr; **The Bridgeman Art Library:** Archives Charmet 8ftl, 10cl, Bibliothèque de l'Institut de France 7tl, The Detroit Institute of Arts, USA / Founders Society purchase with Mr & Mrs Bert L. Smokler & Mr & Mrs Lawrence A. Fleischman funds 189bc, Maas Gallery, London 134c, Peabody Essex Museum, Salem, Massachusetts, USA 172bl, Royal Library, Windsor 174tr; **Vergleichende Lokalisationslehre der Grosshirnrinde, Dr K Brodmann:** 1909, publ: Verlag von Johann Ambrosius Barth, Leipzig 67c; **Dr Peter Brugger:** 173tr; **Caltech Brain Imaging Center:** J. Michael Tyszka & Lynn K. Paul 204ca; **Center for Brain Training (www.centerforbrain.com):** 222bl; **Copyright Clearance Center - Rightslink:** Brain 2008 131(12):3169-3177; doi:10.1093 / brain / awn251, Iris E. C. Sommer et al, Auditory verbal hallucinations predominantly activate the right inferior frontal area. Reprinted by permission of Oxford University Press 193cra, Brain Lang 80: 296-313, 2002, Murray Grossman and, Sentence processing strategies in healthy seniors with poor comprehension: an fMRI study (c) 2002 with permission from Elsevier 215tl, Brain Vol 125, No 8, 1808-1814, Aug 2002, Sterling C. Johnson et al, Neural correlates of self-reflection (c) 2002. Reprinted with permission of Oxford University Press 192bl, Brain, Vol. 122, No. 2, 209-217, Feb 1999, Noam Sobel et al, Blind smell: brain activation induced by an undetected air-borne chemical © 1999 by permission of Oxford University Press 98bl, Current Biology, Vol. 13, December 16, 2003, Nouchine Hadjikhani and Beatrice de Gelder, Seeing Fearful Body Expressions Activates the Fusiform Cortex and Amygdala, 2201-2205, Fig. 1, © 2003, with permission from Elsevier Science Ltd. 144br, Int J Dev Neurosci. 2005 Apr-May;23(2-3):125-41, Robert Schultz, Developmental deficits in social perception in autism: the role of the amygdala and fusiform face area © 2005, with permission from Elsevier 249cr, International Journal of Psychophysiology, V63, No 2 Feb 2007 p214-220, Michael J Wright & Robin C. Jackson, Brain regions concerned with perceptual skills in tennis, An fMRI study (c) 2007 with permission from Elsevier 121, Journal of Neurophysiology 96: 2830-2839, 2006; doi:10.1152 / jn.00628.2006, Arthur Wingfield & Murray Grossman, Language and the Aging Brain: Patterns of Neural Compensation Revealed by Functional Brain Imaging © 2006 The American Physiological Society 215, Journal of Neurophysiology Vol 82 No 3 Sept 1999 1610-1614, 128cl, Journal of Neuroscience, Aug 27, 2008 Vol 28 p8655-8657, Duerden & Laverdure-Dupont, Practice makes cortex, (c) The Society of Neuroscience 157rr, Journal of Neuroscience, May 28, 2008, 28(22):5623-5630. Todd A. Hare et al, Dissociating the Role of the Orbitofrontal Cortex and the Striatum in the Computation of Goal Values and Prediction Errors © 2008. Printed with permission from The Society for Neuroscience 169t, Journal of Neuroscience, Nov 7, 2007, 12190-12197; Hongkeun Kim, Trusting our memories: Dissociating the Neural Correlates of Confidence in Veridical versus Illusory Memories, © 2007, Society for Neuroscience 164c, Michael S Beauchamp & Tony Ro; Adapted with permission from Figure 1, Neural Substrates of Sound-Touch Synesthesia after a Thalamic Lesion; Journal of Neuroscience 2008 28:13696-13702 78bl, The Journal of Neuroscience, December 7, 2005 • 25(49):11489 –11493, Peter Kirsch et al, Oxytocin Modulates Neural Circuitry for Social Cognition and Fear in Humans 127tc, Reprinted from The Lancet, Volume 359, Issue 9305, Page 473, 9 February 2002, Half a Brain, Johannes Borgstein & Caroline Grootendorst, © 2002, with permission from Elsevier 205tr, Nature 373, 607-609 (Feb 16, 1995), Bennett A. Shaywitz et al Yale, Sex differences in the functional organization of the brain for language. Reprinted by permission from Macmillan Publishers Ltd 198cl, Nature 415, 1026-1029 (28 Feb 2002), Antoni Rodriguez-Fornells et al Brain potential and functional MRI evidence for how to handle two languages

with one brain © 2002. Reprinted by permission of Macmillan Publishers Ltd 149tr, Nature 419, 269-270 (Sept 19, 2002), Olaf Blanke et al, Neuropsychology: Stimulating illusory own-body perceptions (c) 2002. Reprinted by permission from Macmillan Publishers Ltd 173cr, Nature Neuroscience 7, 801-802 (18 July 2004) | doi:10.1038 / nn1291, Hélène Gervais et al, Abnormal cortical voice processing in autism © 2004 Reprinted by permission from Macmillan Publishers Ltd / image courtesy Mônica Zilbovicius 249crb, Nature Neuroscience Vol 10, 1 Jan 2007 p119 Figure 3, Yee Joon Kim et al, Attention induces synchronization-based response in steady-state visual evoked potentials © 2007. Reprinted by permission from Macmillan Publishers Ltd. 183tr, Nature Reviews Neuroscience 4, 37-48, Jan 2003 | doi:10.1038 / nrn1009; Arthur W. Toga & Paul M Thompson, Mapping brain asymmetry © 2003. Reprinted by permission from Macmillan Publishers Ltd / image courtesy Dr Arthur W. Toga, Laboratory of Neuro Imaging at UCLA 57cr, Nature Reviews Neuroscience 7, 406-413 (May 2006) | doi:10.1038 / nrn1907, Usha Goswami, Neuroscience and education: from research to practice? © 2006. Reprinted by permission from Macmillan Publishers Ltd / courtesy Dr Guinevere Eden, Georgetown University, Washinton DC 248t, redrawn by DK courtesy Nature Reviews Neuroscience 3, 201-215 (March 2002), Maurizio Corbetta & Gordon L. Shulman, Control of goal-directed and stimulus-driven attention in the brain © 2002 Reprinted by permission from Macmillan Publishers Ltd. 183cb, NeuroImage 15: 302-317, 2002 Murray Grossman et al, Age-related changes in working memory during sentence comprehension: an fMRI study (c) 2002 with permission from Elsevier 215ftl, Neuron 6 March 2013, 77(5): 980-991, fig 6; Charles E. Schroeder et al, "Mechanisms Underlying Selective Neuronal Tracking of Attended Speech at a Cocktail Party" © 2013 with permission from Elsevier (http://dx.doi.org / 10.1016 / j.neuron.2012.12.037) 92tr, Neuron Vol 42 Issue 4, 27 May 2004, p687-695, Jay A. Gottfried et al, Remembrance of Odors Past: Human Olfactory Cortex in Cross-Modal Recognition Memory; with permission from Elsevier 162tr, Neuron, Vol 42, Issue 2, 335-346, Apr 22, 2004, Christian Keysers et al, A Touching Sight (c) 2004 with permission from Elsevier 122bl, Neuron, vol 45 issue 5, 651-660, 3 March 2005, Helen S. Mayberg et al Deep Brain Stimulation for Treatment-Resistant Depression (c) 2005 with permission from Elsevier Science & Technology Journals 239cl, Neuron, Vol 49, Issue 6, 16 Mar 2006, p917-927, Nicholas B Turke-Browne, Do-Joon Yi & Marvin M. Chun, Linking Implicit and Explicit Memory: Common Encoding Factors and Shared Representations © 2006 with permission from Elsevier 159crb, Neuron, Volume 60, Issue 5, 915-929, 10 December 2008, Yoichi Miyawaki et al, Visual Image Reconstruction from Human Brain Activity using a Combination of Multiscale Local Image Decoders, © 2008 with permission from Elsevier 216bl, Psychiatric Times Vol XXII No 7, May 31, 2005, Dean Keith Simonton, PhD, Are Genius and Madness Related: Contemporary Answers to an Ancient Question, (c) 2005 CMPMedica, reproduced with permission of CMPMedica 170br, Science 2010: 329 (5997): 1358-1361 "Prediction of Individual Brain Maturity Using fMRI", fig. 2, Nico U.F. Dosenbach et al (c) 2010 The American Association for the Advancement of Science - Reprinted with permission from AAAS 212cl, Science Feb 20, 2004; © 2004 The American Association for the Advancement of Science, T. Singer, B. Seymour, J. O'Doherty, H. Kaube, R.J. Dolan, C.D. Frith, Empathy for Pain involves the affective but not sensory components of pain 138br, Science Vol 317 No 5841 pp1048, 24 Aug 2007, The Experimental Induction of Out-of-Body Experiences, H. Henrik Ehrsson / photo by H. Henrik Ehrsson © 2007 The American Association for the Advancement of Science 193bl, Science, 13 July 2007, Vol 317. No. 5835, pp.215-219, fig 2, Brendan E. Depue et al, Prefrontal regions orchestrate suppression of emotional memories via a two-phase process. Reprinted with permission from AAAS 158cl, Science, Oct 10, 2003, Vol 302, No 5643 p290-292, Naomi I. Eisenberger et al, Does Rejection Hurt? An fMRI Study of Social Exclusion © 2003 The American Association for the Advancement of Science 139tl, Science, Vol 264, Issue 1502, 1102-1105 (c) 1994 by American Association for the Advancement of Science / H. Damasio, T. Grabowski, R. Frank, A.M. Galaburda & A.R. Damasio, "The return of Phineas Gage: clues about the brain from the skull of a famous patient" / Dept of Image Analysis Facility, University of Iowa 141cr, Trends in Cognitive Sciences, Vol 11 Issue 4, Apr 2007 p158-167 Naotsugu Tsuchiya & Ralph Adolphs, Emotion & consciousness © 2007 Elsevier Ltd / image: Ralph Adolphs 128tr; **Corbis:** Alinari Archives 6tl, Steve Allen 39bc, The Art Archive 8tl, 8cb, Bettmann 6tc, 6tr, 7tc, 8tc, 8bl, 8bc, 9ca, 9br, 11tr, 75br, 136cl, 136c, 136fcl, 147bc, 173cra, 193br, 204-205, 205cra, Bernd Vogel 215c, Bloomimage 186bl, Keith Brofsky 144tr, Fabio Cardoso 157c, Peter Carlsson / Etsa 96br, Christophe Boisvieux 118bl, 187r, Creasource 183bc, 183br, Gianni Dagli Orti 85bl, Kevin Dodge 140l, Ecoscene / Angela Hampton 39cr, EPA 186tl, 190t, 248cla, ER Productions 222cr, Fancy / Veer 159tc, Peter M. Fisher 179tr, Rick Friedman 216ca, Robert Garvey 134tl, Rune Hellestad 196cl, Hulton Collection 99cr, Hutchings Stock Photography 104c, Image 100 157bl, Tracy Kahn 168c, Ed Kashi 151tr, Helen King 183cr, 183cr (Man using computer), Brooks Kraft 199tl, Elisa Lazo de Valdez 180tl, Walter Lockwood 182ca, Tim McGuire 39t, MedicalRF.com 9tr, Mediscan 197cra, Moodboard 38br, 123tr, 157br, 182cr, Greg Newton 186fbr, Tim Pannell 186br, PoodlesRock 7tr, Premium Stock 157cr, Louie Psihoyos 99bl, Radius Images 185b, Redlink 182tr, Reuters 196-197, 217bl, Lynda Richardson 159cl, Chuck Savage 138bc, 198tr, Ken Seet 135t, George Shelley 168b, Sunset Boulevard 57t, Sygma 84br, 180bc, Tim Tadder 38tr, 139br, William Taufic 172tl, 184c, 189br, TempSport 118-119, Thinkstock 38c, Visuals Unlimited 212bc, Franco Vogt 193c, Zefa 101br, 182ftr, 186bc, 192r, 214cr; **Luc De Nil, PhD:** & Kroll, R. (2000). Nieuwe inzichten in de rol van de hersenen tijdens het stotteren van volwassenen aan de hand van recent onderzoek met Positron Emission Tomography (PET). Signaal 32, 13-20. 149cr; **Dr Jean Decety:** Neuropsychologia, Vol 46, Issue 11, Sep 2008, 2607-2614, Jean Decety, Kalina J. Michalska & Yoko Akitsuki, Who caused the pain? An fMRI investigation of empathy and intentionality in children. © 2008 with permission from Elsevier. 140tr; **Dr José Delgado :** 10bl; **Brendan E. Depue:** 164b; **DACS (Design And Artists Copyright Society):** 191; **Dorling Kindersley:** Bethany Dawn 138clb, Colin Keates /

Courtesy of the Natural History Museum, London 49cr; **Dreamstime.com:** Photoeuphoria 152tl; **Henrik Ehrsson et al:** Neural substrate of body size: illusory feeling of shrinking of the waist; PLoS Biol 3(12): e412, 2005 174cr; © **2012 The M.C. Escher Company - Holland. All rights reserved. www.mcescher.com:** 175br; **Alan Evans and the McConnell Brain Imaging Center McGill University:** Ultra high resolution 3D Human Brain Model, Katrin Amunts et al (http: // vimeo.com / 69248914) 75cla; **Explore-At-Bristol:** 87c; **eyevine:** 11cl; **Dr Anthony Feinstein, Professor of Psychiatry, University of Toronto:** 242crb; **Professor John Gabrieli:** Stanford Report, Tuesday February 25, 2003, Remediation training improves reading ability of dyslexic children 153cr; **Getty Images:** AFP 145t, 202bl, John W. Banagan 240fbl, Blend Images 247t, The Bridgeman Art Library / National Portrait Gallery, London 205cla, Maren Caruso 100cr, Comstock Images 134tr, Digital Vision 144tc, ElementalImaging 116-117, 153bl, 170bl, 185cr, Gazimal 182crb, Tim Graham 162br, Louisa Gouliamaki 153bc, Hulton Archive 11bl, 93cr, 129b, 160-161 (girls icecream), 162-163t, 190b, 201tr, 202br, 205c, 222tl, 222tr, 242bl, Masayasu Ikeda 135br, International Rescue 105, Lifestock 144cb, Tanya Little 184br, Don Mason 135cb, Michael Orenstein 136cr, Victoria Pearson 215tr, Peter Ginter 243t, Photo and Co 127cra, Photodisc 215cr, 241cr, Popperfoto 241tr, Louie Psihoyos 239tr, Purestock 215tc, Juergen Richter 175tr, Charlie Schuck 162bl, Chad Slattery 131, Henrik Sorensen 189bl, Sozaijiten / Datacraft 247cr, Tom Stoddart 119br, David Sutherland 191b, Time & Life Pictures 8crb, WireImage 240clb, Elis Years 240bl; **Jordan Grafman PhD:** 141tl; **Dr Hunter Hoffman, U.W.:** 109t, 109c, 109cr; **Courtesy of the Laboratory of Neuro Imaging at UCLA and Martinos Center for Biomedical Imaging at MGH, Consortium of the Human Connectome Project - www.humanconnectomeproject.org ; Courtesy of the Laboratory of Neuro Imaging at UCLA and Martinos Center for Biomedical Imaging at MGH, Consortium of the Human Connectome Project - www.humanconnectomeproject.org ; Courtesy of the Laboratory of Neuro Imaging at UCLA and Martinos Center for Biomedical Imaging at MGH, Consortium of the Human Connectome Project - www.humanconnectomeproject.org ; :** 74r; **Imprint Academic:** The Volitional Brain: Towards a neuroscience of free will, Ed Benjamin Libet, Anthony Freeman & Keith Sutherland © 1999 / Cover illustration by Nicholas Gilbert Scott, Cover design by J.K.B. Sutherland 11cr; **Photographic Unit, The Institute of Psychiatry, London:** 24tl; **iStockphoto.com:** BMPix 175cl, 175c, Jens Carsten Rosemann 85t, Kiyoshi Takahase Segundo 181bcr; **R.C. James:** 199cra; **Frances Kelly :** Lorna Selfe 174tc; **Pilyoung Kim et al:** Fig. 1 from "The Plasticity of Human Maternal Brain: Longitudinal Changes in Brain Anatomy During the Early Postpartum Period", Behavioural Neuroscience 2010, Vol 124, No. 5 695-700 (c) 2010 American Psychological Association DOI: 10.1037 / a0020884 213br; **The Kobal Collection:** 20th Century Fox / Digital Domain 217t; © **2008 Little et al. This is an open-access article distributed under the terms of the Creative Commons Attribution License, which permits unrestricted use, distribution, and reproduction in any medium, provided the original author and source are credited (see http://creativecommons.org/licenses/by/2.5/).; :** Little AC, Jones BC, Waitt C, Tiddeman BP, Feinberg DR, et al. (2008) Symmetry Is Related to Sexual Dimorphism in Faces: Data Across Culture and Species. PLoS ONE 3(5): e2106. doi:10.1371 / journal.pone.0002106 134bl; **Ian Loxley / TORRO / The Cloud Appreciation Society:** 172-173t; **Professor Gary Lynch:** 197br; **Mairéad MacSweeney:** Brain. 2002 Jul;125(Pt 7):1583-93, B Woll, R Campbell, PK McGuire, AS David, SC Williams, J Suckling, GA Calvert, MJ Brammer; Neural systems underlying British Sign Language & audio-visual English processing in native users © 2002. Reprinted by permission of Oxford University Press 78cl; **Rogier B. Mars:** Rogier B. Mars, Franz-Xaver Neubert, MaryAnn P. Noonan, Jerome Sallet, Ivan Toni and Matthew F. S. Rushworth, On the relationship between the 'default mode network" and the 'social brain'; Front. Hum. Neurosci., 21 June 2012 | doi: 10.3389 / fnhum.2012.00189 184bl; **Mediscan:** 246tl; **Pierre Metivier:** 178tc; **MIT Press Journals:** Journal of Cognitive Neuroscience Nov 2006, Vol 18, No 11, p1789-1798, Angela Bartolo et al, Humor Comprehension and Appreciation: A FMRI study, © 2006 Massachusetts Institute of Technology 171crb, Journal of Cognitive Neuroscience, Fall 1997, V9, No 5 p664-686, D. Bavelier et al, Sentence reading: a functional MRI study at 4 Tesla, © 1997 Massachusetts Institute of Technology 148c; **The National Gallery, London:** Applied Vision Research Unit / Professor Alastair Gale, Dr David Wooding, Dr Mark Mugglestone & Kevin Purdy with support of Derby University / Telling Time exhibition at National Gallery 86-87; **The Natural History Museum, London:** 103cr; **Neuramatix (www.neuramatix.com):** 75bl; **Louis N. Vinke, Bowling Green State University, Ohio:** 79bc, 79br; **Oregon Brain Aging Study, Portland VAMC and Oregon Health & Science University:** 214-215b; **Oxford University Press:** 19tr; **Professor Eraldo Paulesu:** 153cl; **Pearson Asset Library:** Pearson Education Ltd / Jules Selmes 122br; **Pearson Group:** © 1991 Pearson Assessment. Reproduced with permission. 85br; **Dr Michael Persinger:** Dr Paul Valliant 173br; **Jack Pettigrew, FRS:** 87br; **(c) Philips:** Philips Design concept dress 'Bubelle' 129cl, 129c; **Photolibrary:** David M. Dennis 8t; **PLoS Biology:** Cantlon JF, Brannon EM, Carter EJ, Pelphrey KA (2006) Functional Imaging of Numerical Processing in Adults and 4-y-Old Children. PLoS Biol 4(5): e125 doi:10.1371 / journal. pbio.0040125 169b, Gross L (2006) Evolution of Neonatal Imitation. PLoS Biol 4(9): e311, Sept 5, 2006 doi:10.1371 / journal.pbio.0040311. © 2006 Public Library of Science 11br; **PNAS:** 103;15623-15628, Oct 17 2006, Jordan Grafman et al, Human fronto–mesolimbic networks guide decisions about charitable donation © 2006 National Academy of Sciences, USA 114tc, June 16, 2008 (DOI: 10.1073 / pnas.0801566105) Ivanka Savic & Per Lindstrom, PET and MRI show differences in cerebral asymmetry and functional connectivity between homo- and heterosexual subjects © 2008 National Academy of Sciences, USA 198bl, March 19, 2002 V99, No 6 4115-4120, Jeremy R. Gray et al, Integration of emotion & cognition in the lateral prefrontal cortex © 2002 National Academy of Sciences, USA 169c, Vol 105 no. 39 15106-15111, Sept 30, 2008, Jean-Claude Dreher et al, Age-related changes in midbrain dopaminergic regulation of the human reward system, © 2008 National

Academy of Sciences, USA 130bl; **Press Association Images:** 182b, AP Photo 147br; **Alice Mado Proverbio:** Biological Psychology Vol 80 Issue 1, Jan 2009 p52-63, A.M. Proverbio, R. Adorni, A. Zani, Inferring native language from early bio-electrical activity © 2009 with permission from Elsevier 153tr; **Public Health Image Library:** Sherif Zaki, MD, PhD; Wun-Ju Shieh, MD, PhD, MPH 231b; **Marcus E. Raichle, Department of Radiology, Washington University School of Medicine, St. Louis, Missouri:** 148bl; **The Random House Group Ltd:** Vintage Books, Ian McEwan, Enduring Love, 2004 244br; **Courtesy of the Rehabilitation Institute of Chicago:** 218-219b; **M. Reisert:** University Medical Center Freiburg; based on the algorithm in M. Reisert et al, Global fiber reconstruction becomes practical, NeuroImage Volume 54, Issue 2, 15 January 2011 pages 955-962 (http: // www.ncbi.nlm.nih.gov / pubmed / 20854913) 204cl; **Courtesy of Professor Katya Rubia:** based on data published in the American Journal of Psychiatry, 2009; 166: 83-94 248b; **Kosha Ruparel & Daniel Langleben, University of Pennsylvania:** 216br; **Science Photo Library:** 12c, 14, 16, 17, 18, 19, 20, 21, 22, 23, 24, 25, 26, 27, 28, 29, 30, 31, 32, 33, 34, 35, 51r, 113cl, 125r, 126cl, 174cl, 215cl, 228tr, 238bc, AJ Photo / Hop American 181b, 193cla, Anatomical Travelogue 177r, Tom Barrick, Chris Clark, SGHMS 13tr, Dr Lewis Baxter 239bl, David Becker 81tl, Tim Beddow 244cl, Juergen Berger 218bl, Biophoto Associates 67bc, Dr Goran Bredberg 90br, BSIP VEM 238br, BSIP, Asteier-Chru, Lille 232cl, BSIP, Ducloux 96cl, BSIP, SEEMME 12br, Oscar Burriel 188cr, 193crb, Scott Camazine 12bc, CNRI 230l, 245tr, 245cr, Custom Medical Stock Photo 248cl, Thomas Deerinck, Ncmir 59, 67fbl, 126bc, 155r, Department of Nuclear Medicine, Charing Cross Hospital 224bl, Eye of Science 69c, 197crb, 218bc, Don Fawcett 111r, 119tl, Simon Fraser 146tr, 210-211, 237t, Simon Fraser / Royal Victoria Infirmary, Newcastle Upon Tyne 9tc, 207r, Dr David Furness, Keele University 67br, GJLP 7bl, Pascal Goetgheluck 104br, Steve Gschmeissner 58l, 61cr, 67bl, 96t, 107bl, C.J. Guerin, PhD, MRC Toxicology Unit 57br, 60l, 63cr, 65cr, 238t, Dr M O Habert, Pitie-Salpetriere, ISM 181cl, Prof J J Hauw 234cl, Innerspace Imaging 9bl, 9-241 (sidebar), ISM 46, Nancy Kedersha 4-5, 8-256 (sidebar), 36-37, 50-51, 76-77, 110-111, 124-125, 132-133, 142-143, 154-155, 166-167, 176-177, 194-195, 206-207, 220-221, Nancy Kedersha / UCLA 70-71, James King-Holmes 91c, 109b, 232-233, Mehau Kulyk 223cl, 227tr, Living Art Enterprises, LCC 12bl, 44br, 126br, Dr Kari Lounatmaa 227tl, 228tc, Dr John Mazziotta Et Al / Neurology 121tr, 93cl, Duncan Shaw 100tl, Medi-mation 232b, MIT AI Lab / Surgical Planning Lab / Brigham & Women's Hospital 10br, Hank Morgan 12cr, 181fcl, 189cl, 189cr, 189fcl, John Greim 112cr, Paul Parker 81br, Prof. P. Motta / Dept. of Anatomy / University 'La Sapienza', Rome 81bl, 91tr, National Institutes of Health 230r, National Library of Medicine 9cr, Susumu Nishinaga 94br, David Parker 77r, Alfred Pasieka 61cl, 80t, 133r, 135bc, 167r, 197tr, 231t, 234t, Pasieka 170cla, Alain Pol, ISM 47, Dr Huntington Potter 231cr, C. Pouedras 58cr, Philippe Psaila 7br, 107tl, John Reader 100tr, Jean-Claude Revy ISM 12cl, Sovereign, ISM 6bl, 6bc, 6br, 13cra, 13c, 37r, 62tl, 64t, 208t, Dr Linda Stannard 228tl, Volker Steger 216cl, Andrew Syred 195r, Sheila Terry 102l, 153cra, Alexander Tsiaras 7bc, 13br, US National Library of Medicine 10tr, Wellcome Dept. of Cognitive Neurology 57bl, 127cr, 143r, 241br, Professor Tony Wright 91bc, Dr John Zajicek 69cr, 221r, Zephyr 13cr, 57bc, 119crb, 218tl, 225cra, 225cb, 227br, 228cl, 229bl, 237c; **seeingwithsound.com:** Peter B L Meijer 89br; **Selmer Bringsjord and collaborating researchers, Rensselaer AI & Reasoning Laboratory:** 217bc; **Roger Shepard:** Adapted from L'egs-istential Quandry, 1974, pen and ink; Published in artist's book, Mind Sights, 1990 W.H. Freeman 173bc; **Stephen Wiltshire Gallery, London:** Stephen Wiltshire, Aerial view of Houses of Parliament and Westminster Abbey, 23 June 2008 164-165; **Li-Hai Tan, PhD:** PNAS March 11, 2008 vol. 105 no. 10 4004-4009 / Paul Kay et al 147t; © **2009 Michael J Tarr:** 83cra; **Taylor & Francis Books (UK):** Riddoch MJ, Humphreys GW. Birmingham Object Recognition Battery (BORB). Lawrence Erlbaum Associates, 1993 85crb; **The Art Archive:** Musée Condé Chantilly / Gianni Dagli OrtiAA 11tl; **TopFoto.co.uk:** 173bl, Imageworks 83bl; **Peter Turkeltaub, MD, PhD:** 152cr; **UCLA Health:** 203t; **Dept of Neurology, University Hospital of Geneva :** paper, ref: Seeck et al (1998) Electroeneph 226t; **University of California, Los Angeles:** 242tl; **Dr Katy Vincent, University of Oxford:** 108c; **Image: Tor Wager:** from H. Kober et al, Neuroimage 2008 Aug 15;42(2): 998-1031, Functional grouping and cortical-subcortical interactions in emotion: a meta-analysis of neuroimaging studies, fig. 7 (http: // www.ncbi.nlm.nih.gov / pubmed / 18579414) 127cla; **Wellcome Images:** 222cra, Wellcome Photo Library 91br, Wessex Reg. Genetics Centre 236bl, 236bc; **Susan Whitfield-Gabrieli, McGovern Institute for Brain Research at MIT:** 185cl; **Wikimedia Commons:** Thomasbg 243br, Van Gogh, Starry Night, MoMA, New York 170-171t; **Wikipedia:** 10c, Histologie du Systeme Nerveux de l'Homme et des Vertebretes, Vols 1 & 2, A. Maloine. Paris 1911 9c, Sternberg, Robert J. (1986). "A triangular theory of love", Psychological Review 93 (2): 119–135, doi:10.1037 / 0033-295X.93.2.119 134ca; **John Wiley & Sons Ltd:** Chris Frith, Making up the Mind – How the brain creates our mental world, 2007 Blackwell Publishing © 2007 John Wiley & Sons Ltd / image courtesy Chiara Portas 13bc, Psychological Science, Vol 19 Issue 1, p12-17, Trey Hedden et al, Cultural Influences on Neural Substrates of Attentional Control, © 2009 Association of Psychological Science 199br, Zygon Vol 28 Issue 2, p177-200, Andrew Newberg, Religious & Mystical States: A Neuropsychological model © 1993 John Wiley & Sons Ltd 187cl; **David Williams, University of Rochester:** 81tr; **Dr Daniel R. Winberger:** 244cb; **Adapted with permission of S.F. Witelson:** Reprinted from The Lancet, Vol 353 Issue 9170, p2150, (19 June 1999), Sandra F. Witelson et al, The exceptional brain of Albert Einstein, (c) 1999 with permission from Elsevier & S.F. Witelson 205br; **Jason Wolff, PhD, UNC:** 249tr; **Professor Michael J Wright:** International Journal of Psychophysiology, V63, No 2 Feb 2007 p214-220, Michael J. Wright & Robin C. Jackson, Brain regions concerned with perceptual skills in tennis, An fMRI study © 2007 with permission from Elsevier 121t; **Professor Semir Zeki:** 128br

Front & Back Endpapers: **Science Photo Library:** Innerspace Imaging

All other images © Dorling Kindersley
For further information see: **www.dkimages.com**